Pharmacology for Health Professionals

Pharmacology for Health Professionals

Edited by **Ned Burnett**

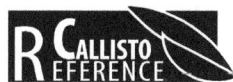

R CALLISTO
REFERENCE

New York

Published by Callisto Reference,
106 Park Avenue, Suite 200,
New York, NY 10016, USA
www.callistoreference.com

Pharmacology for Health Professionals
Edited by Ned Burnett

International Standard Book Number: 978-1-63239-746-1 (Hardback)

Printed in the United States of America.

Contents

Preface

This book has been an outcome of determined endeavour from a group of educationists in the field. The primary objective was to involve a broad spectrum of professionals from diverse cultural background involved in the field for developing new researches. The book not only targets students but also scholars pursuing higher research for further enhancement of the theoretical and practical applications of the subject.

Pharmacology refers to a branch of medicinal science which deals with the study of any artificial, natural and endogenous molecule which has a biochemical or physiological effect on the tissues, cells and organs of any living body. It studies the interactions between drugs and organs. Health professionals like physicians and pharmacists need a deep understanding of the drugs and their administration as they need to provide patients with the correct dosage and efficient medicines. This book gives comprehensive insights into the field of pharmacology. It elucidates the formations and applications of various new and existing drugs in a detailed manner. The objective of this text is to provide in-depth knowledge of the different uses and areas of pharmacology. It will serve as a valuable source of reference for professionals, students and researchers alike.

It was an honour to edit such a profound book and also a challenging task to compile and examine all the relevant data for accuracy and originality. I wish to acknowledge the efforts of the contributors for submitting such brilliant and diverse chapters in the field and for endlessly working for the completion of the book. Last, but not the least; I thank my family for being a constant source of support in all my research endeavours.

Editor

Bioequivalence Study of Two Oral Doxycycline Formulations (Doxysol® and Doxymed®) in Healthy Broiler Chickens

Ahmed M. Soliman[1]*, Mohamed Aboubakr[2], Mohamed El-Hewaity[3]

[1]Department of Pharmacology, Faculty of Veterinary Medicine, Cairo University, Giza, Egypt
[2]Department of Pharmacology, Faculty of Veterinary Medicine, Benha University, Qaliobiya, Egypt
[3]Department of Pharmacology, Faculty of Veterinary Medicine, University of Sadat City, Minoufiya, Egypt
Email: *galalpharma@hotmail.com, *galalpharma@cu.edu.eg

Abstract

Aims: The present study was designed to assess the comparative bio-equivalence of Doxysol® and Doxymed® in healthy broiler chickens after oral administration of both products in a dose of 20 mg doxycycline/kg.b.wt. Materials and Methods: Twenty broiler chickens were divided into two groups. The first group was designed to study the pharmacokinetics of Doxysol, while the 2nd group was designed to study the pharmacokinetics of Doxymed. Each broiler chickens in both groups were injected intravenously with 20 mg doxycycline/kg.b.wt. Blood samples were obtained from the wing vein and collected immediately before and at 5, 15, 30 minute, 1, 2, 4, 6, 8, 12 and 24 hours after a single intravenous or oral administration. Results: Doxycycline in both products obeyed a two compartments open model following I.V. injection in a dose of 20 mg/kg.b.wt. The disposition kinetics of Doxysol® and Doxymed® following oral administration of 20 mg doxycycline base/kg.b.wt. revealed that the maximum blood concentration [$C_{max.}$] were 4.70 and 4.65 μg/ml and attained at [$t_{max.}$] of 1.30 and 1.40 hours, respectively. Doxycycline in Doxysol® and Doxymed® was eliminated with half-lives [$t_{0.5(\beta)}$] equal to 1.98 and 2.31 hours, respectively. The mean systemic bioavailability of doxycycline in Doxysol® and Doxymed® after oral administration in healthy chickens was 92.57 and 88.21%, respectively. Conclusion: Doxymed® is bioequivalent to Doxysol® since $C_{max\,test}/C_{max\,reference}$ and $AUC_{test}/AUC_{reference}$ ratios were 99% and 90%, respectively.

Keywords

Bioequivalence, Doxycycline, Broiler Chickens, Pharmacokinetics

---

*Corresponding author.

1. Introduction

Doxycycline is a semi-synthetic bacteriostatic tetracycline and a broad-spectrum antibiotic against Gram-negative and Gram-positive aerobic and anaerobic bacteria, Rickettsiae, Chlamydiae, Mycoplasmas and some protozoa [1] [2]. Pharmacokinetics properties of doxycycline are superior than older tetracycline, in terms of higher lipid solubility, complete *absorption*, better tissue distribution, longer elimination half-life and lower affinity for calcium [3] [4]. The *in vitro* antimicrobial activity of doxycycline is more effective than other tetracycline for the treatment of respiratory, urinary and gastrointestinal tract diseases [5] [6].

The bioavailability and bioequivalence studies play an important role in determining therapeutic efficacy to register the generic drug products according to the Food and Drug Administration (FDA) regulations [7]. Bioavailability is defined as the rate and extent to which an active drug ingredient is absorbed and becomes available at the site of drug action. In case of bioequivalence it is defined as statistically equivalent bioavailability between two products at the same molar dose of the therapeutic moiety under similar experimental conditions [7] [8]. The drug products are said to be bioequivalent if they are pharmaceutical equivalents or pharmaceutical alternatives and if their rate and extent of absorption do not show a significant differences statistically according to the FDA regulations [7].

The aim of this study is to evaluate bioequivalence of two oral doxycycline powder (Doxysol® and Doxymed®) after oral administration of a single dose in broiler chickens.

2. Materials and Methods

2.1. Drugs

Doxysol®: is manufactured by Ascor Chimici, Italy. It is dispended as oral powder. Each 100 g contains 20 g doxycycline hydrochloride.

Doxymed®: is manufactured by Medmac Co., Amman, Jordan, as oral powder. Each 100 g contains 20 g doxycycline hydrochloride.

2.2. Broiler Chickens and Experimental Design

Twenty healthy broiler chickens (40 - 45 days old and weighing 2 - 2.30 kg) were chosen from Tanta Poultry Farm, Egypt. They were kept individually in cages, within a ventilated, heated room (20°C), and 14 hours of day light. They received a standard commercial ration free from any antibiotics for 30 days before starting the experiment to insure complete clearance of any anti-bacterial substances from their bodies. Water was offered *ad-libitum*.

2.3. Bioequivalence Study of Doxysol® and Doxymed®

Twenty broiler chickens were used to study the bio-equivalence of Doxysol® and Doxymed® after oral administration. Broiler chickens were divided into two groups. The first group comprises ten broiler chickens to study the pharmacokinetics of Doxysol®. The 2nd group (10 broiler chickens) was used to study the pharmacokinetics of Doxymed®. Each broiler chickens in both groups were injected intravenously with 20 mg doxycycline standard activity/kg.b.wt. Broiler chickens were left for 15 days to ensure complete excretion of doxycycline from their bodies. Broiler chickens in the 1st group were administered orally (intra-crop) with Doxysol® in a dose of 20 mg doxycycline/kg.b.wt (1 gram of product/1 liter drinking water), while broiler chickens in the 2nd group were administered orally with Doxymed® in a dose of 20 mg doxycycline/kg.b.wt (1 gram of product/1 liter drinking water)/kg.b.wt.

2.4. Blood Samples

Blood samples were obtained from the wing vein (1 ml) and collected in test tubes immediately before and at 5, 15, 30 minute, 1, 2, 4, 6, 8, 12 and 24 hours after a single intravenous or oral administration (groups 1 and 2). Samples were centrifuged at 3000 rpm for 10 minutes and the obtained sera were used for the estimation of doxycycline concentration. The serum samples were stored at −20°C until analysis, and the assay was performed within a week of obtainment.

2.5. Analytical Procedure

Arret *et al.* [9] described a rapid agar-diffusion assay for the quantitative determination of doxycycline in small volumes of blood by using *Bacillus subtilis* (*ATCC* 6633). The used test organism for the microbiological assay was obtained from Microbiology Department, Faculty of Veterinary Medicine, Cairo University, Egypt.

2.6. Pharmacokinetic Analysis

The pharmacokinetic parameters were determined for each individual sample according to Baggot [10]. Serum concentrations of the two formulations of doxycycline after a single oral administration were subjected to a non-compartmental pharmacokinetic analysis using computerized program, WinNonline 4.1 (Pharsight, USA). Values calculated were: AUC, area under the blood concentration (C_{pt}) time (t) curve to infinity, elimination rate constant (k_{el}, calculated as the slope of the terminal phase of the serum concentration curve), terminal half-life ($t_{0.5}$, where $t_{0.5} = 0.693/k_{el}$), volume of distribution at steady state ($Vd_{(ss)}$), body clearance ($Cl_{(B)}$), the peak serum concentration (C_{max}) and the time to peak concentration (t_{max}). The rate of absorption after oral administration was determined by comparing the area under the serum concentration curve (AUC_{oral}) with that obtained following intravenous injection ($AUC_{i.v.}$) in the same chicken.

$$\text{Bioavailability} = \frac{\left(AUC\right)_{oral} \times D_{i.v}}{\left(AUC\right)_{i.v} \times D_{oral}} \times 100$$

where: D_{iv} = Dose of i.v. administration .

D_{oral} = Dose of oral administration.

The following equation according to FDA regulation [7] was performed to prove that the tested product is bioequivalent to the reference product in the study.

$$\frac{AUC_{(test)}}{AUC_{(reference)}} \text{ or } \frac{C_{max(test)}}{C_{max(reference)}}$$

2.7. Statistical Analysis

Obtained data was analyzed by analysis of variance (ANOVA). The differences were considered significant when $p < 0.05$. All the data are expressed as mean ± SE.

3. Results

The mean serum concentration of doxycycline in broiler chickens were determined up to 24 h and were not detected in all chickens 48 h post single oral and intravenous administration. The mean blood concentrations-time profile (µg/ml) of doxycycline in Doxysol® and Doxymed® after intravenous administration of 20 mg doxycycline/kg.b.wt. in broiler chickens are shown in (**Table 1** and **Figure 1**).

The mean pharmacokinetic parameters of doxycycline (Doxysol® and Doxymed®) after intravenous administration of 20 mg doxycycline/kg.b.wt. in broiler chickens are shown in **Table 2**. The systemic bioavailability (F%) was 92.57 and 88.21% for Doxysol® and Doxymed®, respectively.

Doxycycline in both formulations after intravenous administration could be described in a two compartments-open model. Doxycycline intravenous administration in a dose of 20 mg/kg.b.wt. revealed a high volume of distribution (exceeded than one L/kg) calculated by extrapolation [V_{dB}] and steady state [V_{dss}] method, which are factors made doxycycline is highly distributed in all body tissues. A factor revealed that doxycycline is the drug of choice for attacking the systemic infections caused by sensitive organisms.

The mean serum concentrations of doxycycline in Doxysol® and Doxymed® following oral administration of 20 mg doxycycline/kg.b.wt. in broiler chickens are shown in (**Table 3** and **Figure 2**).

The mean pharmacokinetic parameters of doxycycline in Doxysol® and Doxymed® after oral administration of 20 mg doxycycline/kg.b.wt. in broiler chickens are shown in (**Table 4**).

The disposition kinetics of doxycycline in Doxysol® and Doxymed® following oral administration of 20 mg doxycycline base/kg.b.wt. revealed that the maximum blood concentration [$C_{max.}$] were 4.70 and 4.65 µg/ml and attained at [$T_{max.}$] of 1.30 and 1.40 hours, respectively.

The 90% confidence intervals for the mean ratio of C_{max} and AUC of the reference and tested formulations were within bioequivalence range and summarized in **Table 5**.

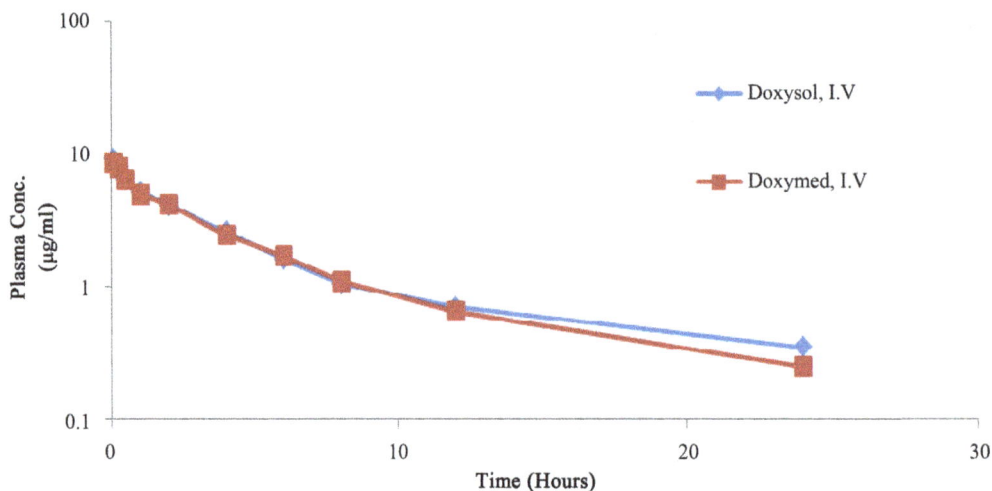

Figure 1. Semilogarthimic plot showing the serum concentrations-time profile of doxycycline in Doxysol® and Doxymed® following intravenous administration at a dose of 20 mg doxycycline/kg.b.wt. in broiler chickens (n = 10).

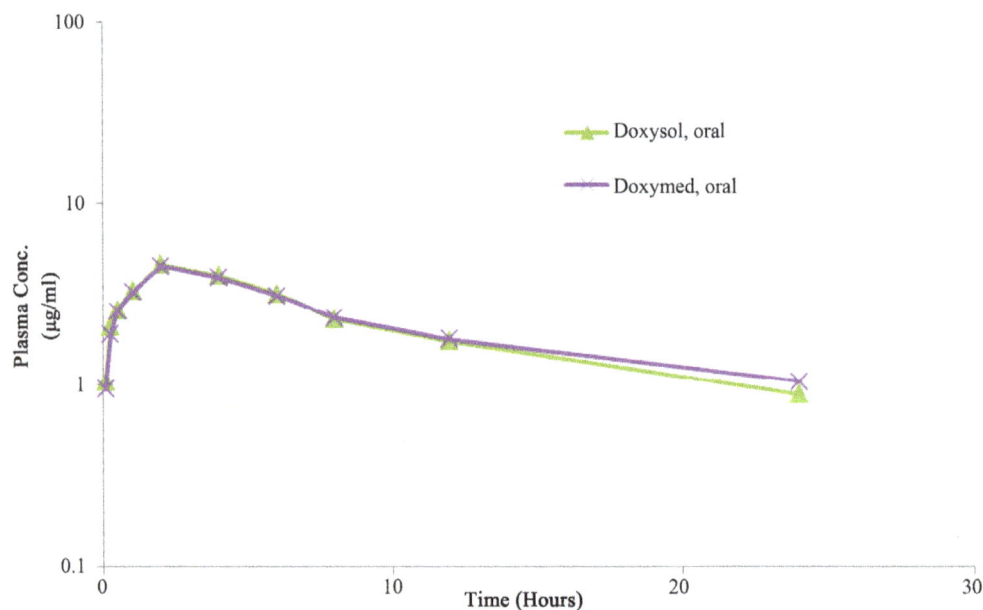

Figure 2. Semilogarthimic plot showing the serum concentrations-time profile of doxycycline in Doxysol® and Doxymed® following oral administration at a dose of 20 mg doxycycline/kg.b.wt. in broiler chickens (n = 10).

4. Discussion

Antibiotics are widely used as veterinary drugs or as feed additives to promote growth [11]-[16]. The pharmacokinetics of doxycycline was reported in chickens following different routes of administrations [17]-[21]. However, the current study was designed to investigate pharmacokinetics and bioequivalence of doxycycline of two powder formulations (Doxysol® and Doxymed®) after oral administration in broiler chickens.

Doxycycline in both formulations after i.v. administration could be described in a two compartments-open model. This indicated that, doxycycline distributed in the body of broiler chickens in two compartments; a central one which represent blood and highly perfused organs (kidney-liver-spleen-heart) and a 2nd peripheral compartment which represented by skin and connective tissues [6]. Doxycycline peak plasma concentration for both formulations was higher than the minimum inhibitory concentrations (MICs) for Mycoplasma gallisepticum (0.2

Table 1. Mean (X ± S.E) serum concentrations (μg/ml) of doxycycline in Doxysol® and Doxymed® following intravenous administration of 20 mg doxycycline/kg.b.wt. in broiler chickens (n = 10).

Time after administration (h)	Doxysol®	Doxymed®
5 min.	9.15 ± 0.60	8.70 ± 0.63
0.25	7.90 ± 0.45	7.90 ± 0.28
0.50	6.40 ± 0.70	6.35 ± 0.63
1	5.20 ± 0.55	5.00 ± 0.90
2	4.10 ± 0.35	4.15 ± 0.35
4	2.60 ± 0.27	2.45 ± 0.60
6	1.60 ± 0.50	1.70 ± 0.35
8	1.05 ± 0.06	1.10 ± 0.08
12	0.70 ± 0.08	0.65 ± 0.07
24	0.35 ± 0.06	0.25 ± 0.04

Table 2. Mean (X ± S.E) pharmacokinetic parameters of doxycycline in Doxysol® and Doxymed® following intravenous administration of 20 mg doxycycline/kg.b.wt. in broiler chickens (n = 10).

Parameter	Unit	Doxysol®	Doxymed®
$°C$	μg/ml	8.95 ± 0.75	8.15 ± 0.50
A	μg/ml	5.35 ± 0.65	4.70 ± 0.29
α	h^{-1}	3.75 ± 0.45	4.10 ± 0.30
$T_{0.5(\alpha)}$	h	0.18 ± 0.09	0.17 ± 0.08
V_c	L/kg	3.40 ± 0.08	3.10 ± 0.06
$V_{d(B)}$	L/kg	4.80 ± 0.07	3.95 ± 0.15
$V_{d(area)}$	L/kg	5.75 ± 0.15	5.15 ± 0.60
V_{dss}	L/kg	5.05 ± 0.13	4.70 ± 0.25
k_{12}	h^{-1}	0.85 ± 0.22	0.90 ± 0.08
k_{21}	h^{-1}	1.25 ± 0.05	1.15 ± 0.07
B	μg/ml	3.60 ± 0.24	3.45 ± 0.23
β	h^{-1}	0.075 ± 0.030	0.065 ± 0.004
$T_{0.5(\beta)}$	h	9.24 ± 0.60	10.66 ± 0.85
k_{13}	h^{-1}	0.37 ± 0.05	0.35 ± 0.05
Cl_B	L/kg/h	0.015 ± 0.002	0.017 ± 0.003
AUC	Mg·h/ml	26.25 ± 1.60	24.60 ± 2.40

Table 3. Mean (X ± S.E) serum concentrations (μg/ml) of doxycycline in Doxysol® and Doxymed® following oral administration of 20 mg doxycycline/kg.b.wt. in broiler chickens (n = 10).

Time after administration (h)	Doxysol®	Doxymed®
5 min.	1.05 ± 0.30	0.95 ± 0.44
0.25	2.10 ± 0.26	1.90 ± 0.60
0.50	2.60 ± 0.70	2.55 ± 0.30
1	3.30 ± 0.39	3.25 ± 0.50
2	4.60 ± 0.80	4.50 ± 0.45
4	4.00 ± 0.45	3.90 ± 0.33
6	3.20 ± 0.50	3.10 ± 0.80
8	2.30 ± 0.60	2.35 ± 0.60
12	1.75 ± 0.85	1.80 ± 0.35
24	0.90 ± 0.06	1.05 ± 0.07

Table 4. Mean (X ± S.E) pharmacokinetic parameters of doxycycline in Doxysol® and Doxymed® following oral administration of 20 mg doxycycline/kg.b.wt. in broiler chickens (n = 10).

Parameter	Unit	Doxysol®	Doxymed®
A	µg/ml	3.75 ± 0.38	3.66 ± 0.40
k_{ab}	h^{-1}	2.65 ± 0.26	2.28 ± 0.30
$T_{0.5(ab)}$	h	0.26 ± 0.07	0.27 ± 0.06
B	µg/ml	3.00 ± 0.36	2.92 ± 0.25
β	h^{-1}	0.04 ± 0.003	0.05 ± 0.002
$T_{0.5(\beta)}$	h	17.32 ± 0.25	13.86 ± 0.35
$T_{max.}$	h	1.30 ± 0.14	1.40 ± 0.18
$C_{max.}$	µg/ml	4.70 ± 0.60	4.65 ± 0.50
AUC	µg·h/ml	24.30 ± 1.60	21.70 ± 1.48
Bioavailability	%	92.57 ± 3.00	88.21 ± 2.62

Table 5. Bioequivalence between Doxysol® (reference) and Doxymed® (test) formulations.

Parameters	Reference	Test	90% CI lower/upper	T/R (%)	Acceptable range (%)	Conclusion
C_{max} (µg/ml)	4.7 ± 0.60	4.65 ± 0.50	88.68 - 112.19	98.93	75 - 133	BE
AUC (µg·h/ml)	24.30 ± 1.60	21.70 ± 1.48	88.98 - 89.57	89.30	80 - 125	BE

BE: Bioequivalence.

Doxycycline in both formulations after i.v. administration could be described in a two compartments-open model. This indicated that, doxycycline distributed in the body of broiler chickens in two compartments; a central one which represent blood and highly perfused organs (kidney-liver-spleen-heart) and a 2nd peripheral compartment which represented by skin and connective tissues [6]. Doxycycline peak plasma concentration for both formulations was higher than the minimum inhibitory concentrations (MICs) for Mycoplasma gallisepticum (0.2 µg/ml) [22], Mycoplasma pneumoniae (<0.5 µg/ml), Staphylococcus aureus (0.25 µg/ml) [23], Streptococcus pneumoniae (<0.4 µg/ml) [24] and E. coli (1 - 4 µg/ml) [25]. However, doxycycline peak plasma concentration for both formulations was lower than the MICs for Pseudomonas aeruginosa (>64 µg/ml) [8] and Enterococcus fecalis (8 to 32 µg/ml) [26]. This emerge the therapeutic usefulness of doxycycline in control many susceptible bacteria. Doxycycline in Doxysol® and Doxymed® was eliminated with half-lives [$t_{0.5(\beta)}$] equal to 17.32 and 13.86 hours, respectively. The long $t_{0.5}$ is a clear characteristic of doxycycline in different species, which range from 4.2 to 16.6 h [1] [17] [18] [27] [28].

The oral bioavailability of Doxysol® and Doxymed® indicated a good absorption from GIT. This is indicated that both products are advised to be given orally in case of acute bacterial attacks in blood and other organs [17] [18]. No significant differences were observed between the pharmacokinetics parameters of the two formulations; these results were showing the bioequivalence of the two formulations were according to the criteria established by FDA [7].

Bioequivalence study is a test to assure the clinical efficacy of a generic versus brand drugs [7]. Bioequivalence refers to a comparison between generic formulations of a drug, or a product in which a change has been made in one or more of the ingredients or in the manufacturing process, and a reference dosage form of the same drug [29].

The 90% confidence intervals for the mean ratio of C_{max} and AUC of the reference and tested formulations were 98.93% and 89.30%, respectively. These values falls within the EMEA bioequivalence acceptance range of 85% - 125% for both T_{max} and AUC and between 75% - 133% for C_{max} [30].

5. Conclusion

Based on the above pharmacokinetic and statistical results that calculated in the current study, we concluded that Doxymed® manufactured by Medmac-Jordan is bioequivalent to Doxysol® manufactured by Ascor Chimici-Italy and both products can be used as interchangeable drug in veterinary medicine practice especially in poultry industrial sector.

References

[1]   Jha, V.K., Jayachandran, C., Singh, M.K. and Singh, S.D. (1989) Pharmacokinetic Data on Doxycycline and Its Distribution in Different Biological Fluids in Female Goats. *Veterinary Research Communications*, **13**, 11-16. http://dx.doi.org/10.1007/BF00366847

[2]   Prats, G., Elkorchi, G., Giralt, M., *et al.* (2005) PK and PK/PD of Doxycycline in Drinking Water after Therapeutic Use in Pigs. *Journal of Veterinary Pharmacology and Therapeutics*, **28**, 525-530. http://dx.doi.org/10.1111/j.1365-2885.2005.00700.x

[3]   Riond, J.L. and Riviere, J.E. (1990) Pharmacokinetics and Metabolic Inertness of Doxycycline in Young Pigs. *American Journal of Veterinary Research*, **51**, 1271-1275.

[4]   Goren, E., De-Jong, W., Doornenbal, P., *et al.* (1988) Therapeutic Efficacy of Doxycycline Hyclate in Experimental *Escherichia coli* Infection in Broilers. *Vet Q*, **10**, 48-52. http://dx.doi.org/10.1080/01652176.1988.9694145

[5]   Croubels, S., Baert, K., De Busser, J. and De Backer, P. (1998) Residue Study of Doxycycline and 4-Epidoxycycline in Pigs Medicated via Drinking Water. *Analyst*, **123**, 2733-2736. http://dx.doi.org/10.1039/a804936j

[6]   Abd El-Aty, A.M., Goudah, A. and Zhou, H.H. (2004) Pharmacokinetics of Doxycycline after Administration as a Single Intravenous Bolus and Intramuscular Doses to Non-Lactating Egyptian Goats. *Pharmacological Research*, **49**, 487-491.

[7]   Chen, M.L., Shah, V., Patnaik, R., *et al.* (2001) Bioavailability and Bioequivalence: An FDA Regulatory Overview, *Pharmaceutical Research*, **18**, 1645-1650. http://dx.doi.org/10.1023/A:1013319408893

[8]   Toutain, P.L. and Bousquet-Melou, A. (2004) Bioavailabilty and Its Assessment. *Journal of Veterinary Pharmacology and Therapeutics*, **27**, 455-466. http://dx.doi.org/10.1111/j.1365-2885.2004.00604.x

[9]   Arret, B., Johnson, D. and Kirshbaum, A. (1971) Outline of Details for Microbiological Assay of Antibiotics. *Journal of Pharmaceutical Sciences*, **60**, 1689-1694. http://dx.doi.org/10.1002/jps.2600601122

[10] Baggot, J. (1978) Some Aspects of Clinical Pharmacokinetics in Veterinary Medicine. *Journal of Veterinary Pharmacology and Therapeutics*, **1**, 5-18. http://dx.doi.org/10.1111/j.1365-2885.1978.tb00300.x

[11] Yoshida, M., Kubota, D., Yonezawa, S., Nakamura, H., Azechi, H. and Terakado, N. (1971) Transfer of Dietary Spiramycin into the Eggs and Its Residue in the Liver of Laying Hen. *Japanese Journal of Antibiotics*, **8**, 103-110.

[12] Yoshida, M., Kubota, D., Yonezawa, S., Nakamura, H., Azechi, H. and Terakado, N. (1973) Transfer of Dietary Doxycycline into the Eggs and Its Residue in the Liver of Laying Hen. *Japanese Journal of Antibiotics*, **10**, 29-36.

[13] Roadaut, B., Moretain, J.P. and Boisseau, J. (1987) Excretion of Oxytetracycline in Eggs after Medication of Laying Hens. *Food Additives and Contaminants*, **4**, 297-307. http://dx.doi.org/10.1080/02652038709373639

[14] Roadaut, B. and Moretain, J.P. (1990) Residues of Macrolide Antibiotics in Eggs Following Medication of Laying Hens. *British Poultry Science*, **31**, 661-675. http://dx.doi.org/10.1080/00071669008417297

[15] Yoshimura, H., Osawa, N., Rasa, F.S.C., Hermawati, D., Werdiningsih, S., Isriyanthi, N.M.R. and Sugimori, T. (1991) Residues of Doxycycline and Oxytetracycline in Eggs after Medication via Drinking Water to Laying Hens. *Food Additives and Contaminants*, **8**, 65-69. http://dx.doi.org/10.1080/02652039109373956

[16] Omija, B., Mitema, E.S. and Maitho, T.E. (1994) Oxytetracycline Residue Levels in Chicken Eggs after Oral Administration of Medicated Drinking Water to Laying Chickens. *Food Additives and Contaminants*, **11**, 641-647. http://dx.doi.org/10.1080/02652039409374265

[17] Anadon, A., Martinez-Larranaga, M.R., Diaz, M.J., Bringas, P., Fernandez, M.C., Fernandez-Cruz, M.L., *et al.* (1994) Pharmacokinetics of Doxycycline in Broiler Chickens. *Avian Pathology*, **23**, 79-90. http://dx.doi.org/10.1080/03079459408418976

[18] Laczay, P., Semjen, G., Lehel, J. and Nagy, G. (2001) Pharmacokinetics and Bioavailability of Doxycycline in Fasted and Non-Fasted Broiler Chickens. *Acta Veterinaria Hungarica*, **49**, 31-37. http://dx.doi.org/10.1556/AVet.49.2001.1.5

[19] Ismail, M.M. and El-Kattan, Y.A. (2004) Disposition Kinetics of Doxycycline in Chickens Naturally Infected with *Mycoplasma gallisepticum*. *British Poultry Science*, **45**, 550-556. http://dx.doi.org/10.1080/00071660400001058

[20] Hantash, T.M., Abu-Basha, E.A., Roussan, D.A. and Abudabos, A.M. (2008) Pharmacokinetics and Bioequivalence of Doxycycline (Providox® and Doxyveto 50 S®) Oral Powder Formulations in Chickens. *International Journal of Poultry Science*, **7**, 161-164. http://dx.doi.org/10.3923/ijps.2008.161.164

[21] El-Gendy, A.Y., Atef, M., Amer, A.M. and Kamel, G.M. (2010) Pharmacokinetics and Tissue Distribution of Doxycycline in Broiler Chickens Pretreated with Either: Diclazuril or Halofuginone. *Food and Chemical Toxicology*, **48**, 3209-3214. http://dx.doi.org/10.1016/j.fct.2010.08.024

[22] Takahashi, I. and Yoshida, T. (1989) Antimycoplasmal Activities of Ofloxacin and Commonly Used Antimicrobial Agents on *Mycoplasma gallisepticum*. *Japanese Journal of Antibiotics*, **42**, 1166-1172.

[23] Bryant, J.E., Brown, M.P., Gronwall, R.R. and Merritt, K.A. (2000) Study of Intra-Gastric Administration of Doxycycline: Pharmacokinetics Including Body Fluid, Endometrial and Minimum Inhibitory Concentrations. Equine Veterinary Journal, **32**, 233-238. http://dx.doi.org/10.2746/042516400776563608

[24] Aronson, A.L. (1980) Pharmacotherapeutics of the Newer Tetracycline. *Journal of the American Veterinary Medical Association*, **176**, 1061-1068.

[25] Moskowitz, S.M., Foster, J.M., Emerson, J. and Burns, J.L. (2004) Clinically Feasible Biofilm Susceptibility Assay for Isolates of *Pseudomonas aeruginosa* from Patients with Cystic Fibrosis. *Journal of Clinical Microbiology*, **42**, 1915-1922. http://dx.doi.org/10.1128/JCM.42.5.1915-1922.2004

[26] Hoelscher, A.A., Bahcall, J.K. and Maki, J.S. (2006) *In Vitro* Evaluation of the Antimicrobial Effects of a Root Canal Sealer-Antibiotic Combination against *Enterococcus faecalis*. *Journal of Endodontics*, **32**, 145-147. http://dx.doi.org/10.1016/j.joen.2005.10.031

[27] Santos, M.D., Vermeersch, H., Remon, J.P., Schelkens, M., De Backer, P., Bree, H.J.J., *et al.* (1996) Pharmacokinetics and Bioavailability of Doxycycline in Turkeys. *Journal of Veterinary Pharmacology and Therapeutics*, **19**, 274-280. http://dx.doi.org/10.1111/j.1365-2885.1996.tb00049.x

[28] Baert, K., Croubels, S., Gasthuys, F., De Busser, J. and De Backer, P. (2000) Pharmacokinetics and Oral Bioavailability of Doxycycline Formulation (Doxycycline 75%) in Non-Fasted Young Pigs. *Journal of Veterinary Pharmacology and Therapeutics*, **23**, 45-48. http://dx.doi.org/10.1046/j.1365-2885.2000.00235.x

[29] Alvinerie, M., Lacoste, E., Sutra, J.F. and Chartier C. (1999) Some Pharmacokinetic Parameters of Eprinomectin in Goats Following Pour-On Administration. *Veterinary Research Communications*, **23**, 449-455. http://dx.doi.org/10.1023/A:1006373609314

[30] Ozdemir, N. and Yildirim, M. (2006) Bioequivalence Study of Two Long-Acting Oxytetracycline Formulations in Sheep. *Veterinary Research Communications*, **30**, 929-934. http://dx.doi.org/10.1007/s11259-006-3235-2

2

Anandamide Depresses Glycinergic and GABAergic Inhibitory Transmissions in Adult Rat Substantia Gelatinosa Neurons

Yasuhiko Kawasaki, Tsugumi Fujita, Kun Yang, Eiichi Kumamoto[*]

Department of Physiology, Saga Medical School, Saga, Japan
Email: [*]kumamote@cc.saga-u.ac.jp

Abstract

Cannabinoid CB1 receptors have been found in the superficial dorsal horn of the spinal cord, particularly the substantia gelatinosa (SG), which is thought to play a pivotal role in modulating nociceptive transmission. Although cannabinoids are known to inhibit excitatory transmission in SG neurons, their effects on inhibitory transmission have not yet been examined fully. In order to know further about a role of cannabinoids in regulating nociceptive transmission, we examined the effects of cannabinoids on inhibitory transmissions in adult rat SG neurons using whole-cell voltage-clamp recordings. Anandamide (10 μM) superfused for 2 min reduced glycinergic and GABAergic electrically-evoked inhibitory postsynaptic current (IPSC) amplitudes; these actions persisted for more than 6 min after washout. Similar actions were produced by cannabinoid-receptor agonist WIN55,212-2 (5 μM) and 2-arachidonoyl glycerol (20 μM). The evoked IPSC amplitudes reduced by anandamide recovered to the control level following superfusion of CB1-receptor antagonist SR141716A (5 μM). A ratio of the second to first evoked IPSC amplitude in paired-pulse experiments was increased by anandamide (10 μM). The frequencies of glycinergic and GABAergic spontaneous IPSCs were reduced by anandamide (10 μM) without a change in their amplitudes. It is concluded that cannabinoids depress inhibitory transmissions in adult rat SG neurons by activating CB1 receptors in nerve terminals. This action could contribute to the modulation of nociceptive transmission by cannabinoids.

Keywords

Spinal Dorsal Horn, Cannabinoid, CB1 Receptor, IPSC, Patch-Clamp, Pain

---

[*]Corresponding author.

1. Introduction

Cannabinoids play an important role in a variety of physiological phenomena including antinociception (for review see [1]-[4]). Cannabinoid receptors are classified into two subtypes, CB1 and CB2, both of which are G-protein coupled receptors [1]. When administered intrathecally, cannabinoids produce antinociception in acute pain models through the activation of the cannabinoid receptors [1] [3] [4]. For instance, applying the prototypical cannabinoid Δ^9-tetrahydrocannabinol resulted in antinociception in the tail-flick test in adult rats [5]. A mixed CB1/CB2 receptor agonist WIN55,212-2 (WIN-2) produced a similar antinociceptive effect [6]. Such behavioral results are possibly due to the activation of the CB1 receptor in the spinal dorsal horn, because expression of this receptor has been demonstrated there by *in situ* hybridization [7], agonist binding [8] and immunohistochemistry [9]-[12]. A selective CB1-receptor antagonist SR141716A enhanced nociceptive responses of rat spinal dorsal horn neurons [13].

The superficial dorsal horn of the spinal cord, particularly the substantia gelatinosa (SG, lamina II of Rexed), is thought to play an important role in regulating nociceptive transmission from the periphery through the modulation of synaptic transmissions in SG neurons (for review see [14]-[16]). In support of this idea, glutamatergic excitatory transmission to SG neurons through primary-afferent fibers is inhibited by various endogenous substances including opioids [17], serotonin [18], nociceptin [19], noradrenaline [20], adenosine [21] and galanin [22] which are thought to act as analgesics in the spinal dorsal horn (for review see [15]). This idea appears to be applied also to the cannabinoid-mediated antinociception, because cannabinoids inhibit glutamatergic transmission in rat SG neurons [23] [24]. A similar inhibition of glutamatergic transmission by cannabinoids has been reported in the spinal trigeminal pars caudalis SG [25].

Glycinergic and GABAergic inhibitory interneurons in the SG are involved in polysynaptic pathways originating in primary-afferent terminals ([26]; for review see [14] [16]), and probably serve to modulate nociceptive transmission [27] [28].Consistent with this idea, the lack of GABA-synthesizing enzyme [29] and also an inhibition of K^+-Cl^- exporter KCC2 expression, which causes inhibitory synaptic response to be excitatory [30], in the rat spinal dorsal horn lead to nociception. There is a difference among endogenous analgesics in modulating inhibitory transmission mediated by the interneurons. For example, noradrenaline [31], acetylcholine ([32]-[34]), serotonin [35] and oxytocin ([36] [37]) enhanced the inhibitory transmission, possibly contributing to antinociception. On the other hand, the inhibitory transmission was unaffected by opioids ([17]), nociceptin ([19]) and galanin ([22]) while being inhibited by adenosine ([38]). The latter action may contribute to nociception rather than antinociception. Depression of inhibitory transmission by cannabinoids has been reported in various CNS regions including the corpus striatum ([39]), the hippocampal CA1 ([40] [41]), the spinal trigeminal pars caudalis SG ([42]) and the substantia nigra pars reticulata (SNR; [43]). However, the effects of cannabinoids on inhibitory transmission in the spinal cord SG have not yet been examined fully. There are no reports about the effects of cannabinoids on glycinergic transmission except for the studies by Jennings *et al.* [42] and Pernía-Andrade *et al.* [44]. Although the latter study revealed an inhibition by WIN-2 of GABAergic and glycinergic transmissions, this was performed in superficial dorsal horn neurons of young (1 - 3 weeks old) mice. An inhibition of inhibitory transmission by cannabinoids may exhibit a developmental change, as seen in the oxytocin actions in rat SG neurons. Oxytocin enhanced spontaneous GABAergic but not glycinergic inhibitory transmission in young (2 - 4 weeks old) rats ([36]) whereas facilitating both of the inhibitory transmissions in adult (6 - 8 weeks old) rats ([37]). The highest concentration of a precursor of an endocannabinoid N-arachidonoylethanolamide (anandamide; ANA) is found in the spinal cord [45]. ANA activates the CB1 receptor more effectively than the CB2 receptor [1]. In the present study, we investigated the effects of ANA on glycinergic and GABAergic inhibitory transmissions in SG neurons of adult rat spinal cord slices by using the whole-cell patch-clamp technique. A part of this study has been reported in abstract form [46].

2. Materials and Methods

All animal experiments were approved by the Animal Care and Use Committee of Saga University, and were conducted in accordance with the Guiding Principles for the Care and Use of Animals in the Field of Physiological Science of the Physiological Society of Japan. All efforts were made to minimize animal suffering and the number of animals used.

2.1. Slice Preparations

Spinal cord slices from adult rats were prepared as described previously [20] [38] [47]. In brief, adult Sprague-

Dawley rats (7 - 8 weeks old; 250 - 300 g) were anesthetized with urethane (1.5 g/kg body weight, i.p.) and a laminectomy was performed to extract a lumbosacral spinal cord segment. The spinal cord was quickly immersed in ice-cold ($1^\circ C$ - $3^\circ C$) Krebs solution (in mM: NaCl 117, KCl 3.6, $CaCl_2$ 1.2, NaH_2PO_4 1.2, $MgCl_2$ 1.2, $NaHCO_3$ 25 and glucose 11) bubbled with 95% O_2-5% CO_2. Rats were killed by exsanguination. A transverse slice (thickness: 500 μm) was cut using a microslicer (DTK-1000, Dousaka, Kyoto, Japan) in oxygenated ice-cold Krebs solution. The slice was then transferred to the recording chamber (volume: 1.5 ml), and continuously perfused with pre-heated ($35^\circ C \pm 1^\circ C$; when measured in the chamber) and oxygenated Krebs solution for at least 1 hr before recordings.

2.2. Whole-Cell Voltage-Clamp Recordings and Focal Stimulation

The SG can be identified under a stereomicroscope as a translucent band across the spinal dorsal horn [20] [38] [47]. Spinal cord slices could be maintained for up to 12 hr when they were superfused at a rate of 15 - 20 ml/min with pre-oxygenated Krebs solution at $35^\circ C \pm 1^\circ C$. The conventional blind whole-cell patch-clamp technique was applied to the SG neurons. The recorded neurons were located at the center of SG to avoid recordings from laminae I and III neurons. Patch-pipettes were filled with solution (in mM): Cs_2SO_4 110, $CaCl_2$ 0.5, $MgCl_2$ 2, EGTA 5, HEPES 5, Mg-ATP 5 and tetraethylammonium (TEA)-Cl 5; and had a resistance of 10 - 15 MΩ. After making a rigid seal (resistance: 5 - 20 GΩ) in the cell-attached mode by a gentle suction into the patch-pipette, the membrane patch was ruptured by a brief period of more powerful suction, resulting in the whole-cell configuration. Only neurons having resting membrane potentials more negative than -55 mV in the current-clamp mode were voltage-clamped and then holding potential (V_H) was shifted to 0 mV used to record IPSCs, as reported previously [17] [38]. K^+-channel blockers (Cs^+ and TEA) were added to the patch-pipette solution to easily perform the shift of V_H and also to shorten the electrotonic length of the dendrites. The recordings of IPSCs started several minutes after the whole-cell mode. Recordings from single neurons under this condition were stable for up to 1 hr.

Electrically-evoked inhibitory postsynaptic currents (IPSCs) were triggered at 0.1 or 0.2 Hz by stimulating SG neurons (somata and axons) with rectangular pulses (duration: 0.1 ms) using an extracellular monopolar silver-wire electrode (50 μm in diameter; isolated except for the tip) located within 150 μm of the recorded neurons; the stimulus intensity was monitored with a digitized output isolator. The amplitude of the evoked IPSC (eIPSC) in response to electrical stimulation varied among the stimuli, possibly because of a fluctuation of the number of quanta released from nerve terminals [see [42] for a similar variation in eIPSC amplitudes]. Paired-pulse stimulation with a short-time interval (15 - 50 ms) was also used to obtain eIPSCs. All signals were amplified by an Axopatch 200B amplifier (Axon Instruments, Foster City, CA, USA), digitized at 333 or 500 kHz with an A/D converter (Digidata 1200A or 1322; Axon Instruments) and stored on a computer using the pCLAMP 6 or 8 data acquisition program (Axon Instruments).

2.3. Data Analysis

The signals were analyzed off-line using an Axograph 4.0 (Axon Instruments). In estimating quantitatively the effects of drugs on evoked transmission at a time, many but not more than six of eIPSC amplitudes were averaged if the amplitudes varied to a large extent in response to individual stimuli. Spontaneous IPSCs (sIPSCs) were automatically analyzed with a variable amplitude template and visually examined to find out whether erroneous sIPSC events were detected; if so, the template was changed and the analysis was repeated. This process was repeated until erroneous sIPSC events were not detected. The frequency and amplitude of sIPSC was calculated from sIPSC events measured for at least 1 min. Data were shown as mean ± S.E.M., and statistical significance was set at $P < 0.05$ using a paired Student's t-test (unless otherwise mentioned) or a Kolmogorov-Smirnov test. In all cases n refers to the number of neurons studied.

2.4. Application of Drugs

All drugs were applied by switching the perfusion solution to one containing the drug at a known concentration using a three-way tap. The perfusion rate or temperature was not altered during the drug application. Drug-containing solutions reached to the recording chamber within 10 s. Drugs used were ANA, R(+)-WIN-2 mesylate (Research Biochemicals International, Natick, MA, USA); 6-cyano-7-nitroquinoxaline-2,3-dione (CNQX) from

Tocris Cookson (Bristol, UK); (-)-bicuculline methiodide and strychnine from Sigma (St. Louis, MO, USA); te-trodotoxin (TTX) from Wako (Osaka, Japan); and SR141716A from the NIMH's Chemical Synthesis and Drug Supply Program. All drugs except TTX, bicuculline and strychnine (where distilled water was used as a solvent) were first dissolved in dimethyl sulfoxide (DMSO) at 1000 times the concentration to be used, and then diluted to the desired concentration in Krebs solution immediately before use. DMSO itself at the highest concentration (0.1%) used in the present study did not significantly affect glycinergic and GABAergic eIPSC amplitudes [92% ± 6% ($n = 3$; $P > 0.05$) and 97%, 112%, respectively, of control around 2 min after the superfusion of DMSO for 2 min].

3. Results

All SG neurons tested exhibited glutamatergic spontaneous excitatory postsynaptic currents (EPSCs) at a V_H of −70 mV where no sIPSCs were observed, since the reversal potential for IPSCs was near −70 mV. On the other hand, when the V_H was shifted to 0 mV, sIPSCs could be encountered in all neurons tested, where no spontane-ous EPSCs were invisible owing to the reversal potential for EPSCs to be close to 0 mV [38]. Neither the fre-quency nor the amplitude of sIPSCs was significantly affected following the application of TTX (0.5 μM; data not shown), indicating that the production of the sIPSCs was independent of the spontaneous activities of neu-rons presynaptic to SG neurons (see [38]).

3.1. ANA Reduces Both Glycinergic and GABAergic eIPSC Amplitudes

Glycinergic and GABAergic eIPSCs were, respectively, evoked in the presence of a $GABA_A$-receptor antagonist bicuculline (10 μM) and a glycine-receptor antagonist strychnine (1 μM) together with a non-NMDA receptor antagonist CNQX (10 μM) which was added to block the activation of glutamatergic interneurons. The glyci-nergic eIPSCs were shorter in duration by about three-fold than the GABAergic ones, as reported previously [17] [38]. The glycinergic and GABAergic eIPSCs were stable in amplitude for at least 7 min after the beginning of their recordings (**Figure 1(A)**).

In 18 (78%) out of 23 neurons examined, ANA (10 μM) superfused for 2 min reduced the amplitude of the glycinergic eIPSC, as seen in **Figure 1(B)**. This action persisted for more than 6 min after washout. The magni-tude of this reduction was measured around 2 min after washout (when a maximal effect of adenosine on eIPSC amplitudes in SG neurons was observed under the same condition as that in the present study; see [38]), al-though the time course of a change in eIPSC amplitudes following ANA superfusion varied among neurons tested, probably due to a difference in their position such as depth from the surface of spinal cord slice. The re-ductive extent was 27% ± 3% ($n = 18$; $P < 0.05$). The remaining five neurons did not exhibit a change (>5%) in the amplitude. GABAergic eIPSC amplitudes also were reduced by ANA (10 μM) in a similar manner, as seen in **Figure 1(C)**. This action was observed in 17 (71%) out of 24 neurons tested with the extent of 42% ± 4% ($n = 17$; $P < 0.05$) around 2 min after washout. In the remaining five neurons, two neurons exhibited a small increase in the amplitude (by 17% and 8% around 2 min in the presence of ANA) while three neurons were not affected by ANA. Since some of the neurons tested did not exhibit the inhibitory action of ANA, the effects of ANA at various concentrations on eIPSCs were examined in single neurons. **Figures 2(A)-(B)** demonstrate, respectively, the effects on glycinergic and GABAergic eIPSCs of ANA which is applied successively at various concentra-tions ranging from 1 to 10 μM. The ANA-induced reductions in glycinergic and GABAergic eIPSC amplitudes were seen at a low concentration such as 1 μM with extents of 33% ± 7% and 20% ± 4% (each $n = 3$), respec-tively, around 2 min after washout. Under the reduction by ANA at a concentration of 5 μM, ANA (10 μM) did not exhibit a further decrease in glycinergic or GABAergic eIPSC amplitudes [103% and 104%; 92% ± 19% ($n = 3$), respectively, of that just before the ANA (10 μM) application], indicating an occlusion of ANA actions.

3.2. The eIPSC Amplitude Reductions Produced by ANA Are Mediated by Cannabinoid Receptors

We first examined whether a cannabinoid-receptor agonist WIN-2 mimicks the depressive action of ANA on evoked inhibitory transmissions. **Figures 3(A)-(B)** demonstrate the effects of WIN-2 (5 μM) superfused for 2 min on evoked glycinergic and GABAergic transmissions, respectively. In 8 (80%) out of 10 neurons tested, WIN-2 reduced glycinergic eIPSC amplitudes in a manner similar to that of ANA, as seen in **Figure 3(A)**.

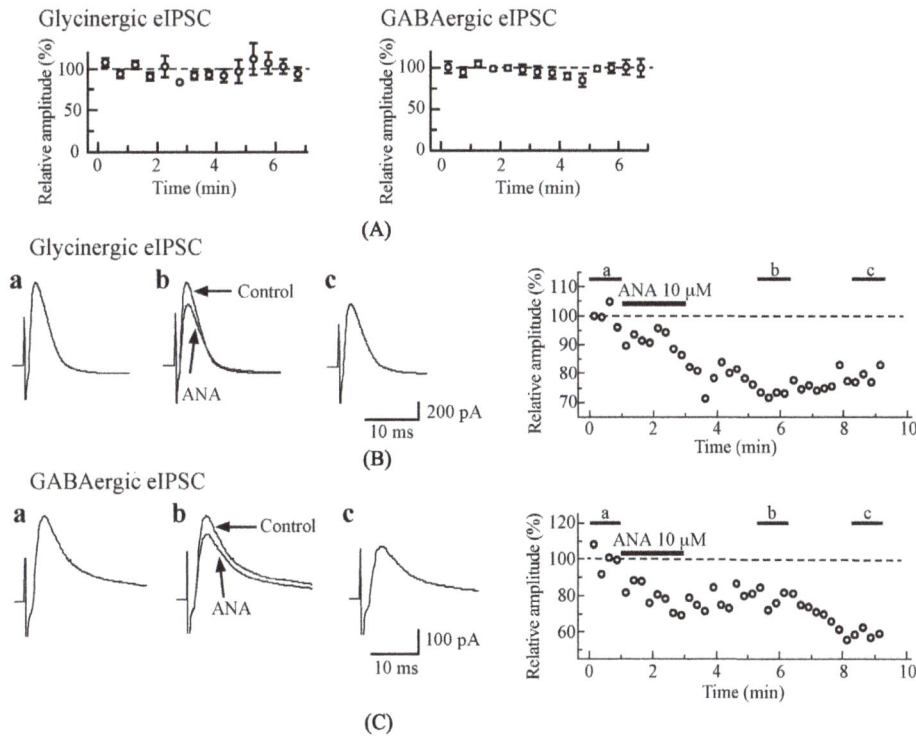

Figure 1. Reductions by anandamide (ANA; 10 μM) of the peak amplitudes of electrically-evoked IPSCs (eIPSCs) recorded from substantia gelatinosa (SG) neurons. (A) Time courses of the peak amplitudes of glycinergic and GABAergic eIPSCs recorded over 7 min under the condition of control. Each point with vertical bars shows the averaged value of the amplitudes of 3 consecutive eIPSCs, and is the mean and S.E.M. of data obtained from 3 - 4 neurons and expressed as a percentage of the mean of all the values for the amplitudes. (B) & (C) Glycinergic and GABAergic eIPSCs, respectively, in the control and under the action of ANA. Left records: averaged traces of 12 consecutive eIPSCs in the control (a) and under the action of ANA [b (where control eIPSC is superimposed for comparison) and c]. Right graphs: time courses of changes in the peak amplitudes of eIPSC under the action of ANA, relative to control. Each point shows the averaged value of the amplitudes of 3 consecutive eIPSCs. In each of (B) and (C), averaged results in time ranges (a, b, c) in the right graph correspond to traces (a, b, c) in the left record, respectively. The glycinergic and GABAergic eIPSCs were observed in the presence of bicuculline (10 μM) and strychnine (1 μM), respectively, together with CNQX (10 μM); holding potential (V_H) = 0 mV.

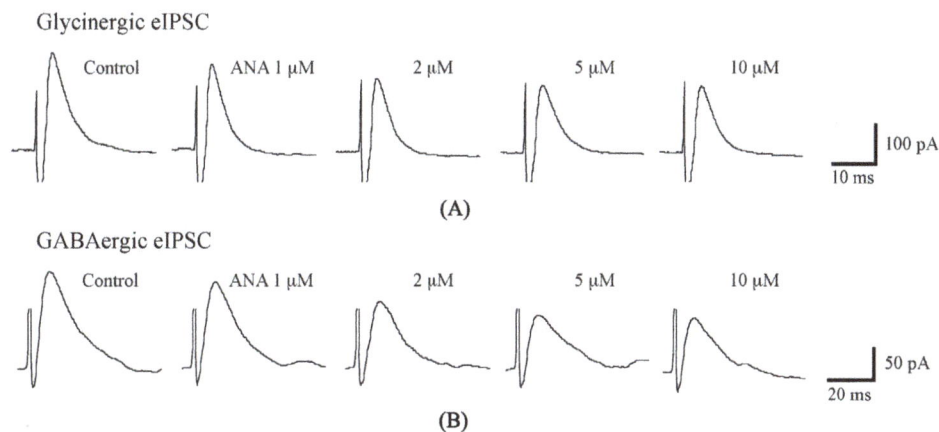

Figure 2. Effects of ANA at various concentrations on evoked inhibitory transmissions in SG neurons. (A) & (B) Averaged traces of three consecutive glycinergic and GABAergic eIPSCs, respectively, in the control and under the action of ANA (around 2 min after washout) at concentrations of 1, 2, 5 and 10 μM, where ANA was superfused successively for 2 min at each concentration in the order of low to high ones in the same neuron. Here, there was a time interval of 2 min between the applications of the different concentrations of ANA. The eIPSCs in (A) and (B) were observed in the presence of bicuculline (10 μM) and strychnine (1 μM), respectively, together with CNQX (10 μM); V_H = 0 mV.

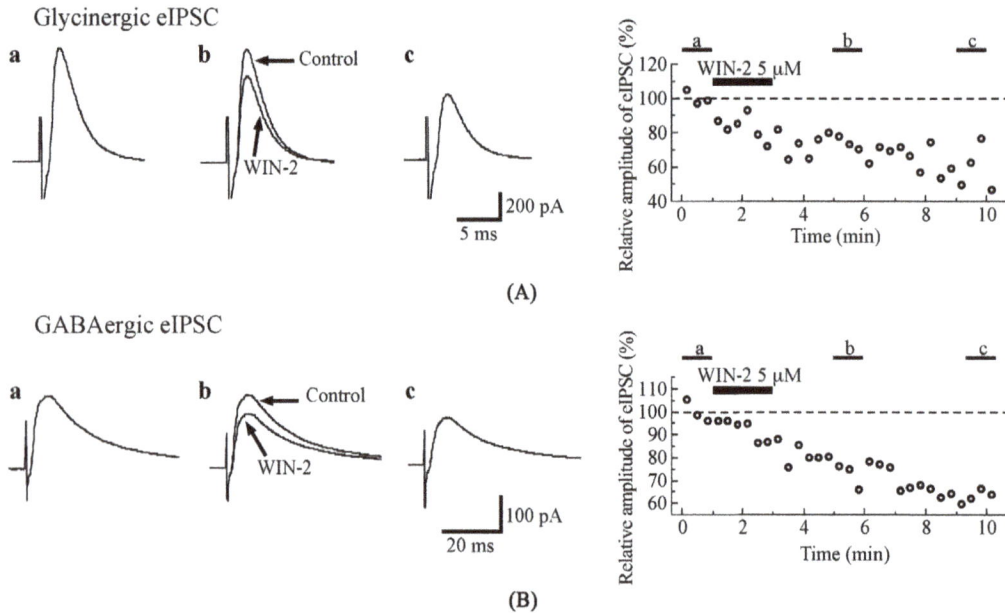

Figure 3. Reductions by WIN55,212-2 (WIN-2; 5 μM) of the peak amplitudes of eIPSCs recorded from SG neurons. (A) & (B) Glycinergic and GABAergic eIPSCs, respectively, in the control and under the action of WIN-2. Left records: averaged traces of 6 consecutive eIPSCs in the control (a) and under the action of WIN-2 [b (where control eIPSC is superimposed for comparison) and c]. Right graphs: time courses of changes in the peak amplitudes of eIPSC under the action of WIN-2, relative to control. Each point shows the averaged value of the amplitudes of two consecutive eIPSCs. In each of (A) and (B), averaged results in time ranges (a, b, c) in the right graph correspond to traces (a, b, c) in the left record, respectively. The eIPSCs in (A) and (B) were observed in the presence of bicuculline (10 μM) and strychnine (1 μM), respectively, together with CNQX (10 μM); $V_H = 0$ mV.

When estimated around 2 min after washout of WIN-2 in a manner similar to that for ANA actions, the magnitude of the reduction was 20% ± 4% ($n = 8$; $P < 0.05$). The remaining two neurons did not exhibit the reduction. GABAergic eIPSC amplitudes also were reduced by WIN-2 (5 μM) in a manner similar to that for glycinergic eIPSCs, as seen in **Figure 3(B)**. This action was observed in 13 (68%) out of 19 neurons tested with the extent of 28% ± 4% ($n = 13$; $P < 0.05$) around 2 min after washout. In the remaining four neurons, two neurons exhibited a small increase in the amplitude (by 25% and 11% around 2 min in the presence of WIN-2) while other two neurons were not affected by WIN-2. An endogenous agonist of cannabinoid receptors, 2-arachydonoyl glycerol (2-AG; 20 μM; [48]), the level of which is considerably higher than that of ANA in the spinal cord [49], also reduced eIPSC amplitudes, as shown in **Figure 4**. The magnitudes of the reductions in glycinergic and GABAergic eIPSC amplitudes were, respectively, 32% ± 11% ($n = 4$; $P < 0.05$) and 30% ± 5% ($n = 4$; $P < 0.05$) around 2 min after washout of 2-AG.

We next examined how a CB1-receptor antagonist SR141716A (5 μM) affects the reductions in eIPSC amplitudes by ANA (10 μM). SR141716A by itself did not significantly affect glycinergic and GABAergic eIPSC amplitudes [90% ± 2% ($n = 6$) and 93% ± 7% ($n = 5$) of control, respectively, about 2 min after the commencement of its superfusion], and following its washout there was not a further change in the amplitudes, as different from ANA and WIN-2 actions. Since the inhibitory effect of ANA on eIPSCs was not observed in some of the neurons tested, we examined whether the inhibition persisting after washout of ANA is reduced by SR141716A, as done for the inhibitory effect of WIN-2 on evoked inhibitory transmissions in spinal trigeminal SG neurons [42]. In neurons where ANA (10 μM) attenuated glycinergic or GABAergic eIPSC amplitude, the amplitude recovered to the control level by SR141716A (5 μM), as seen in **Figure 5**. In neurons which exhibited an amplitude reduction of 46% ± 11% ($n = 4$; $P < 0.05$) around 2 min after washout of ANA, glycinergic eIPSC amplitudes recovered to 84% ± 8% of those before ANA application around 2 min after the beginning of SR141716A superfusion. Following SR141716A superfusion for 2 min, GABAergic eIPSC amplitudes recovered to 109% and 99% of those before ANA application which resulted in a reduction in the amplitude (by 57% and 25% around 2 min after washout).

Glycinergic eIPSC

(A)

GABAergic eIPSC

(B)

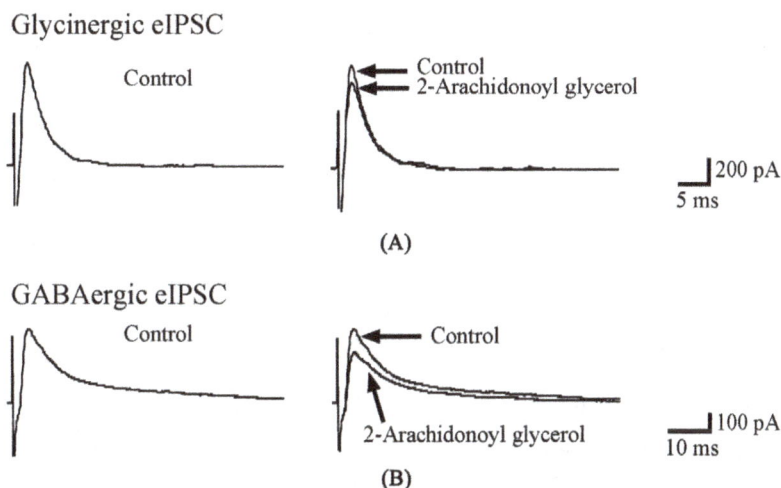

Figure 4. Reductions by 2-arachidonoyl glycerol (20 μM) of the peak amplitudes of eIPSCs recorded from SG neurons. (A) and (B) Averaged traces of 6 consecutive glycinergic and GABAergic eIPSCs, respectively, in the control (left) and under the action of 2-arachidonoyl glycerol (right) where control eIPSC is superimposed for comparison. The eIPSCs in (A) and (B) were observed in the presence of bicuculline (10 μM) and strychnine (1 μM), respectively, together with CNQX (10 μM); $V_H = 0$ mV.

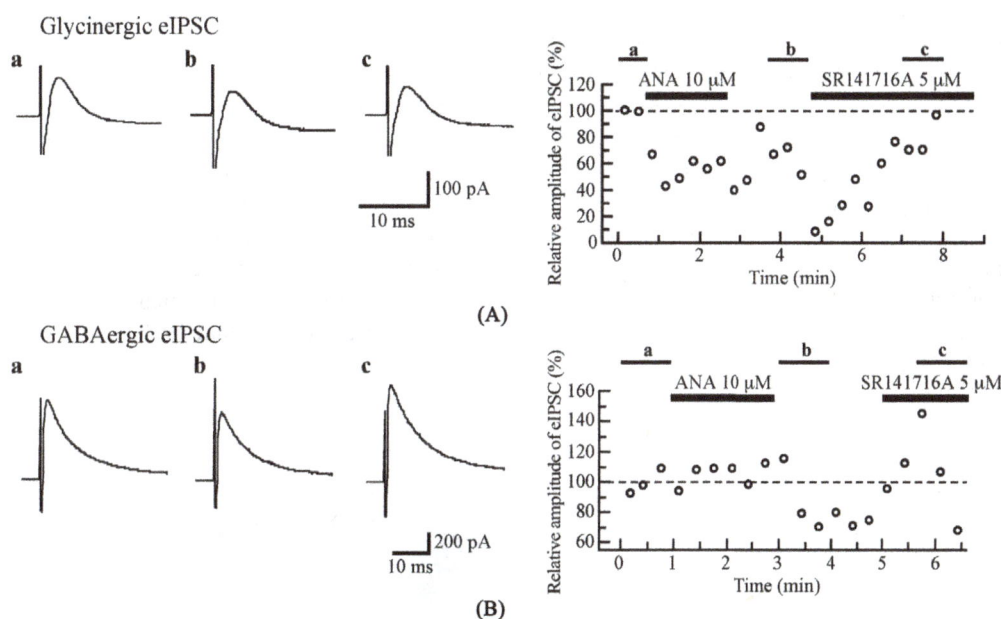

Glycinergic eIPSC

(A)

GABAergic eIPSC

(B)

Figure 5. Reduced eIPSC amplitudes by ANA (10 μM) recovered to the control level by SR141716A (5 μM) in SG neurons. (A) & (B) Glycinergic and GABAergic eIPSCs, respectively, in the control, under the action of ANA and a recovery from its action in the presence of SR141716A. Left records: averaged traces of 4 - 6 consecutive glycinergic and GABAergic eIPSCs in the control (a), under the action of ANA (b) and following superfusion of SR141716A (c). Right graphs: time courses of changes in the peak amplitudes of eIPSC by applying SR141716A under the inhibitory action of ANA, relative to control. Each point shows the averaged value of the amplitudes of two consecutive eIPSCs. In each of (A) and (B), averaged results in time ranges (a, b, c) in the right graph correspond to traces (a, b, c) in the left record, respectively. The eIPSCs in (A) and (B) were observed in the presence of bicuculline (10 μM) and strychnine (1 μM), respectively, together with CNQX (10 μM); $V_H = 0$ mV.

3.3. ANA Increases Paired-Pulse Ratios of eIPSC Amplitudes

To characterize the reductions in eIPSC amplitudes by ANA, we carried out a paired-pulse experiment with a time interval of 15 - 50 ms, where the interval used for glycinergic eIPSCs was shorter than that for GABAergic eIPSCs because the former eIPSCs were shorter in duration than the latter ones, as described above. Glycinergic and GABAergic eIPSCs exhibited a paired-pulse depression (PPD) or paired-pulse facilitation (PPF) in a manner dependent on the paired-pulse intervals used, as seen in the most left traces of **Figure 6**, although these phenomena were not examined here in detail. When examined in neurons exhibiting the ANA-induced reductions in eIPSC amplitudes, a ratio of the second to first eIPSC amplitude in each case of PPD and PPF was increased by ANA (10 μM). The amplitude ratios in the PPD (0.706) and PPF (1.11; see **Figure 6(A)**) of glycinergic eIPSC amplitudes were increased by 21% and 9%, respectively (the first eIPSC amplitude reduction by ANA: 35% and 16%, respectively). The amplitude ratios in the PPD (0.959 and 0.895 [see **Figure 6(B)**]) and PPF (1.18) of GABAergic eIPSC amplitudes were increased by 18%, 65% and 22%, respectively (the first eIPSC amplitude reduction by ANA: 56%, 39% and 14%, respectively).

3.4. ANA Reduces the Frequency but Not Amplitude of sIPSC

Two kinds of glycinergic and GABAergic sIPSCs could be encountered in SG neurons, as reported previously [17] [38]. ANA (10 μM) superfused for 2 min reduced the frequency of glycinergic sIPSCs which were observed in the presence of bicuculline (10 μM). This action persisted several minutes after washout of ANA, as seen in **Figure 7(A)**. **Figure 7(A)** also demonstrates cumulative distributions of the amplitude and inter-event interval of glycinergic sIPSC in the control and under the action of ANA. A proportion of sIPSCs having a longer inter-event interval was increased by ANA while there was not a change in the cumulative distribution of sIPSC amplitude. In 5 out of 7 neurons examined, when estimated around 1 min after washout of ANA (when its inhibitory action on eIPSCs was apparent; see **Figure 1**), glycinergic sIPSC frequency was on average reduced by 46% ± 5% ($n = 5$; $P < 0.01$; control: 2.09 ± 0.27 Hz), whereas the amplitude was unchanged [95% ± 3% ($P > 0.05$) of control (25.4 ± 4.7 pA)]. Remaining two neurons did not respond to ANA. In the presence of strychnine (1 μM), GABAergic sIPSCs, which were longer by about three-fold in duration than glycinergic ones (compare sIPSC traces in a fast time scale in **Figures 7(A)-(B)**; see also [38]) as seen for the corresponding eIPSCs, could be recorded. As seen for glycinergic sIPSCs, ANA (10 μM) superfused for 2 min reduced GABAergic sIPSC frequency (see **Figure 7(B)**). When cumulative distributions of the amplitude and inter-event interval of GABAergic sIPSC were examined as shown in **Figure 7(B)**, ANA increased a proportion of sIPSCs having a longer inter-event interval while unaffecting the cumulative distribution of sIPSC amplitude. In all of five neurons tested, when estimated around 1 min after washout of ANA, the GABAergic sIPSC frequency was decreased by 35% ± 7% ($n = 5$; $P < 0.05$; control: 1.04 ± 0.35 Hz) without a change in the amplitude [93% ± 4% ($P > 0.05$) of control (19.6 ± 3.6 pA)].

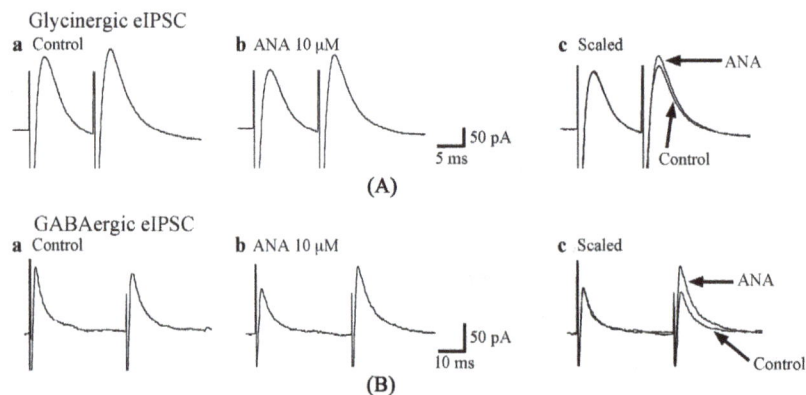

Figure 6. Effects of ANA (10 μM) on evoked glycinergic and GABAergic inhibitory transmissions in response to a paired-pulse stimulus in SG neurons. (A) and (B) Averaged traces of 6 consecutive paired-pulse induced glycinergic and GABAergic eIPSCs, respectively, (with a time interval of 20 and 40 ms, respectively) in the control (a), under the action of ANA (b) and their superimposition (c; where the first eIPSC in the paired eIPSC in the control was scaled to that under the action of ANA). The eIPSCs in (A) and (B) were observed in the presence of bicuculline (10 μM) and strychnine (1 μM), respectively, together with CNQX (10 μM); $V_H = 0$ mV.

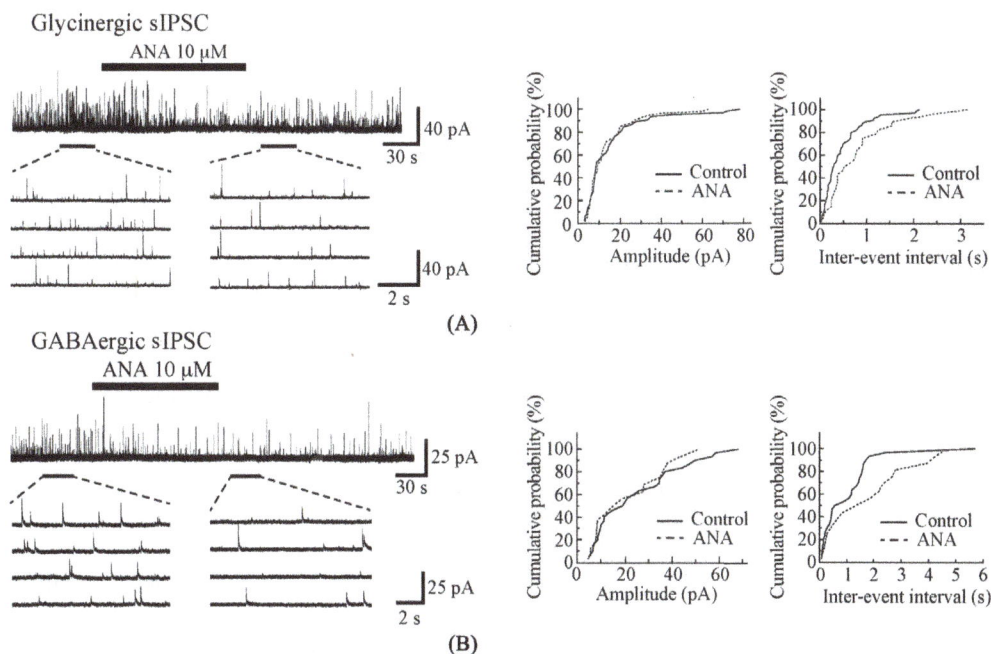

Figure 7. Effects of ANA (10 µM) on glycinergic (A) and GABAergic spontaneous inhibitory transmissions (B) in SG neurons. Continuous chart recordings of glycinergic and GABAergic sIPSCs (upper in (A) and (B)) in the control and under the action of ANA. The horizontal bars above records indicate the period of time during which ANA is applied. Traces given below the chart recordings show sIPSCs, which are shown in an expanded scale in time, recorded consecutively for a period indicated by a bar shown below the recordings. In the right two graphs of (A), are shown cumulative histograms of the amplitude and inter-event interval of glycinergic sIPSC in the control (continuous line) and under the action of ANA (dotted line), where their histograms are made from sIPSCs measured for 1 min (127 and 69 sIPSC events, respectively). ANA had no effect on the amplitude distribution ($P = 0.26$) while shifting the interval distribution to a longer one ($P < 0.05$; Kolmogorov-Smirnov test). In the right two graphs of (B), are shown cumulative histograms of the amplitude and inter-event interval of GABAergic sIPSC in the control (continuous line) and under the action of ANA (dotted line), where their histograms are made from sIPSCs measured for 1 min (51 and 28 sIPSC events, respectively). ANA had no effect on the amplitude distribution ($P = 0.37$) while shifting the interval distribution to a longer one ($P < 0.05$; Kolmogorov-Smirnov test). (A) and (B) were obtained in the presence of bicuculline (10 µM) and strychnine (1 µM), respectively; $V_H = 0$ mV.

4. Discussion

The present study demonstrated that ANA reduces glycinergic and GABAergic eIPSC amplitudes and sIPSC frequencies in many of the adult rat SG neurons examined. These actions were presynaptic in origin, because glycinergic and GABAergic sIPSC amplitudes were not affected by ANA. This idea is supported by paired-pulse experiments, because ANA increases a ratio of the second to first glycinergic or GABAergic eIPSC amplitude. This increase would not be expected if ANA inhibits a sensitivity of postsynaptic neurons to glycine or GABA and as a result the first and second eIPSC amplitudes are reduced by the same extent.

4.1. Depression of Inhibitory Transmission by ANA Is Mediated by CB1 Receptors

The reductions in glycinergic and GABAergic eIPSC amplitudes by ANA were mimicked by the CB1/CB2 receptor agonist WIN-2 and disappeared in the presence of the selective CB1 receptor antagonist SR141716A, indicating an involvement of CB1 receptors. This action of WIN-2 as well as ANA persisted at least 7 min after washout, as seen in the inhibitory action of WIN-2 on GABAergic eIPSCs in the hippocampus [40]. This persistence would be possibly due to a lipophilic nature of the cannabinoids. A similar inhibition by WIN-2 of glycinergic and GABAergic inhibitory transmissions has been reported in superficial dorsal horn neurons in young mice [44].

Since it is known that ANA activates not only CB1 receptors but also transient receptor potential (TRP) vanilloid-1 (TRPV1) channels [50] and that SR141716A inhibits TRPV1 responses [51], the ANA-induced inhibition may have been mediated by both CB1 receptors and TRPV1 channels. This is, however, unlikely in the case of ANA (10 μM) actions in the SG, because ANA at a high concentration such as 20 μM enhances glutamatergic spontaneous transmission in a manner sensitive to a non-selective TRP antagonist ruthenium red [52] while ANA at 10 μM does not affect the transmission [24]. TRPV1 channels in the spinal trigeminal SG are activated by ANA at a higher concentration such as 30 μM [53]. Furthermore, a TRPV1 agonist capsaicin has no effect on glycinergic and GABAergic eIPSCs (and also sIPSCs) in SG neurons ([54] [55]; for review see [56]).

Although 2-AG is known to be more potent than ANA in activating CB1 receptors [57], this fact does not appear to be applied to their depressive effects on inhibitory transmissions in the present study, because the IPSC amplitude reduction produced by 2-AG (20 μM) is comparable in extent to that of ANA (10 μM). This may be due to the fact that 2-AG is more easily degraded than ANA by their inactivating enzymes such as ANA amidohydrolase (for review see [58]) in spinal cord slices.

The presynaptic effect of ANA on GABAergic transmission is consistent with the presence of GABA in CB1 receptor-like immunoreactive SG neurons [11]. The fact that the ANA action was seen in some of the SG neurons examined may be consistent with the observation that a part of CB1 receptor-like immunoreactive SG neurons was labeled for GABA [11] or that GABAergic neuron terminals in the SG originate from not only SG interneurons but also other laminae and medullary neurons (for review see [59]). Even if the descending pathways from the medulla have been disrupted in the slice preparation used in the present study, it is not unlikely that nerve terminals originating from the pathways are intact and thus exhibit the spontaneous and evoked releases of glycine and/or GABA, considering that single neurons isolated using an enzyme-free and mechanical dissociation procedure have adherent functional synaptic terminals (for review see [60]). Since some of SG inhibitory neuron terminals appeared to express CB1 receptors, neurons not responding to cannabinoids were excluded from the statistical analysis of the reductions in eIPSC amplitude and sIPSC frequency by cannabinoids.

Presynaptic inhibition of GABAergic transmission by CB1 receptor activation similar to that in the spinal cord SG has been reported in the corpus striatum [39], the hippocampal CA1 [40] [41], the spinal trigeminal SG [42] and the SNR [43]. Jennings *et al.* [42] have demonstrated CB1 receptor-mediated presynaptic inhibition of glycinergic transmission in the spinal trigeminal SG. Although the superfusion time (2 min) of cannabinoids used in the present study was shorter than those (10 - 20 min) in previous studies and thus the result obtained may not have been in a steady state, the GABAergic eIPSC amplitude reduction produced by WIN-2 was almost similar in extent among different types of neurons [spinal cord SG: 28% at 5 μM (present study); hippocampal CA1: 47% at 5 μM ([40]); spinal trigeminal SG: 35% at 3 μM ([42]); SNR: 43% at 10 μM ([43])]. This may be due to the fact that the superfusion rate (15 - 20 ml/min) used in our study is much larger than those (1 - 2 ml/min) in other studies.

Although a cellular mechanism for the ANA action is not examined here, this would be due to an inhibition of voltage-gated Ca^{2+} channels present in nerve terminals, because WIN-2 inhibits Ca^{2+}-channel currents in AtT20 cells transfected with CB1 receptors [61] and in cultured rat hippocampal neurons [62]. Liang *et al.* [25] have demonstrated a presynaptic inhibition by WIN-2 of glutamatergic transmission in a manner sensitive to N-type Ca^{2+}-channel blockers. This idea about the involvement of Ca^{2+} channels could be applied to the reductions in not only eIPSC amplitude but also sIPSC frequency, because sIPSC frequency in SG neurons is decreased in Ca^{2+}-free Krebs solution and thus presynaptic Ca^{2+} channels are partially open at the resting state, resulting in a tonic Ca^{2+} entry in nerve terminals [38].

It is of interest to note that there is a similarity in cannabinoids-induced inhibition between glycinergic and GABAergic transmissions. This result might be due to the fact that these two kinds of synapses are controlled under a similar release machinery. Spinal dorsal horn, especially SG, neurons contain both glycine and GABA, which might be co-released into the dorsal horn [26]. Similar inhibitions by WIN-2 between glycinergic and GABAergic transmissions have been reported in the rodent spinal cord and trigeminal SG [42] [44]. No difference in presynaptic modulation between glycinergic and GABAergic transmissions is also seen in the action of adenosine in the rat spinal cord SG [38]. On the other hand, the glycinergic and GABAergic transmissions in the SG neurons are affected by a phospholipase A_2 activator melittin in a manner different from each other [34] [63]. Thus, it seems to be unlikely that the glycinergic and GABAergic transmissions in SG neurons are always modulated in a similar manner.

4.2. Physiological Significance of the Depressive Effects of Cannabinoids on Inhibitory Transmissions in SG Neurons

The depressive effects of cannabinoids on inhibitory transmissions are expected to lead to an increase in the excitability of SG neurons, a result different from those of other endogenous analgesics in such that the inhibitory transmissions are facilitated by noradrenaline [31], acetylcholine ([32]-[34]), serotonin ([35]) and oxytocin ([36] [37]) and is not affected by opioids ([17]), nociceptin ([19]) and galanin ([22]) in adult rat SG neurons. On the other hand, adenosine exhibits a disinhibitory effect similar to that of cannabinoids. A part of antinociception produced by intrathecally-administered cannabinoids has been reported to be due to the release of endogenous analgesics such as noradrenaline [5] and opioids ([64]; for review see [1]). The cannabinoid-induced disinhibition may result in the release of the endogenous analgesics which inhibit excitatory transmission in SG neurons. Alternatively, the presynaptic depression of inhibitory transmission as revealed in the present study may lead to the reduction in background noise as a result of a decrease in opening of glycine and $GABA_A$ receptor-channels which in turn could increase input resistance and thus make SG neurons electrically compact, contributing to the modulation of nociceptive transmission, as suggested for the disinhibitory action of adenosine [38]. As different from the above-mentioned idea that the depressions of inhibitory transmissions by cannabinoids are involved in antinociception, Pernía-Andrade et al. [44] have proposed the idea that such depressions mediate primary-afferent C-fiber induced pain sensitization.

The spinal cord contains a high level of ANA and 2-AG ([45] [49]). Wallmichrath and Szabo [43] have reported a continuous inhibition of GABAergic transmission by endocannabinoids in the SNR. Therefore, inhibitory transmissions in SG neurons may have been tonically depressed by the endocannabinoids. However, this is not the case in the present study, because SR141716A alone does not affect glycinergic and GABAergic eIPSC amplitudes in SG neurons.

With respect to the origin of endocannabinoids, ANA and 2-AG appear to be released from neurons as a result of an increase in neuronal activities including the activation of voltage-gated Ca^{2+} channels and of metabotropic glutamate receptors, probably through a hydrolysis of phospholipid precursors from membrane phosphoglycerides. The endocannabinoids may mediate signals from postsynaptic neurons to presynaptic terminals in a retrograde manner, resulting in the reduction in the release of glycine and/or GABA, as shown in the hippocampus ([41]; for review see [65] [66]). It remains to be examined what kinds of neuronal activity induce the endocannabinoid-mediated modulation of inhibitory transmission in the SG. Since Hashimotodani et al. [67] have demonstrated that neuronal proteinase-activated receptor 1 (PAR-1) drives synaptic retrograde signaling of an eIPSC inhibition mediated by 2-AG in cultured rat hippocampal neurons, PAR-1 activation in postsynaptic neurons may be one candidate for retrograde one in the SG. It remains to be examined how PAR-1 activation affects inhibitory transmissions in SG neurons, although this activation facilitates glutamatergic spontaneous excitatory transmission in SG neurons [47].

5. Conclusion

The present study demonstrated that ANA depressed glycinergic and GABAeregic transmissions in adult rat SG neurons by activating CB1 receptors in nerve terminals. This depression could contribute to the modulation of nociceptive transmission by ANA together with its inhibitory action on excitatory transmission as reported previously [23] [24].

Acknowledgements

This work was supported by Grants-in-aid for Scientific Research from the Ministry of Education, Science, Sports and Culture of Japan (KAKENHI: 14580790).

References

[1]　Pertwee, R.G. (2001) Cannabinoid Receptors and Pain. *Progress in Neurobiology*, **63**, 569-611. http://dx.doi.org/10.1016/S0301-0082(00)00031-9

[2]　Freund, T.F., Katona, I. and Piomelli, D. (2003) Role of Endogenous Cannabinoids in Synaptic Signaling. *Physiological Reviews*, **83**, 1017-1066. http://dx.doi.org/10.1152/physrev.00004.2003

[3]　Walker, J.M. and Hohmann, A.G. (2005) Cannabinoid Mechanisms of Pain Suppression. *Handbook of Experimental*

Pharmacology, **168**, 509-554. http://dx.doi.org/10.1007/3-540-26573-2_17

[4]   Manzanares, J., Julian, M.D. and Carrascosa, A. (2006) Role of the Cannabinoid System in Pain Control and Therapeutic Implications for the Management of Acute and Chronic Pain Episodes. *Current Neuropharmacology*, **4**, 239-257. http://dx.doi.org/10.2174/157015906778019527

[5]   Lichtman, A.H. and Martin, B.R. (1991) Cannabinoid-Induced Antinociception Is Mediated by a Spinal α_2-Noradrenergic Mechanism. *Brain Research*, **559**, 309-314. http://dx.doi.org/10.1016/0006-8993(91)90017-P

[6]   Hohmann, A.G., Tsou, K. and Walker, J.M. (1998) Cannabinoid Modulation of Wide Dynamic Range Neurons in the Lumbar Dorsal Horn of the Rat by Spinally Administered WIN55,212-2. *Neuroscience Letters*, **257**, 119-122. http://dx.doi.org/10.1016/S0304-3940(98)00802-7

[7]   Mailleux, P. and Vanderhaeghen, J.-J. (1992) Distribution of Neuronal Cannabinoid Receptor in the Adult Rat Brain: A Comparative Receptor Binding Radioautography and *in Situ* Hybridization Histochemistry. *Neuroscience*, **48**, 655-668. http://dx.doi.org/10.1016/0306-4522(92)90409-U

[8]   Hohmann, A.G., Briley, E.M. and Herkenham, M. (1999) Pre- and Postsynaptic Distribution of Cannabinoid and Mu Opioid Receptors in Rat Spinal Cord. *Brain Research*, **822**, 17-25. http://dx.doi.org/10.1016/S0006-8993(98)01321-3

[9]   Tsou, K., Brown, S., Sañudo-Peña, M.C., Mackie, K. and Walker, J.M. (1998) Immunohistochemical Distribution of Cannabinoid CB1 Receptors in the Rat Central Nervous System. *Neuroscience*, **83**, 393-411. http://dx.doi.org/10.1016/S0306-4522(97)00436-3

[10] Farquhar-Smith, W.P., Egertová, M., Bradbury, E.J., McMahon, S.B., Rice, A.S.C. and Elphick, M.R. (2000) Cannabinoid CB_1 Receptor Expression in Rat Spinal Cord. *Molecular and Cellular Neuroscience*, **15**, 510-521. http://dx.doi.org/10.1006/mcne.2000.0844

[11] Salio, C., Fischer, J., Franzoni, M.F. and Conrath, M. (2002) Pre- and Postsynaptic Localizations of the CB1 Cannabinoid Receptor in the Dorsal Horn of the Rat Spinal Cord. *Neuroscience*, **110**, 755-764. http://dx.doi.org/10.1016/S0306-4522(01)00584-X

[12] Hegyi, Z., Kis, G., Holló, K., Ledent, C. and Antal, M. (2009) Neuronal and Glial Localization of the Cannabinoid-1 Receptor in the Superficial Spinal Dorsal Horn of the Rodent Spinal Cord. *European Journal of Neuroscience*, **30**, 251-262. http://dx.doi.org/10.1111/j.1460-9568.2009.06816.x

[13] Chapman, V. (1999) The Cannabinoid CB_1 Receptor Antagonist, SR141716A, Selectively Facilitates Nociceptive Responses of Dorsal Horn Neurones in the Rat. *British Journal of Pharmacology*, **127**, 1765-1767. http://dx.doi.org/10.1038/sj.bjp.0702758

[14] Willis Jr., W.D. and Coggeshall, R.E. (1991) Sensory Mechanisms of the Spinal Cord. 2nd Edition, Plenum Press, New York. http://dx.doi.org/10.1007/978-1-4899-0597-0

[15] Fürst, S. (1999) Transmitters Involved in Antinociception in the Spinal Cord. *Brain Research Bulletin*, **48**, 129-141. http://dx.doi.org/10.1016/S0361-9230(98)00159-2

[16] Todd, A.J. (2010) Neuronal Circuitry for Pain Processing in the Dorsal Horn. *Nature Reviews Neuroscience*, **11**, 823-836. http://dx.doi.org/10.1038/nrn2947

[17] Kohno, T., Kumamoto, E., Higashi, H., Shimoji, K. and Yoshimura, M. (1999) Actions of Opioids on Excitatory and Inhibitory Transmission in Substantia Gelatinosa of Adult Rat Spinal Cord. *Journal of Physiology* (*London*), **518**, 803-813. http://dx.doi.org/10.1111/j.1469-7793.1999.0803p.x

[18] Ito, A., Kumamoto, E., Takeda, M., Takeda, M., Shibata, K., Sagai, H. and Yoshimura, M. (2000) Mechanisms for Ovariectomy-Induced Hyperalgesia and Its Relief by Calcitonin: Participation of 5-HT$_{1A}$-Like Receptor on C-Afferent Terminals in Substantia Gelatinosa of the Rat Spinal Cord. *Journal of Neuroscience*, **20**, 6302-6308.

[19] Luo, C., Kumamoto, E., Furue, H., Chen, J. and Yoshimura, M. (2002) Nociceptin Inhibits Excitatory but Not Inhibitory Transmission to Substantia Gelatinosa Neurones of Adult Rat Spinal Cord. *Neuroscience*, **109**, 349-358. http://dx.doi.org/10.1016/S0306-4522(01)00459-6

[20] Kawasaki, Y., Kumamoto, E., Furue, H. and Yoshimura, M. (2003) α_2 Adrenoceptor-Mediated Presynaptic Inhibition of Primary Afferent Glutamatergic Transmission in Rat Substantia Gelatinosa Neurons. *Anesthesiology*, **98**, 682-689. http://dx.doi.org/10.1097/00000542-200303000-00016

[21] Lao, L.J., Kawasaki, Y., Yang, K., Fujita, T. and Kumamoto, E. (2004) Modulation by Adenosine of Aδ and C Primary-Afferent Glutamatergic Transmission in Adult Rat Substantia Gelatinosa Neurons. *Neuroscience*, **125**, 221-231. http://dx.doi.org/10.1016/j.neuroscience.2004.01.029

[22] Yue, H.Y., Fujita, T. and Kumamoto, E. (2011) Biphasic Modulation by Galanin of Excitatory Synaptic Transmission in Substantia Gelatinosa Neurons of Adult Rat Spinal Cord Slices. *Journal of Neurophysiology*, **105**, 2337-2349. http://dx.doi.org/10.1152/jn.00991.2010

[23] Morisset, V. and Urban, L. (2001) Cannabinoid-Induced Presynaptic Inhibition of Glutamatergic EPSCs in Substantia

Gelatinosa Neurons of the Rat Spinal Cord. *Journal of Neurophysiology*, **86**, 40-48.

[24] Luo, C., Kumamoto, E., Furue, H., Chen, J. and Yoshimura, M. (2002) Anandamide Inhibits Excitatory Transmission to Rat Substantia Gelatinosa Neurones in a Manner Different from that of Capsaicin. *Neuroscience Letters*, **321**, 17-20. http://dx.doi.org/10.1016/S0304-3940(01)02471-5

[25] Liang, Y.C., Huang, C.C., Hsu, K.S. and Takahashi, T. (2004) Cannabinoid-Induced Presynaptic Inhibition at the Primary Afferent Trigeminal Synapse of Juvenile Rat Brainstem Slices. *Journal of Physiology* (*London*), **555**, 85-96. http://dx.doi.org/10.1113/jphysiol.2003.056986

[26] Todd, A.J., Watt, C., Spike, R.C. and Sieghart, W. (1996) Colocalization of GABA, Glycine, and Their Receptors at Synapses in the Rat Spinal Cord. *Journal of Neuroscience*, **16**, 974-982.

[27] Sandkühler, J. (2009) Models and Mechanisms of Hyperalgesia and Allodynia. *Physiological Reviews*, **89**, 707-758. http://dx.doi.org/10.1152/physrev.00025.2008

[28] Zeilhofer, H.U., Wildner, H. and Yévenes, G.E. (2012) Fast Synaptic Inhibition in Spinal Sensory Processing and Pain Control. *Physiological Reviews*, **92**, 193-235. http://dx.doi.org/10.1152/physrev.00043.2010

[29] Moore, K.A., Kohno, T., Karchewski, L.A., Scholz, J., Baba, H. and Woolf, C.J. (2002) Partial Peripheral Nerve Injury Promotes a Selective Loss of GABAergic Inhibition in the Superficial Dorsal Horn of the Spinal Cord. *Journal of Neuroscience*, **22**, 6724-6731.

[30] Coull, J.A.M., Boudreau, D., Bachand, K., Prescott, S.A., Nault, F., Sik, A., de Koninck, P. and de Koninck, Y. (2003) Trans-Synaptic Shift in Anion Gradient in Spinal Lamina I Neurons as a Mechanism of Neuropathic Pain. *Nature*, **424**, 938-942. http://dx.doi.org/10.1038/nature01868

[31] Baba, H., Shimoji, K. and Yoshimura, M. (2000) Norepinephrine Facilitates Inhibitory Transmission in Substantia Gelatinosa of Adult Rat Spinal Cord (Part 1): Effects on Axon Terminals of GABAergic and Glycinergic Neurons. *Anesthesiology*, **92**, 473-484. http://dx.doi.org/10.1097/00000542-200002000-00030

[32] Baba, H., Kohno, T., Okamoto, M., Goldstein, P.A., Shimoji, K. and Yoshimura, M. (1998) Muscarinic Facilitation of GABA Release in Substantia Gelatinosa of the Rat Spinal Dorsal Horn. *Journal of Physiology* (*London*), **508**, 83-93. http://dx.doi.org/10.1111/j.1469-7793.1998.083br.x

[33] Takeda, D., Nakatsuka, T., Papke, R. and Gu, J.G. (2003) Modulation of Inhibitory Synaptic Activity by a Non-$\alpha4\beta2$, Non-$\alpha7$ Subtype of Nicotinic Receptors in the Substantia Gelatinosa of Adult Rat Spinal Cord. *Pain*, **101**, 13-23. http://dx.doi.org/10.1016/S0304-3959(02)00074-X

[34] Liu, T., Fujita, T. and Kumamoto, E. (2011) Acetylcholine and Norepinephrine Mediate GABAergic but Not Glycinergic Transmission Enhancement by Melittin in Adult Rat Substantia Gelatinosa Neurons. *Journal of Neurophysiology*, **106**, 233-246. http://dx.doi.org/10.1152/jn.00838.2010

[35] Fukushima, T., Ohtsubo, T., Tsuda, M., Yanagawa, Y. and Hori, Y. (2009) Facilitatory Actions of Serotonin Type 3 Receptors on GABAergic Inhibitory Synaptic Transmission in the Spinal Superficial Dorsal Horn. *Journal of Neurophysiology*, **102**, 1459-1471. http://dx.doi.org/10.1152/jn.91160.2008

[36] Breton, J.D., Veinante, P., Uhl-Bronner, S., Vergnano, A.M., Freund-Mercier, M.J., Schlichter, R. and Poisbeau, P. (2008) Oxytocin-Induced Antinociception in the Spinal Cord Is Mediated by a Subpopulation of Glutamatergic Neurons in Lamina I-II Which Amplify GABAergic Inhibition. *Molecular Pain*, **4**, 19. http://dx.doi.org/10.1186/1744-8069-4-19

[37] Jiang, C.Y., Fujita, T. and Kumamoto, E. (2014) Synaptic Modulation and Inward Current Produced by Oxytocin in Substantia Gelatinosa Neurons of Adult Rat Spinal Cord Slices. *Journal of Neurophysiology*, **111**, 991-1007. http://dx.doi.org/10.1152/jn.00609.2013

[38] Yang, K., Fujita, T. and Kumamoto, E. (2004) Adenosine Inhibits GABAergic and Glycinergic Transmission in Adult Rat Substantia Gelatinosa Neurons. *Journal of Neurophysiology*, **92**, 2867-2877. http://dx.doi.org/10.1152/jn.00291.2004

[39] Szabo, B., Dörner, L., Pfreundtner, C., Nörenberg, W. and Starke, K. (1998) Inhibition of GABAergic Inhibitory Postsynaptic Currents by Cannabinoids in Rat Corpus Striatum. *Neuroscience*, **85**, 395-403. http://dx.doi.org/10.1016/S0306-4522(97)00597-6

[40] Hoffman, A.F. and Lupica, C.R. (2000) Mechanisms of Cannabinoid Inhibition of $GABA_A$ Synaptic Transmission in the Hippocampus. *Journal of Neuroscience*, **20**, 2470-2479.

[41] Wilson, R.I. and Nicoll, R.A. (2001) Endogenous Cannabinoids Mediate Retrograde Signalling at Hippocampal Synapses. *Nature*, **410**, 588-592. http://dx.doi.org/10.1038/35069076

[42] Jennings, E.A., Vaughan, C.W. and Christie, M.J. (2001) Cannabinoid Actions on Rat Superficial Medullary Dorsal Horn Neurons *in Vitro*. *Journal of Physiology* (*London*), **534**, 805-812. http://dx.doi.org/10.1111/j.1469-7793.2001.00805.x

[43] Wallmichrath, I. and Szabo, B. (2002) Analysis of the Effect of Cannabinoids on GABAergic Neurotransmission in the Substantia Nigra Pars Reticulata. *Naunyn-Schmiedeberg's Archives of Pharmacology*, **365**, 326-334. http://dx.doi.org/10.1007/s00210-001-0520-z

[44] Pernía-Andrade, A.J., Kato, A., Witschi, R., Nyilas, R., Katona, I., Freund, T.F., Watanabe, M., Filitz, J., Koppert, W., Schüttler, J., Ji, G., Neugebauer, V., Marsicano, G., Lutz, B., Vanegas, H. and Zeilhofer, H.U. (2009) Spinal Endocannabinoids and CB_1 Receptors Mediate C-Fiber-Induced Heterosynaptic Pain Sensitization. *Science*, **325**, 760-764. http://dx.doi.org/10.1126/science.1171870

[45] Yang, H.Y.T., Karoum, F., Felder, C., Badger, H., Wang, T.C.L. and Markey, S.P. (1999) GC/MS Analysis of Anandamide and Quantification of *N*-Arachidonoylphosphatidylethanolamides in Various Brain Regions, Spinal Cord, Testis, and Spleen of the Rat. *Journal of Neurochemistry*, **72**, 1959-1968. http://dx.doi.org/10.1046/j.1471-4159.1999.0721959.x

[46] Kawasaki, Y., Yang, K., Lao, L.J., Matsumoto, N., Fujita, T., Kumamoto, E. and Hasuo, H. (2002) Action of Anandamide on Inhibitory Transmission to Substantia Gelatinosa Neurons in the Rat Spinal Cord. Society for Neuroscience Abstract, 453.4.

[47] Fujita, T., Liu, T., Nakatsuka, T. and Kumamoto, E. (2009) Proteinase-Activated Receptor-1 Activation Presynaptically Enhances Spontaneous Glutamatergic Excitatory Transmission in Adult Rat Substantia Gelatinosa Neurons. *Journal of Neurophysiology*, **102**, 312-319. http://dx.doi.org/10.1152/jn.91117.2008

[48] Sugiura, T., Kondo, S., Sukagawa, A., Nakane, S., Shinoda, A., Itoh, K., Yamashita, A. and Waku, K. (1995) 2-Arachidonoylglycerol: A Possible Endogenous Cannabinoid Receptor Ligand in Brain. *Biochemical and Biophysical Research Communications*, **215**, 89-97. http://dx.doi.org/10.1006/bbrc.1995.2437

[49] Di Marzo, V., Breivogel, C.S., Tao, Q., Bridgen, D.T., Razdan, R.K., Zimmer, A.M., Zimmer, A. and Martin, B.R. (2000) Levels, Metabolism, and Pharmacological Activity of Anandamide in CB_1 Cannabinoid Receptor Knockout Mice: Evidence for Non-CB_1, Non-CB_2 Receptor-Mediated Actions of Anandamide in Mouse Brain. *Journal of Neurochemistry*, **75**, 2434-2444. http://dx.doi.org/10.1046/j.1471-4159.2000.0752434.x

[50] Zygmunt, P.M., Petersson, J., Andersson, D.A., Chuang, H.H., Sørgård, M., Di Marzo, V., Julius, D. and Högestätt, E.D. (1999) Vanilloid Receptors on Sensory Nerves Mediate the Vasodilator Action of Anandamide. *Nature*, **400**, 452-457. http://dx.doi.org/10.1038/22761

[51] De Petrocellis, L., Bisogno, T., Maccarrone, M., Davis, J.B., Finazzi-Agrò, A. and Di Marzo, V. (2001) The Activity of Anandamide at Vanilloid VR1 Receptors Requires Facilitated Transport across the Cell Membrane and Is Limited by Intracellular Metabolism. *Journal of Biological Chemistry*, **276**, 12856-12863. http://dx.doi.org/10.1074/jbc.M008555200

[52] Morisset, V., Ahluwalia, J., Nagy, I. and Urban, L. (2001) Possible Mechanisms of Cannabinoid-Induced Antinociception in the Spinal Cord. *European Journal of Pharmacology*, **429**, 93-100. http://dx.doi.org/10.1016/S0014-2999(01)01309-7

[53] Jennings, E.A., Vaughan, C.W., Roberts, L.A. and Christie, M.J. (2003) The Actions of Anandamide on Rat Superficial Medullary Dorsal Horn Neurons *in Vitro*. *Journal of Physiology* (*London*), **548**, 121-129. http://dx.doi.org/10.1113/jphysiol.2002.035063

[54] Yang, K., Kumamoto, E., Furue, H. and Yoshimura, M. (1998) Capsaicin Facilitates Excitatory but Not Inhibitory Synaptic Transmission in Substantia Gelatinosa of the Rat Spinal Cord. *Neuroscience Letters*, **255**, 135-138. http://dx.doi.org/10.1016/S0304-3940(98)00730-7

[55] Yang, K., Kumamoto, E., Furue, H., Li, Y.Q. and Yoshimura, M. (1999) Action of Capsaicin on Dorsal Root-Evoked Synaptic Transmission to Substantia Gelatinosa Neurons in Adult Rat Spinal Cord Slices. *Brain Research*, **830**, 268-273. http://dx.doi.org/10.1016/S0006-8993(99)01408-0

[56] Kumamoto, E., Fujita, T. and Jiang, C.Y. (2014) TRP Channels Involved in Spontaneous L-Glutamate Release Enhancement in the Adult Rat Spinal Substantia Gelatinosa. *Cells*, **3**, 331-362. http://dx.doi.org/10.3390/cells3020331

[57] Savinainen, J.R., Järvinen, T., Laine, K. and Laitinen, J.T. (2001) Despite Substantial Degradation, 2-Arachidonoylglycerol Is a Potent Full Efficacy Agonist Mediating CB_1 Receptor-Dependent G-Protein Activation in Rat Cerebellar Membranes. *British Journal of Pharmacology*, **134**, 664-672. http://dx.doi.org/10.1038/sj.bjp.0704297

[58] Ueda, N., Goparaju, S.K., Katayama, K., Kurahashi, Y., Suzuki, H. and Yamamoto, S. (1998) A Hydrolase Enzyme Inactivating Endogenous Ligands for Cannabinoid Receptors. *Journal of Medical Investigation*, **45**, 27-36.

[59] Todd, A.J. and Spike, R.C. (1993) The Localization of Classical Transmitters and Neuropeptides within Neurons in Laminae I-III of the Mammalian Spinal Dorsal Horn. *Progress in Neurobiology*, **41**, 609-645. http://dx.doi.org/10.1016/0301-0082(93)90045-T

[60] Akaike, N. and Moorhouse, A.J. (2003) Techniques: Applications of the Nerve-Bouton Preparation in Neuropharmacology. *Trends in Pharmacological Sciences*, **24**, 44-47. http://dx.doi.org/10.1016/S0165-6147(02)00010-X

[61] Mackie, K., Lai, Y., Westenbroek, R. and Mitchell, R. (1995) Cannabinoids Activate an Inwardly Rectifying Potassium Conductance and Inhibit Q-Type Calcium Currents in AtT20 Cells Transfected with Rat Brain Cannabinoid Receptor. *Journal of Neuroscience*, **15**, 6552-6561.

[62] Twitchell, W., Brown, S. and Mackie, K. (1997) Cannabinoids Inhibit N- and P/Q-Type Calcium Channels in Cultured Rat Hippocampal Neurons. *Journal of Neurophysiology*, **78**, 43-50.

[63] Liu, T., Fujita, T., Nakatsuka, T. and Kumamoto, E. (2008) Phospholipase A_2 Activation Enhances Inhibitory Synaptic Transmission in Rat Substantia Gelatinosa Neurons. *Journal of Neurophysiology*, **99**, 1274-1284. http://dx.doi.org/10.1152/jn.01292.2007

[64] Mason Jr., D.J., Lowe, J. and Welch, S.P. (1999) Cannabinoid Modulation of Dynorphin A: Correlation to Cannabinoid-Induced Antinociception. *European Journal of Pharmacology*, **378**, 237-248. http://dx.doi.org/10.1016/S0014-2999(99)00479-3

[65] Kano, M., Ohno-Shosaku, T., Hashimotodani, Y., Uchigashima, M. and Watanabe, M. (2009) Endocannabinoid-Mediated Control of Synaptic Transmission. *Physiological Reviews*, **89**, 309-380. http://dx.doi.org/10.1152/physrev.00019.2008

[66] Ohno-Shosaku, T. and Kano, M. (2014) Endocannabinoid-Mediated Retrograde Modulation of Synaptic Transmission. *Current Opinion in Neurobiology*, **29**, 1-8. http://dx.doi.org/10.1016/j.conb.2014.03.017

[67] Hashimotodani, Y., Ohno-Shosaku, T., Yamazaki, M., Sakimura, K. and Kano, M. (2011) Neuronal Protease-Activated Receptor 1 Drives Synaptic Retrograde Signaling Mediated by the Endocannabinoid 2-Arachidonoylglycerol. *Journal of Neuroscience*, **31**, 3104-3109. http://dx.doi.org/10.1523/JNEUROSCI.6000-10.2011

3

Interaction of Flomazenil with Anxiolytic Effects of *Citrus aurantium* L. Essential Oil on Male Mice

Leila Adibi[1], Maryam Khosravi[1], Shahrzad Khakpour[2], Hedayat Sahraei[3],
Mahsa Hadipour Jahromy[2*]

[1]Biology Department, Faculty of Biological Sciences, Islamic Azad University North Tehran Branch, Tehran, Iran
[2]Herbal Pharmacology Research Center, Tehran Medical Sciences Branch, Faculty of Medicine, Islamic Azad University, Tehran, Iran
[3]Neuroscience Research Center, Baghiatallah University of Medical, Tehran, Iran
Email: *jahromymh@yahoo.com

Abstract

Due to our previous findings about the role of GABAegic neurotransmission in anxiolytic effects of *Citrus aurantium* L. essential oil, we are now presenting flomazenil interaction with this herb, as an antagonist of benzodiazepines at GABA receptor. The study was performed on 84 male albino mice assigned to 14 groups of six. The animals were injected intraperitoneally with the *Citrus aurantium* L. essential oil for 5 days. On the fifth day, either normal saline or flomazenil (0.1 mg/kg) was injected to the experimental groups. Thirty minutes after the injection, all the groups were assessed for anxiety-related behavior by elevated plus-maze test. In groups receiving *Citrus aurantium* L. essential oil at doses of 2.5 and 5 percent, the time spent in the open arms increased significantly (P < 0.001). The injection of flumazenil alone induced anxiety quite clearly observed by decreasing the time or number of entries in open arms. As an antagonist of benzodiazepines at GABA receptor, flumazenil acted as a competitive antagonist for *Citrus aurantium* L. essential oil regarding the increment in the number of entries to the open arms and the time spent in the open arms (P < 0.001) compared to flumazenil. It can then be concluded that *Citrus aurantium* L. essential oil induces its anxiolytic effects like benzodiazepines, in the same site at GABA receptor.

Keywords

Anxiety, *Citrus aurantium* L., Flomazenil

---

*Corresponding author.

1. Introduction

Anxiety is common psychopathies that involve many persons [1]. Various neurotransmitter systems such as GABAergic, noradrenergic and serotonergic systems are responsible for anxiety symptoms [2]. GABA is the most important neurotransmitter in the brain affecting such behaviors as learning, pain, memory, paroxysm, and anxiety [3].

Anxiety occurs along with some biochemical changes and reactions in the brain such as increase in adrenalin (that quickens the heart beat) and reduction in dopamine (dopamine pain). Excessive anxiety makes the body ready for fight or running away.

It is normal to have some levels of anxiety in daily life which can be managed. An increase in levels of anxiety affects one's ability to enjoy life. Today, anxiety is considered one of the inability factors among the elderly [3].

The brain is the central organ for producing and coping with stress, because it establishes behavioral and physiological responses against stressors. In an adult, as the brain develops, the ability to cope with the stressors and responding to them also develops. Structural changes such as neuronal replacement, dendrite status change, and synopsis return are among brain responses features to the environment [4].

GABA as an important inhibitory neurotransmitter system plays a significant role, whether directly or indirectly, in neurological disorders. Among disorders that are affiliated with GABAA receptor, we can name anxiety, cognitive impairment, hysteria, mental disorder, schizophrenia, and sleep disorder (insomnia). GABA is a neurotransmitter system which can reduce anxiety with an inhibitory effect. It has been observed that stress increases glutamate in prefrontal cortex and hippocampus [5].

GABA hyperpolarizes post-synaptic neurons and has an important role in balancing excitation and neurons inhibition. Excessive inhibition or weak excitation will lead to coma, depression, reduction in blood pressure, calmness, and sleep. Excessive excitation or weak inhibition will lead to restlessness, anxiety, high blood pressure and insomnia. Disorders' symptoms depend on the region of the brain that is out of balance [6].

Many herbal medicines have been reported to pose anxiolytic effects.

Reasons to use southern (Shirazian) *Citrus aurantium* L. are that there are more alkanes in southern *Citrus aurantium* L. compared to the northern type. Besides an amount of aldehyde in the essential oil, a sign of the better quality of the product has been reported to be more in southern *Citrus aurantium* L.

There are oxides in northern *Citrus aurantium* L. essential oil, and not in the southern one. Also, alcoholic compounds in the northern oil are more frequent than those in the southern one. These compounds, because of having hydroxylic group, are able to make hydrogen bond with water. Therefore they bond with vapor drops and enter the water-cooler along with water and enter the essential oil after condensation. The findings also show that, oxygen monoterpenes, which are among aromatic hydrocarbons, are more frequent in northern *Citrus aurantium* L. This sesquiterpene, which has anti-bacterial effects of terpenic hydrocarbons which are responsible for the aroma and healing effects of the essential oil, has a higher percentage in the southern essential oil. In sum, southern *Citrus aurantium* L. is richer in basic components of essential oil, so it has a better quality in terms of aroma [7].

2. Materials and Methods

This study was done on 84 male albino mice weighed 25 g supplied by Pasteur Institute. The mice were assigned to 14 groups of 6 for the experiment. The animals were kept in temperature of 22°C to 24°C with a 12/12 hour light-dark cycle. Except for the actual time of the experiment, the mice had complete access to sufficient food and water. The study started after an acclimation period of 1 week. The terms and conditions of keeping laboratory animals were followed completely during the experiment.

2.1. Preparation of the Essential Oil and the Medicine

Collected *Citrus aurantium* L. flowers were dried and then grinded by an electric mill. 300 g of the dried powder of *Citrus aurantium* L. were put in a 1000 cc balloon and distilled water was added to make up the volume to 1000 cc. Next, the balloon was put on the heater and connected to the Clevenger apparatus for 2 hours. 2 drops of n-hexane was added to the tube. Essential oil, which was yellow in color and had a strong odor, was then collected and dewatered using sodium sulfate. The vials were completely covered by aluminum foil and kept in a cool place. The essential oil using olive oil was obtained at different densities of 0.5, 2.5, and 5 percent.

Flomazenil (1 mg/kg) was supplied by Kimiadarou Company. Flomazenil was injected using saline sterile 9% (normal saline).

2.2. Method

After an acclimation period of 1 week, the animals were injected intraperitoneally with the *Citrus aurantium* L. essential oil at a certain hour for 5 days. On the fifth day and thirty minutes before applying *Citrus aurantium* L. essential oil, flomazenil (0.1 mg/kg) was injected to the experimental groups. Thirty minutes after the injection, all the groups were assessed for anxiety-related behavior by elevated plus-maze test.

3. Findings

Figure 1 shows how the intraperitoneal injection of the essential oil of *Citrus aurantium* L. (at doses of 0.5, 2.5, and 5 percent) resulted in the increase of the time spent in the open arms. In terms of the time spent in the open arms, there was a significant difference between the groups that were injected with doses of 2.5 and 5 percent and the control groups ($P < 0.001$)

Figure 2 shows that the intraperitoneal injection of the essential oil of *Citrus aurantium* L. (at doses of 0.5, 2.5, and 5 percent) does not make a significant difference in the number of entries to open arms, although the number of the entries to open arms in recipient groups of 2/5 and 5 percent of doses was higher than the 0.5 percent group.

Figure 3 shows that the intraperitoneal injection of flomazenil as compared to the control and sham leads to a significant reduction in the time spent on open arms.

Figure 4 shows that the intraperitoneal injection of flomazenil (1 mg/kg) leads to a significant reduction in the number of open arms as compared to the control group ($p < 0.001$). Applying flomazenil and *Citrus aurantium* L. at doses of 0.5, 2.5, and 5 percent simultaneously leads to an increase in the number of entries to the open arms with flomazenil group ($p < 0.01$) and ($p < 0.001$).

4. Discussion

The results of this study show that essential oil of *Citrus aurantium* L., in terms of applied dose, can reduce the anxiety in mice significantly. Sedative and anti-anxiety effects of this plant have been mentioned in previous studies [8]. It is possible that these effects are the result of an interaction with GABAergic pathways and subsequent impacts on GABAA receptors. One of the essential compounds of *Citrus aurantium* L. is limonene which reduces the activity of neurons in central nervous system [8]. After researching the brain, limonene attaches itself

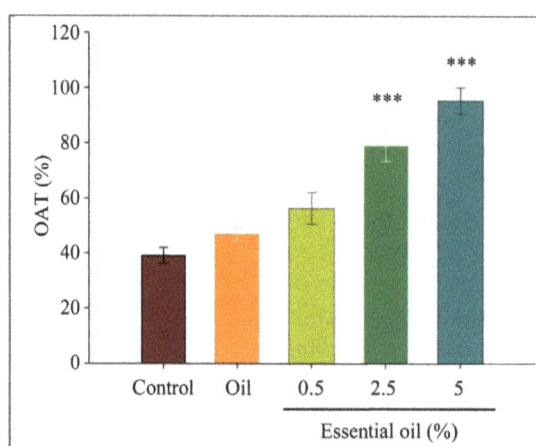

Figure 1. Comparison between experimental group (received essential oil of *Citrus aurantium* L. at doses of 0.5, 2.5, and 5 percent), control group and sham group (received olive oil) in anti-anxiety effect of *Citrus aurantium* L. essential oil. Mean ± S.E.M. n = 7. ***P < 0.001 versus control and sham groups. OAT is the spent time in open arms.

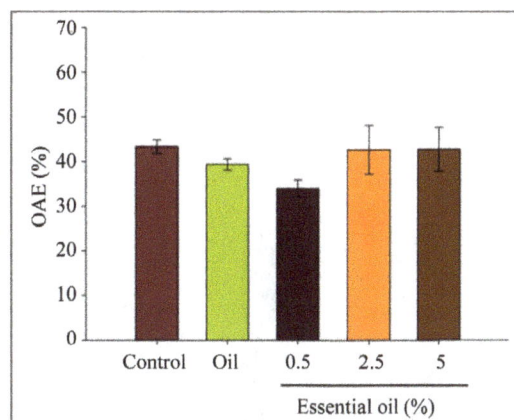

Figure 2. Comparison between experimental group (received essential oil of *Citrus aurantium* L. at doses of 0.5, 2.5, and 5 percent), control group and sham group (received olive oil) in anti-anxiety effect of *Citrus aurantium* L. essential oil. Mean ± S.E.M. n = 6.

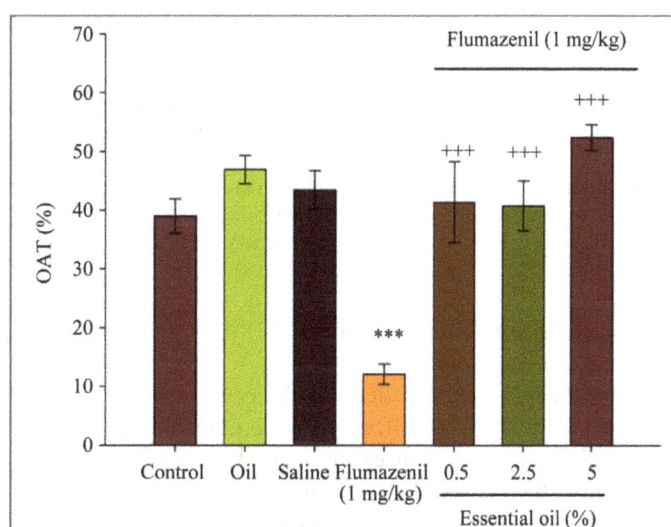

Figure 3. Effect of *Citrus aurantium* L. essential oil in experimental groups (received essential oil of *Citrus aurantium* L. at doses of 0.5, 2.5, and 5 percent), control and sham group (received olive oil), flomazenil and its combination with essential oils on the percent of time spent in open arms. Mean ± S.E.M. n = 6. ***P < 0.001 versus control and sham groups. +P < 0.05 versus flomazenil group. OAT% is the percent time spent in open arms.

to GABAA receptors and reduces anxiety-related activities [8]. Another study shows how limonene, by acting on GABAA receptors, increases the density of gamma-aminobutyric acid and reduces stress [9]. Limonene is therefore one of the compounds in *Citrus aurantium* L. which has anti-anxiety effects.

Coumarin is another compound in *Citrus aurantium* L. which has similar sedative effects. A study done by Pereira (2009) demonstrates how acute administration of coumarin to prefrontal cortex and hippocampus of mice can help preventing seizures by effecting GABAA receptors and therefore releasing more gamma-aminobutyric acid in prefrontal cortex. Linalool is also another compound in *Citrus aurantium* L. which exert inhibitory effects in the nervous system through pre-synaptic inhibition and prevention of acetylcholine release [10]. Linalool is a competitive antagonist for glutamate receptors; consequently, by blocking these receptors, it reduces the effect of this neurotransmitter system and prevents epileptic and anxiety-related fits [11].

In this study flomazenil (1 mg/kg) was used as the antagonist of GABA receptors. Flomazenil reverses the

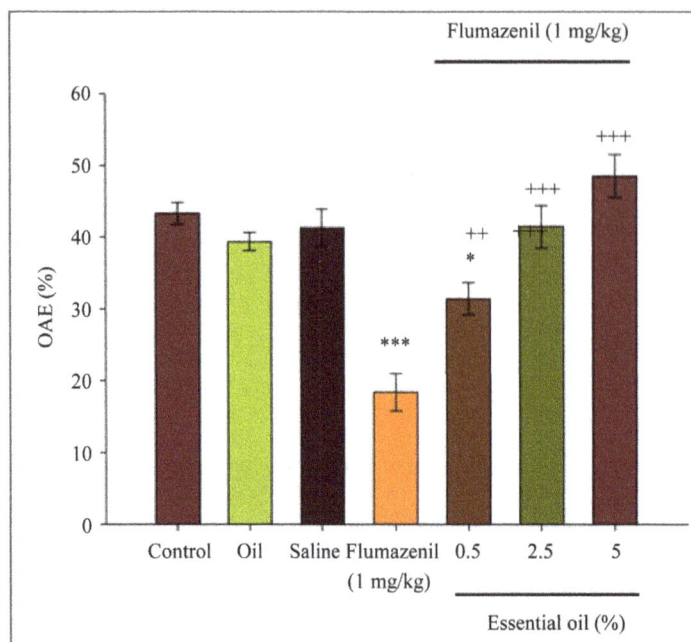

Figure 4. Effect of *Citrus aurantium* L. essential oil in experimental groups (received essential oil of *Citrus aurantium* L. at doses of 0.5, 2.5, and 5 percent), control and sham group (received olive oil), flomazenil and its combination with essential oils on the percent of number of entries in open arms. Mean ± S.E.M. n = 6. Mean ± S.E.M. n = 6. ***P < 0.001 versus control and sham groups. +P < 0.05 versus flomazenil group. OAE% is the number of entries in open arms.

inhibition effect of benzodiazepines by competing them [12]. Flomazenil leaves its antagonistic effect by attaching on the benzodiazepines on GABA receptors [13].

Flomazenil antagonizes the benzodiazepine effects in the central nervous system, but it is not able to antagonize the effects of the medicines which are effective on the GABAergic neurons. Also flomazenil is not able to reverse the epioids effects [13]. Some evidences show that flomazenil separates benzodiazepine from the receptor. Flomazenil attachment to the benzodiazepine place on the receptor will lead to a change in the receptors sensitivity and changes the receptors attachment tendency to benzodiazepines [13]. The intraperitoneal injection of flomazenil increases the anxiety behavior of the mice and reduces the time spent on open arms and time of the open arms entry.

In this study, simultaneous injection of *Citrus aurantium* L. essential oil and flomazenil leads to inhibition of flomazenil effect and an increase in the open arms entry and staying in open arms.

5. Conclusion

It can then be concluded that *Citrus aurantium* L. essential oil induces its anxiolytic effects like benzodiazepines, in the same site at GABA receptor due to the blockade of its anxiolytic effects by flomazenil.

References

[1] Bueno, C.H., Zangrossi Jr., H. and Viana, M.B. (2005) The Inactivation of the Basolateral Nucleus of the Rat Amygdala Has an Anxiolytic Effect in the Elevated T-Maze and Light/Dark Transition Tests. *Brazilian Journal of Medical and Biological Research*, **38**, 1697-1701. http://dx.doi.org/10.1590/S0100-879X2005001100019

[2] Zarrindast, M.R., Torabi, M., Rostami, P. and Fazli-Tabaei, S. (2006) The Effects of Histaminergic Agents in the Dorsal Hippocampus of Rats in the Elevated Plus-Maze Test of Anxiety. *Pharmacology Biochemistry and Behavior*, **85**, 501-506. http://dx.doi.org/10.1016/j.pbb.2006.09.019

[3] Andreasen, N.C. (2004) Acute and Delayed Posttraumatic Stress Disorder: A History and Some Issues. *American Journal of Psychiatry*, **161**, 1321-1323. http://dx.doi.org/10.1176/appi.ajp.161.8.1321

[4] Gray, J.A. and McNaughton, N. (2000) The Neuropsychology of Anxiety. 2nd Edition, Oxford Medical Publications, Oxford.

[5] Taylor, M, Bhagwagar, Z., Cowen, P.J. and Sharp, T. (2003) GABA and Mood Disorders. *Psychological Medicine*, **33**, 3873-3893. http://dx.doi.org/10.1017/S0033291702006876

[6] Chebib, M. and Johnston, G.A.R. (2000) GABA-Activated Ligand Gated Ion Channels: Medicinal Chemistry and Molecular Biology. *Journal of Medicinal Chemistry*, **43**, 1427-1447. http://dx.doi.org/10.1021/jm9904349

[7] Carvalho-Freitas, M.I. and Costa, M. (2002) Anxiolytic and Sedative Effects of Extracts and Essential Oil from *Citrus aurantium* L. *Biological & Pharmaceutical Bulletin*, **25**, 1629-1633. http://dx.doi.org/10.1248/bpb.25.1629

[8] Re, L., Barocci, S., Sonnino, S., *et al.* (2000) Linalool Modifies the Nicotinic Receptor-Ion Channel Kinetics at the Mouse Neuromuscular Junction. *Neurochemical Research*, **42**, 177-181.

[9] Silva Brum, L.F., Emanuelli, T., Souza, D.O., *et al.* (2001) Effects of Linalool on Glutamate Release and Uptake in Mouse Cortical Synaptosomes. *Neurochemical Research*, **26**, 191-194. http://dx.doi.org/10.1023/A:1010904214482

[10] Fuster, J.M. (2000) The Prefrontal Cortex—An Update: Time Is of the Essence. *Neuron*, **30**, 319-333. http://dx.doi.org/10.1016/S0896-6273(01)00285-9

[11] Johnston, G.A.R. (2005) GABA$_A$ Receptor Channel Pharmacology. *Current Pharmaceutical Design*, **11**, 1867-1885. http://dx.doi.org/10.2174/1381612054021024

[12] Lader, M.B. and Morton, S.V. (1992) A Pilot Study of the Effects of Flumazenil on Symptoms Persisting after Benzodiazepine Withdrawal. *Journal of Psychopharmacology*, **6**, 19-28. http://dx.doi.org/10.1177/026988119200600303

[13] Votey, S.R., Bosse, G.M., Bayer, M.J. and Hoffman, J.R. (1991) Flumazenil: A New Benzodiazepine Antagonist. *Annals of Emergency Medicine*, **20**, 181-188. http://dx.doi.org/10.1016/S0196-0644(05)81219-3

4

The Adverse Event Profile in Patients Treated with Transferon™ (Dialyzable Leukocyte Extracts): A Preliminary Report

4

Toni Homberg[1], Violeta Sáenz[2], Jorge Galicia-Carreón[2], Iván Lara[2],
Edgar Cervantes-Trujano[1,2], Maria C. Andaluz[1,2], Erika Vera[1], Oscar Pineda[1],
Julio Ayala-Balboa[1], Alejandro Estrada-García[3], Sergio Estrada-Parra[3],
Mayra Pérez-Tapia[4], Maria C. Jiménez-Martínez[5*]

[1]Clinical Trials Branch and Clinical Immunology Service, Unit of External Services and Clinical Research (USEIC), National School of Biological Sciences, National Polytechnic Institute, Mexico City, Mexico
[2]Unit of Pharmacovigilance, Unit of External Services and Clinical Research (USEIC), National School of Biological Sciences, National Polytechnic Institute, Mexico City, Mexico
[3]Department of Immunology, National School of Biological Sciences, National Polytechnic Institute, Mexico City, Mexico
[4]Unit of R&D in Bioprocesses (UDIBI), National School of Biological Sciences, National Polytechnic Institute, Mexico City, Mexico
[5]Department of Biochemistry, Faculty of Medicine, National Autonomous University of Mexico, Mexico City, Mexico
Email: *mcjimenezm@bq.unam.mx

Abstract

Background: Dialyzable leukocyte extracts (DLE) are heterogeneous mixtures of peptides less than 10 kDa in size that are used as immunomodulatory adjuvants in immune-mediated diseases. Transferon™ is DLE manufactured by National Polytechnic Institute (IPN), and is registered by Mexican health-regulatory authorities as an immunomodulatory drug and commercialized nationally. The proposed mechanism of action of Transferon™ is induction of a Th1 immunoregulatory response. Despite that it is widely used, to date there are no reports of adverse events related to the clinical safety of human DLE or Transferon™. Objective: To assess the safety of Transferon™ in a large group of patients exposed to DLE as adjuvant treatment. Methods: We included in this study 3844 patients from our Clinical Immunology Service at the Unit of External Services and Clinical Research (USEIC), IPN. Analysis was performed from January 2014 to November 2014, searching for clinical adverse events in patients with immune-mediated diseases and treated with

---

*Corresponding author.

Transferon™ as an adjuvant. Results: In this work we observed clinical nonserious adverse events (AE) in 1.9% of patients treated with Transferon™ (MD 1.9, IQR 1.7 - 2.0). AE were 2.8 times more frequently observed in female than in male patients. The most common AE were headache in 15.7%, followed by rash in 11.4%, increased disease-related symptomatology in 10%, rhinorrhea in 7.1%, cough in 5.7%, and fatigue in 5.7% of patients with AE. 63% of adverse event presentation occurred from day 1 to day 4 of treatment with Transferon™, and mean time resolution of adverse events was 14 days. In 23 cases, the therapy was stopped because of adverse events and no serious adverse events were observed in this study. Conclusion: Transferon™ induced low frequency of nonserious adverse events during adjuvant treatment. Further monitoring is advisable for different age and disease groups of patients.

Keywords

Dialyzable Leukocyte Extracts, Adverse Events, Monitoring, Drug Safety, Adjuvant Therapy, Immunoregulation, Guidelines, Transfer Factor, Pharmacovigilance

1. Introduction

Dialyzable leukocyte extracts (DLE) are heterogeneous mixtures of peptides under 10 kDa, released after disruption of peripheral blood leukocytes from healthy donors [1]. It has been reported that administration of DLE improves clinical responses in allergies [2], in infections and immunodeficiency syndromes [3]-[5], and in some other immune-mediated diseases (reviewed in [6]). The therapeutic adjuvant effect of DLE is associated with their ability to modulate immune responses changing innate signaling pathways, such as TLRs [7], NF-kB, and cyclic adenosine monophosphate (cAMP) in cultured cells [8] [9]; DLE could modulate production of cytokines, including TNF-a, IL-6 [10] [11], and induce IFN-g secretion, driving immune response to a Th1 immune-regulatory response [12] [13].

Transferon^{TM} is a human dialyzable leukocyte extract manufactured by National Polytechnic Institute (IPN), Mexico, at Good Manufacturing Practice (GMP) facilities. Transferon^{TM} is registered by Mexican health authorities as a drug and is commercialized nationally. Although Transferon^{TM} is a mixture of peptides, it has been demonstrated that there is a high batch-to-batch reproducibility in the chromatographic profile and also in the biological efficacy, demonstrated *in vitro* by up-regulation of IFN-g in a lymphocytic cell line (Jurkat clone E6-1) [1].

DLEs have been widely used since the 1970s due to their immune-regulatory functions for various clinical purposes [6] [14] [15]; to date, there are no current reports about the safety of Transferon^{TM}; thus, it was the aim of our study.

2. Methods

2.1. Patients

We included a total of 3844 patients in this study. The medical staff from the Clinical Immunology Service, Unit of External Services and Clinical Research (USEIC) at IPN, was responsible for clinical evaluation. Analysis was performed from January 2014 to November 2014, searching for clinical adverse events in patients who received oral formulation of Transferon^{TM} (Pharma-ft, UDIMEB formerly Laboratorio de Investigación Científica, IPN, MEX) as adjuvant therapy in immune-mediated diseases.

Patients selected for the use of DLE as an adjuvant treatment were those with immune-related disease, and whose symptoms remained in spite of standard treatment for that specific disease. DLE dosing was indicated based on the guidelines suggested by Berrón-Pérez *et al.* [6]. Adverse events were evaluated in the population with the following selection criteria: all patients who were treated with DLE during the period of January 2014-November 2014 who took at least one dose of DLE, and followed dosing instructions as indicated. Pediatric patients were considered those younger than 11 years. Patients signed an informed consent as part of running clinical protocols IC 12-001, IC 12-002, IC-12-003 designed to determine the safety of Transferon^{TM}. Patients aged between 8 and 17 years also gave their verbal assent to participate in these protocols. Adverse events were defined in this study according to local law regulation in drug safety [16], and to the international regulation [17]. Serious adverse events were considered as any drug effect that results in death, life-threatening events, hospitalization, and disability; while nonserious adverse events were defined as drug related signs or symptoms that are tolerable, not life-threatening, sometimes needing additional treatment and/or require stopping the drug. The clinical terms used to describe each adverse event were based on terminology of the Medline Plus medical dictionary, from the National Institutes of Health [18]. As part of the national pharmacovigilance program, both serious and nonserious adverse events need to be reported to the federal authorities as stated by the Mexican Official Standard [16]. Adverse event surveillance was performed by the medical staff, and the pharmacovigilance unit helped to classify and report each event according to [16], defined in numeral 6.1.3. "Clinical Investigation Notification Method" of the Mexican Official Standard. All involved personnel were properly trained for reporting adverse events and knowledgeable in all relevant Mexican regulation.

2.2. Statistical Analysis

Statistical analyses were performed using the GraphPad Prism software, version 6.0f (San Diego, CA). Demographic variables were analyzed with descriptive statistics, and results are presented in tables and plots. In order to determine differences between groups, T test and X^2 were used, and a $p < 0.05$ was considered as statistically significant.

3. Results

3.1. Characteristics of Patients

From a total of 3844 patients that were included in this study, 42 patients of them developed 70 nonserious adverse events (AE). Incidence of nonserious adverse events was observed in 1.9% of patients treated with Transferon™ (MD 1.9%, IQR 1.7 - 2.0). AE were 2.8-times more frequently observed in female than in male patients ($p < 0.0001$); the mean age of adverse event presentation in adult patients was 47 ± 15 years old; while in children it was 5 ± 2.8 years old. AE were 3.2-times more frequent in adults than in children ($p = 0.0002$) (**Figure 1**). No serious AE were reported in patients treated with Transferon™.

3.2. Immune-Mediated Diseases and Adverse Events

Immune-mediated diseases in which adjuvant treatment with Transferon™ is indicated were classified into one of three types: Allergic Diseases, Infectious Diseases and Autoimmune Diseases. From a total of 42 patients that developed an AE, 41.4% were observed in patients with diagnosis of allergic diseases, 24.3% were observed in patients with diagnosis of autoimmune diseases, and 34.3% were observed in patients with diagnosis of infectious disease. Frequency of immune-mediated diseases and frequency of adverse events are depicted in **Table 1**.

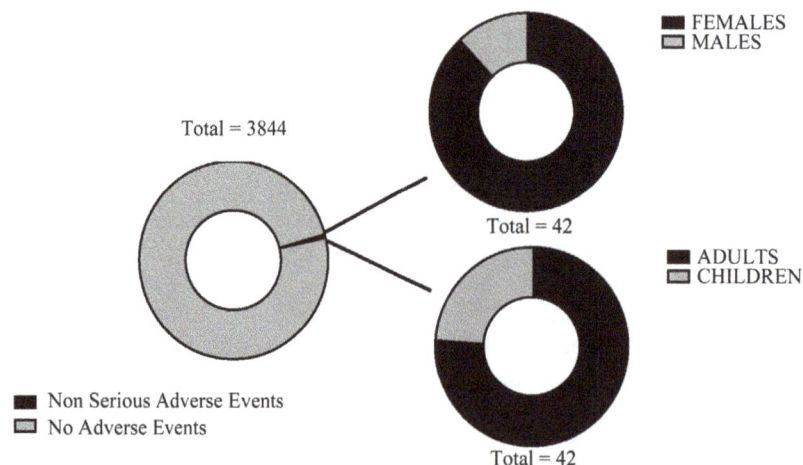

Figure 1. Distribution of adverse events and demographic data of patients treated with Transferon™.

Table 1. Immune-mediated diseases in which Transferon^{TM} is indicated and adverse events observed.

Adverse events (AE) in different diseases	Patients	
	Number of patients with AE	Frequency of patients with AE (%)
Allergic diseases		
Allergic rhinitis	14	20
Asthma	11	15.6
Urticaria	2	2.9
Atopic dermatitis	2	2.9
Infectious diseases		
Upper respiratory infection	5	7.1
Infection by human papillomavirus	5	7.1
Herpes simplex virus infection	4	5.7
Infection by hepatitis C virus	2	2.9
Herpes zoster virus infection	1	1.4
Autoimmune diseases		
Rheumatoid arthritis	10	14.3
Systemic lupus erythematosus	5	7.1
Inflammatory bowel disease	3	4.3
Mixed connective tissue disease	2	2.9
Multiple sclerosis	2	2.9
Fibromyalgia	2	2.9

3.3. Adverse Events

The most common AE observed with DLE was headache in 15.7% of patients, followed by rash in 11.4%, increased disease-related symptomatology in 10%, rhinorrhea in 7.1%, cough in 5.7%, and fatigue in 5.7% of patients (**Figure 2**). The remaining adverse events in patients treated with DLE are described in **Table 2**.

3.4. Patterns of Onset and Resolution of Adverse Events

Transferon^{TM} was administered in units, in a dose-reduction scheme, as suggested by Berrón-Pérez *et al*. [6]. One unit of Transferon^{TM} is a standardized vial containing 2 mg of dialyzed peptides/5mL [1]. Total units received per patient were dependent of the diagnosis, and patients who developed AE were at different stages of treatment: 27.14% of patients were taking 1 U every day for the first week, 20% of patients were taking 2 U/week, 28.6% of patients were taking 1 U once a week, 2.3% of patients were taking 1 U every 10 days, and 21.3% of patients were taking 1 U every 2 weeks. We did not find a significant correlation between higher dosage and higher frequency of AE.

The majority of AE (63%) appeared between 1 - 4 days of treatment with Transferon^{TM}. AE lasted from 15 min to 14 days, and 77.1% of AE were resolved within the next 72 h after onset (**Figure 3**). In 32.9% of patients, Transferon^{TM} was stopped because of adverse events; in 14.3% of patients, Transferon^{TM} dosage was decreased after AE onset; and 2.86% of patients continued treatment with DLE without changes.

3.5. Drug Interactions

Although AE were more frequently observed in patients taking thyroid hormone or estrogen substitution, and/or

Frequent Adverse Events

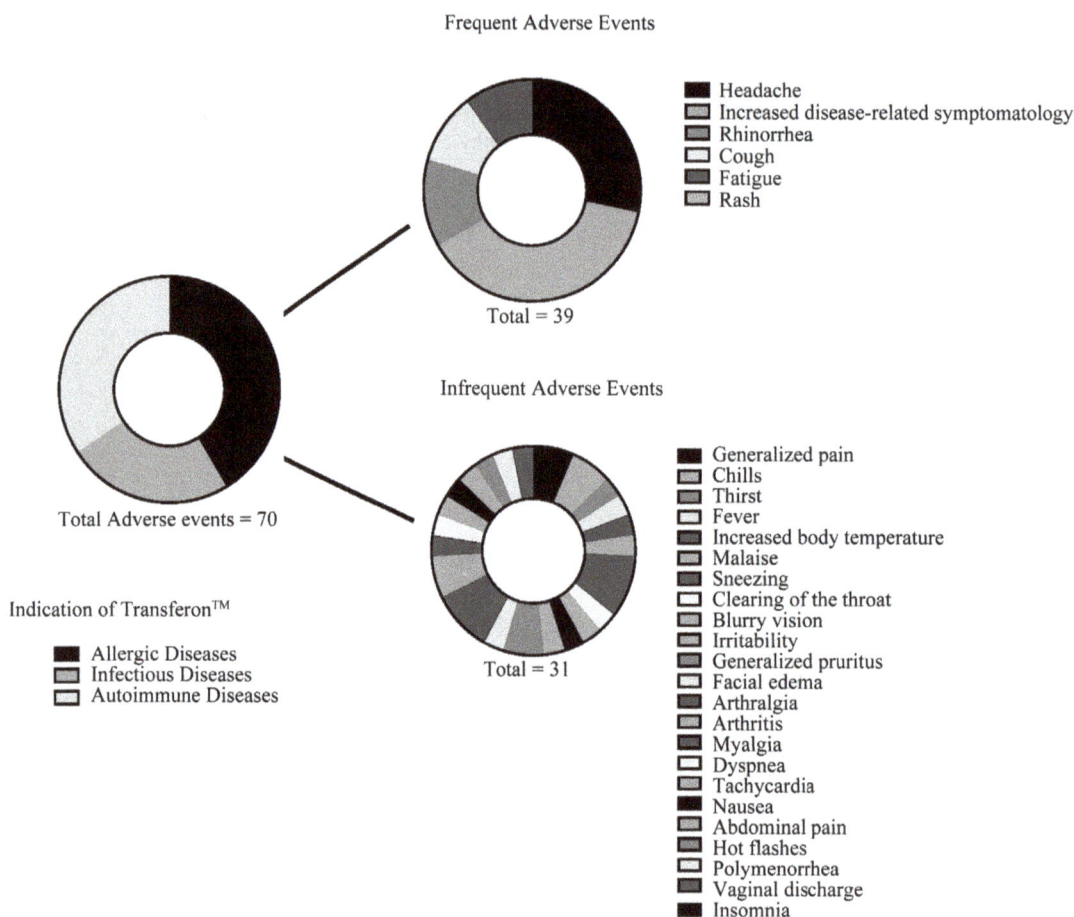

■ Headache
▨ Increased disease-related symptomatology
▨ Rhinorrhea
☐ Cough
▨ Fatigue
▨ Rash

Total = 39

Total Adverse events = 70

Indication of Transferon™

■ Allergic Diseases
▨ Infectious Diseases
☐ Autoimmune Diseases

Infrequent Adverse Events

Total = 31

■ Generalized pain
▨ Chills
▨ Thirst
☐ Fever
▨ Increased body temperature
▨ Malaise
▨ Sneezing
☐ Clearing of the throat
▨ Blurry vision
▨ Irritability
▨ Generalized pruritus
☐ Facial edema
▨ Arthralgia
▨ Arthritis
▨ Myalgia
☐ Dyspnea
▨ Tachycardia
■ Nausea
▨ Abdominal pain
▨ Hot flashes
☐ Polymenorrhea
▨ Vaginal discharge
■ Insomnia

Figure 2. Distribution of type of adverse events in patients treated with Transferon™.

glucocorticoid therapy, no significant interactions between Transferon™ and other concomitant medication were identified.

4. Discussion

Dialyzable leukocyte extracts are heterogeneous mixtures of polar and hydrophilic peptides under 10 kDa, released after disruption of peripheral blood leukocytes from healthy donors [1]. DLE have been used to modulate immune response [1] [10]-[13] in patients suffering immune-mediated diseases [6] [14] [15]. Transferon™ is a human dialyzable leukocyte extract manufactured by National Polytechnic Institute (IPN), Mexico, at GMP facilities. The use of Transferon™ is widely extended in our country [6]; but despite their broad clinical use, to our knowledge no adverse events have been studied before.

In this work, we observed a low frequency of AE with the use of DLE. A significant adverse effect is usually considered as a reaction present in at least 2% of the studied population [19]. Of all included patients, only 1.9% of them developed adverse events. These results suggest that DLE is a safe and tolerable substance, but the unexpected low incidence of adverse events also opens the possibility of Transferon™-related adverse events may remain under-diagnosed.

Comparing our adverse event profile with adverse effects of glatiramer acetate (GA), a four peptide-based product with 5 - 9 kDa in size [19]-[21], we did not find similarities. GA is an injectable synthetic amino acid-based product with immune regulatory properties, reported incidence of adverse effects is at least 10%, mostly related to injection-site reaction. DLE is an oral peptide mixture lower than 10 kDa in size, and even though oral and injectable formulations cannot be fully compared, we expected to find some similar adverse effects between Transferon™ and GA. Nevertheless, some interesting patterns in adverse events presentation with the use of

Table 2. Adverse events identified in patients using Transferon™.

Type of clinical adverse event (AE)	Patients	
	Number of patients with AE	Frequency of patients with AE (%)
General symptoms		
Fatigue	4	5.71
Generalized pain	2	2.86
Chills	2	2.86
Thirst	1	1.43
Fever	1	1.43
Increased body temperature	1	1.43
Malaise	1	1.43
Ear, nose and throat		
Rhinorrhea	5	7.14
Cough	4	5.71
Sneezing	3	4.29
Clearing of the throat	1	1.43
Eyes		
Blurry vision	1	1.43
Neurologic		
Headache	11	15.71
Psychiatric		
Insomnia	1	1.43
Irritability	1	1.43
Skin		
Rash	8	11.43
Generalized pruritus	2	2.86
Facial edema	1	1.43
Bones, joints and muscles		
Arthralgia	3	4.26
Arthritis	2	2.86
Myalgia	1	1.43
Cardiopulmonary		
Dyspnea	1	1.43
Tachycardia	1	1.43
Gastrointestinal		
Nausea	1	1.43
Abdominal pain	1	1.43
Gynecology/Endocrine		
Hot flashes	1	1.43
Polymenorrhea	1	1.43
Vaginal discharge	1	1.43
Other		
Increased disease-related symptomatology	7	10
TOTAL	70	100

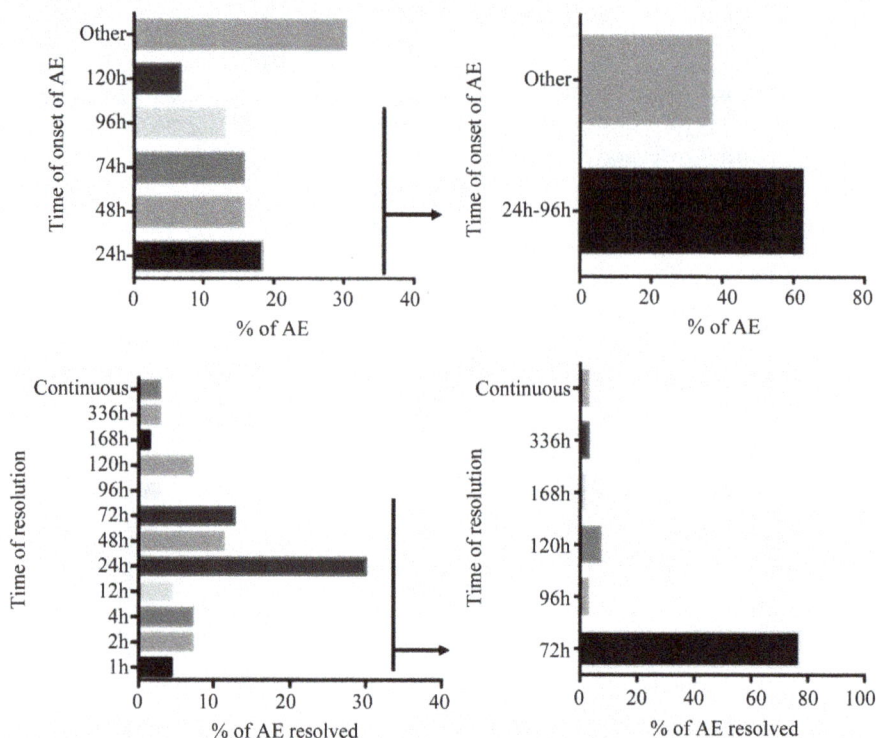

Figure 3. Time of onset and resolution of adverse events in patients treated with Transferon[TM].

Transferon[TM] are worth analyzing, *i.e.* AE were more frequent in females, and we detected 2 vulnerable age groups: ages 1 to 10, and 40 - 60 years old; this suggests that dosing should be reevaluated in order to reduce adverse events in both groups, and physicians need to increase clinical supervision to opportunely detect AE in children. It is unknown if hormonal factors may be involved in the female predominant adverse event profile showed in our study, but it is recognized that hormones may influence drug metabolism. Gender differences in adverse drug events have been observed before [22] [23], and factors other than hormonal effects such as body weight and differences in pharmacokinetics may be involved. In order to determine if hormonal factors are related in this pattern, it would be desirable to further study adverse event incidence in different female groups, such as before menarche and after menopause.

In this study we observed that most common AE were headache, followed by rash, increased disease-related symptomatology, rhinorrhea, cough and fatigue. In line with our results, the most common side effects of IFN-gamma include fever, chills, fatigue, myalgia, and headache [24]-[26], and it is well known that Transferon[TM] induces IFN-g *in vivo* [12] [13], and *in vitro* [1]. On the other hand, some DLE have been associated to an *in vitro* transient elevation of cAMP [8] [9], and increased concentrations of cAMP are related with headache [27]-[29], rhinorrhea [30] [31], and fatigue [32]-[34]. If Transferon[TM] is able to increase cAMP it is unknown, and needs further investigation. Importantly, no serious AE were observed in this study.

Limitations

The study population was heterogeneous, involving an extensive age group and patients presenting various different diseases as well as varied concomitant treatments for these diseases. Additional studies should be conducted in a controlled population. The low incidence of adverse events elevates the possibility that adverse events may be under-reported, and strengthening our pharmacovigilance protocols will aide in this matter. Finally, the lack of other adverse reaction reports associated to human DLE limits our possibility of comparison.

5. Conclusion

To our knowledge, no data on the adverse event profile of other DLEs have been published, and this study is an adequate first step to describe adverse events associated with DLE and Transferon™; Transferon™ induced low frequency of nonserious adverse events during adjuvant treatment; however, further monitoring is advisable for different age and disease groups of patients.

Conflicts of Interest

S. E-P and M. P-T have been compensated for their work by UDIMEB, the producer of Transferon™. All other authors declare no conflict of interest.

Author Contributions

T.H.—performed clinical evaluation, analyzed and interpreted clinical immunological data, and wrote the paper; V.S.—trained medical staff in pharmacovigilance and developed pharmacovigilance procedures according to Mexican regulation. V.S., J.G.-C.; I.L.—collected clinical information, and analyzed data; E.C.-T., M.C.A., E.V., O.P., J.A.-B.—performed clinical-immunological evaluation of patients; A.E-G.—analyzed data, wrote paper; S.E.-P.—contributed with critical criticism of paper and wrote paper; M.P.-T. and M.C.J.-M.—designed the study, analyzed data, wrote paper and conducted research. A.E.-G. received a PhD scholarship from CONACyT number 164000.

References

[1] Medina-Rivero, E., Merchand-Reyes, G., Pavón, L., Vázquez-Leyva, S., Pérez-Sánchez, G., Salinas-Jazmín, N., Estrada-Parra, S., Velasco-Velázquez, M. and Pérez-Tapia, S.M. (2014) Batch-to-Batch Reproducibility of Transferon™. *Journal of Pharmaceutical and Biomedical Analysis*, **88**, 289-294. http://dx.doi.org/10.1016/j.jpba.2013.09.004

[2] Navarro Cruz, D., Serrano Miranda, E., Orea, M., Estrada Parra, S., Teran-Ortiz, L., Gomez-Vera, J. and Flores-Sandoval, G. (1996) Transfer Factor in Moderate and Severe Atopic Dermatitis. *Revista Alergia México*, **43**, 116-123.

[3] Byston, J., Cech, K., Pekarek, J. and Jilkova, J. (1996) Effect of Anti-Herpes Specific Transfer Factor. *Biotherapy*, **9**, 73-75. http://dx.doi.org/10.1007/BF02628660

[4] Masi, M., De Vinci, C. and Baricordi, O.R. (1996) Transfer Factor in Chronic Mucocutaneous Candidiasis. *Biotherapy*, **9**, 97-103. http://dx.doi.org/10.1007/BF02628665

[5] Viza, D., Fudenberg, H.H., Palareti, A., Ablashi, D., De Vinci, C. and Pizza, G. (2013) Transfer Factor: An Overlooked Potential for the Prevention And Treatment of Infectious Diseases. *Folia Biologica* (*Prague*), **59**, 53–67.

[6] Berron-Perez, R., Chavez-Sanchez, R., Estrada-Garcia, I., Espinosa-Padilla, S., Cortez-Gomez, R., Serrano-Miranda, E., Ondarza-Aguilera, R., Perez-Tapia, M., Pineda Olvera, B., Jimenez-Martinez, M.C., Portugues, A., Rodriguez, A., Cano, L., Pacheco, P.U., Barrientos, J., Chacon, R., Serafin, J., Mendez, P., Monges, A., Cervantes, E. and Estrada-Parra, S. (2007) Indications Usage, and Dosage of the Transfer Factor. *Revista Alergia México*, **54**, 134–139.

[7] García-Hernández, U., Robledo-Avila, F.H., Alvarez-Jiménez, V.D., Rodríguez-Cortés, O., Wong-Baeza, I., Serafín-López, J., Aguilar-Anguiano, L.M., Estrada-Parra, S., Estrada-García, I., Pérez-Tapia, S.M. and Chacón-Salinas, R. (2014) Dialyzable Leukocyte Extracts Activate TLR-2 on Monocytes. *Natural Product Communications*, **9**, 853-856.

[8] Herlin, T., Jensen, J.R., Thestrup-Pedersen, K. and Zachariae, H. (1981) Dialyzable Leukocyte Extract Stimulates cAMP in T Gamma Lymphocytes. *Allergy*, **36**, 337-343. http://dx.doi.org/10.1111/j.1398-9995.1981.tb01585.x

[9] Tsuneta, H. (1984) The Role of Cultured Thymic Epithelium and Dialyzable Leukocyte Extracts on the Maturation Process of T Cell. Study of Their Effects on Cyclic Nucleotides Levels in Thymocytes. *Hokkaido Igaku Zasshi*, **59**, 128-139.

[10] Franco-Molina, M.A., Mendoza-Gamboa, E., Castillo-Leon, L., Tamez-Guerra, R.S. and Rodriguez-Padilla, C. (2005) Bovine Dialyzable Leukocyte Extract Modulates the Nitric Oxide and Pro-Inflammatory Cytokine Production in Lipopolysaccharide-Stimulated Murine Peritoneal Macrophages *in Vitro*. *Journal of Medicinal Food*, **8**, 20-26. http://dx.doi.org/10.1089/jmf.2005.8.20

[11] Hernandez, M.E., Mendieta, D., Pérez-Tapia, M., Bojalil, R., Estrada-Garcia, I., Estrada-Parra, S. and Pavon, L. (2013) Effect of Selective Serotonin Reuptake Inhibitors and Immunomodulator on Cytokines Levels: An Alternative Therapy for Patients with Major Depressive Disorder. *Clinical and Developmental Immunology*, Article ID: 267871. http://dx.doi.org/10.1155/2013/267871

[12] Estrada-Parra, S., Nagaya, A., Serrano, E., Rodriguez, O., Santamaria, V., Ondarza, R., Chavez, R., Correa, B., Monges, A., Cabeza, R., Calva, C. and Estrada-Garcia, I. (1998) Comparative Study of Transfer Factor and Acyclovir in the Treatment of Herpes Zoster. *International Journal of Immunopharmacology*, **20**, 521-535. http://dx.doi.org/10.1016/S0192-0561(98)00031-9

[13] Luna-Baca, G.A., Linares, M., Santacruz-Valdes, C., Aguilar-Velazquez, G., Chavez, R., Perez-Tapia, M., Estrada-Garcia, I., Estrada-Parra, S. and Jimenez-Martinez, M.C. (2007) Immunological Study of Patients with Herpetic Stromal Keratitis Treated with Dialyzable Leukocyte Extracts. 13th International Congress of Immunology-ICI, Proceedings Immunology, Rio de Janeiro, 21-25 August 2007, 67-70.

[14] Kirkpatrick, C.H. and Smith, T.K. (1976) The Nature of Transfer Factor and Its Clinical Efficacy in the Management of Cutaneous Disorders. Journal of Investigative Dermatology, 67, 425-430. http://dx.doi.org/10.1111/1523-1747.ep12514723

[15] Nekam, K., Kalmar, L., Gergely, P., Kelemen, G., Fekete, B., Lang, I., Levai, J. and Petranyi, G.Y. (1977) In Vitro Effect of Transfer Factor on Active Rosettes and Leucocyte Migration of Patients with Cancer. Clinical & Experimental Immunology, 27, 416-420.

[16] Mexican Official Standard NOM-220-SSA1-2012, Installation and Operation of Pharmacovigilance.

[17] US Department of Health and Human Services Food and Drug Administration, Office of the Commissioner, Center for Drug Evaluation and Research, Center for Biologics Evaluation and Research, Center for Devices and Radiological Health, Office of Good Clinical Practice (2009) Guidance for Clinical Investigators, Sponsors, and IRBs Adverse Event Reporting to IRBs—Improving Human Subject Protection.

[18] Reviewed on Line (2014). www.nlm.nih.gov/medlineplus/mplusdictionary.html

[19] Copaxone Product Monograph (2011).

[20] Johnson, K.P., Brooks, B.R., Cohen, J.A., Ford, C.C., Goldstein, J., Lisak, R.P., Myers, L.W., Panitch, H.S., Rose, J.W., Schiffer, R.B., Vollmer, T., Weiner, L.P. and Wolinsky, J.S. (1998) Extended Use of Glatiramer Acetate (Copaxone) Is Well Tolerated and Maintains Its Clinical Effect on Multiple Sclerosis Relapse Rate and Degree of Disability. Copolymer 1 Multiple Sclerosis Study Group. Neurology, 50, 701-708. http://dx.doi.org/10.1212/WNL.50.3.701

[21] Bornstein, M.B., Miller, A., Slagle, S., Weitzman, M., Crystal, H., Drexler, E., Keilson, M., Merriam, A., Wassertheil-Smoller, S., Spada, V., et al. (1987) A Pilot Trial of COP 1 in Exacerbating-Remitting Multiple Sclerosis. The New England Journal of Medicine, 317, 408-414. http://dx.doi.org/10.1056/NEJM198708133170703

[22] Tran, C.L., Knowles, S.R., Liu, B.A. and Shear, N.H. (1998) Gender Differences in Adverse Drug Reactions. Journal of Clinical Pharmacology, 38, 1003-1009. http://dx.doi.org/10.1177/009127009803801103

[23] Pistone, G., Gurreri, R., Alaimo, R., Curiale, S. and Bongiorno, M.R. (2014) Gender Differences in Adverse Drug Reactions in Dermatological Patients in West Sicily: An Epidemiological Study. Journal of Dermatolog Treat, 25, 510-512. http://dx.doi.org/10.3109/09546634.2013.814755

[24] Murray, H.W. (1994) Interferon-Gamma and Host Antimicrobial Defense: Current and Future Clinical Applications. The American Journal of Medicine, 97, 459-467. http://dx.doi.org/10.1016/0002-9343(94)90326-3

[25] Gallin, J.L., Farber, J.M., Holland, S.M. and Nutman, T.B. (1995) Interferon-γ in the Management of Infectious Diseases. Annals of Internal Medicine, 123, 216-224. http://dx.doi.org/10.7326/0003-4819-123-3-199508010-00009

[26] Hübel, K.K., Dale, D.C. and Liles, W.C. (2002) Therapeutic Use of Cytokines to Modulate Phagocyte Function for the Treatment of Infectious Diseases: Current Status of Granulocyte Colony-Stimulating Factor, Granulocyte-Macrophage Colony-Stimulating factor, macrophage Colony-Stimulating Factor, and Interferon-γ. The Joural of Infectious Diseases, 185, 1490-1501. http://dx.doi.org/10.1086/340221

[27] Birk, S., Kruuse, C., Petersen, K.A.T., Felt-Hansen, P. and Olesen, J. (2006) The Headache-Inducing Effect of Cilostazol in Human Volunteers. Cephalalgia, 26, 1304-1309. http://dx.doi.org/10.1111/j.1468-2982.2006.01218.x

[28] DeSantana, J.M. and Sluka, K.A. (2008) Central Mechanisms in the Maintenance of Chronic Widespread Noninflammatory Muscle Pain. Current Pain and Headache Reports, 12, 338-343. http://dx.doi.org/10.1007/s11916-008-0057-7

[29] Guo, S., Olesen, J. and Ashina, M. (2014) Phosphodiesterase 3 Inhibitor Cilostazol Induces Migraine-Like Attacks via Cyclic AMP Increase. Brain, 137, 2951-2959. http://dx.doi.org/10.1093/brain/awu244

[30] Schmidt, B.M., Kusma, M., Feuring, M., Timmer, W.E., Neuhäuser, M., Bethke, T., Stuck, B.A., Hörmann, K. and Wehling, M. (2001) The Phosphodiesterase 4 Inhibitor Roflumilast Is Effective in the Treatment of Allergic Rhinitis. Journal of Allergy and Clinical Immunology, 108, 530-536. http://dx.doi.org/10.1067/mai.2001.118596

[31] Lee, R.J., Chen, B., Doghramji, L., Adappa, N.D., Palmer, J.N., Kennedy, D.W. and Cohen, N.A. (2013) Vasoactive Intestinal Peptide Regulates Sinonasal Mucociliary Clearance and Synergizes with Histamine in Stimulating Sinonasal Fluid Secretion. The FASEB Joural, 27, 5094-103. http://dx.doi.org/10.1096/fj.13-234476

[32] Kolbeck, R.C. and Speir, W.A. (1991) Theophylline, Fatigue, and Diaphragm Contractility: Cellular Levels of 45Ca and cAMP. Journal of Applied Physiology, 70, 1933-1937.

[33] Staines, D.R. (2006) Phosphodiesterase Inhibitors May Be Indicated in the Treatment of Postulated Vasoactive Neuro-

peptide Autoimmune Fatigue-Related Disorders. *Medical Hypotheses*, **66**, 203-204.
http://dx.doi.org/10.1016/j.mehy.2005.08.006

[34] Staines, D.R., Brenu, E.W. and Marshall-Gradisnik, S. (2009) Postulated Vasoactive Neuropeptide Immunopathology Affecting the Blood-Brain/Blood-Spinal Barrier in Certain Neuropsychiatric Fatigue-Related Conditions: A Role for Phosphodiesterase Inhibitors in Treatment? *Neuropsychiatric Disease and Treatment*, **5**, 81-89.

5

Toxicological Evaluation of Disulfiram, Copper Gluconate and Disulfiram/Copper Gluconate Combination on Renal Function in Rodents

Udeme Owunari Georgewill, Iyeopu Minakiri Siminialayi,
Atuboyedia Wolfe Obianime

Department of Pharmacology, Faculty of Basic Medical Sciences, College of Health Sciences, University of Port Harcourt, Port Harcourt, Nigeria
Email: udgeorgewill@yahoo.com

Abstract

This research work investigated and compared the chronic renal toxicological profile of disulfiram, copper gluconate and disulfiram/copper gluconate combination, in a 90-day time- and dose-dependent study in rodents. 88 rats weighing an average of 280 g divided into eleven groups consisting of 8 rats each were used for this experiment. The control groups received normal saline as placebo and 99.5% dimethyl sulfoxide (DMSO) (solvent control). Three oral doses (low, medium and high) of disulfiram (18.65 mg/kg, 37.3 mg/kg and 74.6 mg/kg), copper gluconate (3.75 mg/kg, 7.5 mg/kg and 15 mg/kg) and both drugs in combination were administered daily with those of the combination given 12 hours apart. Blood samples were collected via cardiac puncture in heparinised bottles and centrifuged, and the serum was decanted on 30, 45, 60 and 90 days for analysis. Renal function parameters—electrolytes (Na^+, K^+), urea and creatinine were evaluated. Results showed significant ($p < 0.05$) dose- and time-dependent increase in electrolyte level (Na^+, K^+), blood urea and creatinine respectively. The results are all pointers to the development of renal failure. It therefore appears that the DSF/CG combination is nephrotoxic and this effect is dose-dependent and synergistic.

Keywords

Disulfiram, Copper Gluconate, Renal Function

1. Introduction

Cancer, also termed malignant tumour or neoplasm, is a group of diseases involving abnormal cell growth with a potential to invade or spread to other parts of the body. In Nigeria, breast cancer, cervical cancer and prostate cancer are most prevalent amongst women and men respectively [1]. Added to this, is the burden cancer imposes on the Niger delta region of Nigeria where this study is sited. Researchers attest to the fact that individuals in this region are at increasing risk of developing cancers as a result of oil exploration activities [2]. This underscores the interest of the researchers in new drug treatment for cancers that would be readily available to low-income economies and affordable. Disulfiram is an old drug hitherto used for alcoholism. The addition of copper gluconate makes the combination a potentially effective and cheap means of treating cancer and is therefore being repurposed for use in cancer chemotherapy. Repurposing non-cancer related drugs with possible anti-tumoral activities is a promising strategy for identifying prospective new anti-cancer drugs in a cost-efficient and time-saving way [3]-[5]. Repurposing disulfiram has recently become of interest because of its pre-clinically described anti-cancer effects against various human cancers, which include breast, cervical, colorectal, lung, melanoma, prostate as well as myeloma and leukaemia [6] [7]. Disulfiram, a member of the dithiocarbamate family, possesses metal-binding properties [8] and is thought to inhibit superoxide dismutase resulting in inhibition of the angiogenic potential [9]. In the presence of Cu (II), disulfiram is converted to the two-electron oxidized form of diethyldithiocarbamate, which is the active form in inducing cell death [10]. Chen *et al.* [11] have reported that disulfiram could bind to cellular copper or zinc to form a complex that has a proteasome-inhibitory effect, which might contribute to its apoptosis-inducing effect. Diethyldithiocarbamate is a main physiological metabolite found after gastrointestinal uptake of disulfiram [12]-[14]. Disulfiram and diethyldithiocarbamate are convertible into each other via a copper containing intermediate complex. Cen *et al.* [10] also proposed that the complex of two diethyldithiocarbamate molecules formed by redox active Cu (II), could be mainly responsible for the proapoptotic response to disulfiram. In a study on ovarian cancer cell lines, Papaioannou *et al.* [15] reported that when cell lines were tested using disulfiram alone and disulfiram with copper supplementation, disulfiram alone reduced cell survival of ovarian cancer cells at an optimum concentration even in the absence of copper supplementation, but supplementation with 1 µM copper chloride, increased the cytotoxic effect of disulfiram in all other ovarian cancer cells tested.

A major problem with most antineoplastic agents is the adverse effects that occur following their use. Renal failure in cancer patients is a common problem in oncology and this complication is frequently multifactorial in origin. Several antineoplastic agents are potentially nephrotoxic; previous renal impairment as well as combinations with other nephrotoxic drugs may increase the risk of nephrotoxicity during administration of chemotherapy [16]. Also, exposure to heavy metals is potentially harmful. Because of its ability to reabsorb and accumulate divalent metals, the kidney is the first target organ of heavy metal toxicity. The extent of renal damage by heavy metals depends on the nature, the dose, the route and the duration of exposure [17]. We set out to study the effect of disulfiram, copper gluconate and disulfiram/copper gluconate combination on the kidneys in rodents.

2. Methodology

88 male albino Swiss rats weighing an average of 280 g obtained from the Department of Pharmacology animal house were used for this study. The rats were bred and maintained under suitable conditions, allowed an acclimatization period of two (2) weeks, housed in hygienic cages in groups of four and allowed free access to feed obtained from vital feeds UAC PLC and water *ad libitum*. The beddings were changed and cages cleaned out on alternate days. Animals were handled according to Helsinki declaration on animal care. The animals were divided into 11 groups, each consisting of 8 rats each. The groups included those for treatment and the control groups. Drugs were administered orally via a 1ml syringe.

3. Chronic Toxicity Tests

This study spanned 3 months and was domiciled in the Department of Pharmacology, University of Port Harcourt, Animal House and Laboratory. A dose and time dependent toxicological evaluation of the effects of these individual drugs and their combinations on the renal profiles of rodents was evaluated. The rats were divided into eleven groups consisting of 8 rats each. Groups 1 and 2 served as control groups and the rats received normal saline as placebo and 99.5% DMSO (solvent control) respectively. Drugs were administered orally via a 1 ml syringe as $1/5^{th}$, $1/10^{th}$ and $1/20^{th}$ of the LD_{50} of disulfiram and copper gluconate at 373 mg/kg and 75 mg/kg respectively [18].

4. Drug Administration

Control group 1: Had 8 rats and received 1 ml of normal saline orally daily;
Control group 2/Solvent control: Had 8 rats and received 0.5 ml of (DMSO) dimethyl sulfoxide;
Group 3a: Had 8 rats and received 15 mg/kg of copper gluconate daily orally;
Group 3b: Had 8 rats and received 7.5 mg/kg of copper gluconate daily orally;
Group 3c: Had 8 rats and received 3.75 mg/kg of copper gluconate daily orally;
Group 4a: Had 8 rats and received 74.6 mg/kg of DSF and 15 mg/kg of copper gluconate daily orally;
Group 4b: Had 8 rats and received 37.3 mg/kg of DSF and 7.5 mg/kg of copper gluconate daily orally;
Group 4c: Had 8 rats and received 18.65 mg/kg of DSF and 3.75 mg/kg of copper gluconate daily orally;
N/B The drug combination was given following the protocol of Grossman *et al.* [19];
Group 5a: Had 8 rats and received 74.6 mg/kg of DSF daily orally;
Group 5b: Had 8 rats and received 37.3 mg/kg of DSF daily orally;
Group 5c: Had 8 rats and received 18.65 mg/kg of DSF daily orally.

5. Collection of Samples

Two animals per group were sacrificed using diethyl ether anaesthesia and blood samples were obtained on days 30, 45, 60 and 90 for analysis via cardiac puncture. Blood samples were centrifuged at 3000 rpm for 15 minutes and serum separated from the cells. The samples were then assayed for Na^+, K^+, by flame photometry [20] and urea and creatinine using the Clinical Chemistry Autoanalyser RX Series by Randox Laboratories Limited, United Kingdom.

6. Stock Solutions

Stock solutions were prepared from 99.5% DMSO for disulfiram and distilled water for copper gluconate. Pure analytical grade samples, CAS No. 527-09-3 (98% min purity) and CAS No. 97-77-8 (98% min purity) obtained from Shijiazhuang Aopharm Import and Export Co. Limited China were used for the study.

7. Ethical Approval

Ethical approval was obtained from the University of Port Harcourt Research Ethics Committee.

8. Statistical Analysis

Statistical analysis was done using graph pad prism 5 statistical package and ANOVA for comparison of the means of the various groups. Results are expressed as means ± SEM. Test group results were compared with that of the control groups. A p-value < 0.05 was considered significant.

9. Results and Discussion

Anticancer agents are frequently associated with a variety of renal and electrolyte disorders. These drugs could affect the kidneys manifesting as an asymptomatic elevation of serum creatinine or acute renal failure. The kidneys are the major pathway for elimination of many antineoplastic agents as well as their metabolites. Therefore, renal impairment can result in delayed drug excretion and metabolism of anticancer agents resulting to increased systemic toxicity. Potassium, an essential intracellular, positively charged ion, is actively "pumped" in to the cell from surrounding extracellular fluid, while, sodium, is pumped out. This is necessary for proper fluid balance, and creates an electrical charge across the cell membrane. This is also the fundamental principle which allows nerves to conduct impulses and so communicate between cells and muscles to contract. Potassium is important to proper heart functioning. Hypokalaemia or hyperkalaemia quickly leads to electrolyte imbalance which affects all muscles, nerves and numerous key body functions. Increased potassium levels could be as a result of damage to the kidneys resulting in extrusion of the ions into the extracellular space [21]. Results of the present study revealed that low dose disulfiram, copper gluconate and disulfiram/copper gluconate combination revealed significantly increased (p < 0.05) sodium ion levels (**Table 1**). Medium and high doses of all three therapeutic agents significantly increased (p < 0.05) sodium levels (**Table 2** and **Table 3**). Low, medium and high doses of

Table 1. Effect of low dose DSF (18.65 mg/kg), CG (3.75 mg/kg) and DSF/CG (18.65/3.75 mg/kg) on Na^+ (mEq/l).

	30 Days	45 Days	60 Days	90 Days
CONTROL 1	146.7 ± 0.882	145.3 ± 2.667	142.0 ± 1.528	143.7 ± 0.882
DSF	151.3 ± 0.333*	156.3 ± 1.202*	153.0 ± 1.000*	153.7 ± 1.856*
CG	154.3 ± 0.333*	155.3 ± 1.333*	155.7 ± 1.202*	157.0 ± 1.000*
DSF/CG	157.0 ± 0.577*	157.7 ± 0.333*	158.3 ± 0.333*	158.7 ± 0.333*

Results are expressed as mean ± SEM, the superscript (*) means significant difference with respect to control at $p < 0.05$ (ANOVA).

Table 2. Effect of medium dose DSF (37.3 mg/kg), CG (7.5 mg/kg) and DSF/CG (37.3/7.5 mg/kg) combination on Na^+ (mEq/l).

	30 Days	45 Days	60 Days	90 Days
CONTROL 1	144.3 ± 2.186	144.3 ± 2.186	145.7 ± 2.603	146.3 ± 2.186
DSF	155.0 ± 1.528*	155.7 ± 0.882*	156.0 ± 2.309*	156.3 ± 2.333*
CG	158.3 ± 1.202*	160.3 ± 0.882*	158.7 ± 1.453*	159.3 ± 1.202*
DSF/CG	160.0 ± 0.577*	160.7 ± 1.202*	160.3 ± 0.882*	161.3 ± 0.333*

Results are expressed as mean ± SEM, the superscript (*) means significant difference with respect to control at $p < 0.05$ (ANOVA).

Table 3. Effect of high dose DSF (74.6 mg/kg), CG (15 mg/kg) and DSF/CG (74.6/15 mg/kg) combination on Na^+ (mEq/l).

	30 Days	45 Days	60 Days	90 Days
CONTROL 1	146.3 ± 3.180	160.3 ± 1.202	146.3 ± 3.180	146.3 ± 3.180
DSF	164.0 ± 2.309*	160.3 ± 1.202*	162.0 ± 1.155*	164.0 ± 2.309*
CG	165.3 ± 1.764*	162.7 ± 0.667*	162.7 ± 0.667*	165.3 ± 1.764*
DSF/CG	169.0 ± 2.082*	163.3 ± 0.333*	163.3 ± 0.333*	169.0 ± 2.082*

Results are expressed as mean ± SEM, the superscript (*) means significant difference with respect to control at $p < 0.05$ (ANOVA).

all three therapeutic agents increased potassium levels significantly ($p < 0.05$) (**Tables 4-6**). This results point to an increased risk for the development of kidney failure perhaps due to direct toxic effects of the agents on the kidneys.

The blood urea nitrogen (BUN) test is a measure of the amount of nitrogen in the blood that comes from urea. It is used as a marker of renal function, though it is inferior to other markers such as creatinine because blood urea levels are influenced by other factors such as diet and dehydration [22]. On urea levels, disulfiram at low dose showed no significant effect ($p > 0.05$) while copper gluconate and the disulfiram and copper gluconate combination caused a significant increase ($p < 0.05$) when compared to the control (**Table 7**). At the medium and high doses, our results revealed significant increase ($p < 0.05$) for disulfiram alone, copper gluconate alone and the disulfiram and copper gluconate combination when compared with the control (**Table 8** and **Table 9**).

Effect of low, medium and high dose disulfiram, copper gluconate and their combination on creatinine levels were significantly increased ($p < 0.05$) when compared with the control (**Tables 10-12**). Serum creatinine is an important indicator of renal health because it is an easily measured by-product of muscle metabolism that is excreted unchanged by the kidneys. Plasma creatinine concentration is the most widely used measure for estimation of the glomerular filtration rate (GFR) [23]. Creatinine is synthesized primarily in the liver from the methylation of glycocyamine (guanidino acetate, synthesized in the kidney from the amino acids arginine and glycine) by S-adenosyl methionine and is removed from the blood chiefly by the kidneys, via glomerular filtration and proximal tubular secretion. A rise in blood creatinine level is observed only with marked damage to functioning nephrons. A persistent rise in both urea and creatinine is a sign of kidney failure. Kidney failure and death can occur with as little as 1 gram of copper sulphate [24]. Heavy metals such as cadmium (Cd), mercury (Hg), lead

Table 4. Effect of low dose DSF (18.65 mg/kg), CG (3.5 mg/kg) and DSF/CG (18.65/3.75 mg/kg) combination on K$^+$ (mEq/l).

	30 Days	45 Days	60 Days	90 Days
CONTROL 1	4.433 ± 0.667	4.800 ± 0.404	4.833 ± 0.203	4.833 ± 0.167
DSF	5.810 ± 0.021*	5.993 ± 0.121*	5.877 ± 0.065*	5.877 ± 0.065*
CG	6.167 ± 0.088*	6.233 ± 0.145*	6.233 ± 0.145*	6.500 ± 0.289*
DSF/CG	6.340 ± 0.170*	6.387 ± 0.199*	6.500 ± 0.289*	6.900 ± 0.208*

Results are expressed as mean ± SEM, the superscript (*) means significant difference with respect to control at p < 0.05 (ANOVA).

Table 5. Effect of medium dose DSF (37.3 mg/kg), CG (7.5 mg/kg), DSF/CG (37.3/7.5 mg/kg) combination on K$^+$ (mEq/l).

	30 Days	45 Days	60 Days	90 Days
CONTROL 1	5.100 ± 0.322	5.100 ± 0.322	5.033 ± 0.384	5.100 ± 0.306
DSF	6.610 ± 0.427*	6.100 ± 0.126*	6.200 ± 0.116*	6.200 ± 0.058*
CG	6.767 ± 0.145*	6.867 ± 0.186*	7.067 ± 0.176*	7.133 ± 0.176*
DSF/CG	7.033 ± 0.273*	7.100 ± 0.300*	7.133 ± 0.318*	7.300 ± 0.153*

Results are expressed as mean ± SEM, the superscript (*) means significant difference with respect to control at p < 0.05 (ANOVA).

Table 6. Effect of high dose DSF (74.6 mg/kg), CG (15 mg/kg) and DSF/CG (74.6/15 mg/kg) combination on K$^+$ (mEq/l).

	30 Days	45 Days	60 Days	90 Days
CONTROL 1	5.200 ± 0.351	6.300 ± 0.384	4.900 ± 0.379	4.900 ± 0.379
DSF	6.200 ± 0.058*	6.300 ± 0.058*	6.367 ± 0.033*	6.967 ± 0.338*
CG	7.133 ± 0.176*	7.333 ± 0.067*	7.700 ± 0.252*	7.833 ± 0.203*
DSF/CG	7.633 ± 0.088*	7.867 ± 0.067*	7.867 ± 0.067*	12.60 ± 3.754

Results are expressed as mean ± SEM, the superscript (*) means significant difference with respect to control at p < 0.05 (ANOVA).

Table 7. Effect of low dose DSF (18.65 mg/kg), CG (3.75 mg/kg) and DSF/CG (18.65/3.75 mg/kg) combination on urea (mmol/l).

	30 Days	45 Days	60 Days	90 Days
CONTROL 1	16.83 ± 0.601	18.67 ± 1.856	18.33 ± 1.667	19.00 ± 2.000
DSF	21.33 ± 1.764	22.67 ± 0.882	23.00 ± 0.577	23.00 ± 0.577
CG	24.83 ± 0.601*	25.17 ± 0.441*	25.33 ± 0.333*	25.33 ± 0.333*
DSF/CG	26.00 ± 0.289*	26.67 ± 0.601*	27.00 ± 0.866*	27.50 ± 1.041*

Results are expressed as mean ± SEM, the superscript (*) means significant difference with respect to control at p < 0.05 (ANOVA).

Table 8. Effect of medium dose DSF (37.3 mg/kg), CG (7.5 mg/kg), DSF/CG (37.3/7.5 mg/kg) combination on urea (mmol/l).

	30 Days	45 Days	60 Days	90 Days
CONTROL 1	19.00 ± 1.528	19.00 ± 1.528	18.67 ± 2.333	18.33 ± 2.186
DSF	23.67 ± 0.333*	23.67 ± 0.333*	25.83 ± 0.833*	24.90 ± 0.208*
CG	25.33 ± 0.333*	25.77 ± 0.433*	25.67 ± 0.333*	26.33 ± 0.333*
DSF/CG	28.00 ± 0.764*	28.33 ± 0.882*	28.67 ± 0.833*	29.33 ± 0.167*

Results are expressed as mean ± SEM, the superscript (*) means significant difference with respect to control at p < 0.05 (ANOVA).

Table 9. Effect of high dose DSF (74.6 mg/kg), CG (15 mg/kg) and DSF/CG (74.6/15 mg/kg) combination on urea (mmol/l).

	30 Days	45 Days	60 Days	90 Days
CONTROL 1	18.00 ± 2.082	18.33 ± 2.186	18.33 ± 2.186	18.67 ± 1.856
DSF	25.43 ± 0.233*	26.00 ± 0.289*	26.33 ± 0.441*	26.83 ± 0.727*
CG	26.83 ± 0.167*	27.00 ± 0.289*	27.50 ± 0.189*	27.83 ± 0.441*
DSF/CG	29.50 ± 0.289*	29.77 ± 0.145*	30.50 ± 0.764*	34.17 ± 2.489*

Results are expressed as mean ± SEM, the superscript (*) means significant difference with respect to control at p < 0.05 (ANOVA).

Table 10. Effect of low dose DSF (18.65 mg/kg), CG (3.75 mg/kg) and DSF/CG (18.65/3.75 mg/kg) combination on creatinine (mmol/l).

	30 Days	45 Days	60 Days	90 Days
CONTROL 1	0.533 ± 0.333	0.667 ± 0.067	0.733 ± 0.067	0.733 ± 0.067
DSF	0.883 ± 0.020*	0.927 ± 0.039*	0.957 ± 0.035*	0.977 ± 0.003*
CG	0.927 ± 0.019*	0.927 ± 0.019*	0.943 ± 0.029*	0.970 ± 0.012*
DSF/CG	0.960 ± 0.021*	0.963 ± 0.023*	0.990 ± 0.010*	1.023 ± 0.039*

Results are expressed as mean ± SEM, the superscript (*) means significant difference with respect to control at p < 0.05 (ANOVA).

Table 11. Effect of medium dose DSF (37.3 mg/kg), CG (7.5 mg/kg), DSF/CG (37.3/7.5 mg/kg) combination on creatinine (mmol/l).

	30 Days	45 Days	60 Days	90 Days
CONTROL 1	0.733 ± 0.044	0.733 ± 0.044	0.767 ± 0.033	0.700 ± 0.577
DSF	1.017 ± 0.042*	1.093 ± 0.064*	1.023 ± 0.039*	1.100 ± 0.577*
CG	1.030 ± 0.061*	1.033 ± 0.060*	1.033 ± 0.060*	1.223 ± 0.099*
DSF/CG	1.107 ± 0.081*	1.197 ± 0.048*	1.200 ± 0.050*	1.250 ± 0.050*

Results are expressed as mean ± SEM, the superscript (*) means significant difference with respect to control at p < 0.05 (ANOVA).

Table 12. Effect of high dose DSF (74.6 mg/kg), CG (15 mg/kg) and DSF/CG (74.6/15 mg/kg) combination on creatinine (mmol/l).

	30 Days	45 Days	60 Days	90 Days
CONTROL 1	0.667 ± 0.088	0.700 ± 0.058	0.700 ± 0.058	0.700 ± 0.058
DSF	1.183 ± 0.044*	1.283 ± 0.060*	1.467 ± 0.033*	1.467 ± 0.033*
CG	1.257 ± 0.092*	1.340 ± 0.122*	1.417 ± 0.164*	1.417 ± 0.164*
DSF/CG	1.400 ± 0.076*	1.423 ± 0.087*	1.670 ± 0.215*	2.817 ± 0.217*

Results are expressed as mean ± SEM, the superscript (*) means significant difference with respect to control at p < 0.05 (ANOVA).

(Pb), chromium (Cr) and platinum (Pt) are a major environmental and occupational hazard. Unfortunately, these non-essential elements are toxic at very low doses and non-biodegradable with a very long biological half-life. Thus, exposure to heavy metals is potentially harmful. Because of its ability to reabsorb and accumulate divalent metals, the kidney is the first target organ of heavy metal toxicity. The extent of renal damage by heavy metals depends on the nature, the dose, route and duration of exposure. Both acute and chronic intoxication have been demonstrated to cause nephropathies, with various levels of severity ranging from tubular dysfunctions like acquired Fanconi syndrome to severe renal failure leading occasionally to death [17].

10. Conclusion

Disulfiram and copper gluconate as single agents are nephrotoxic as seen from our results. Administered as a combination, disulfiram/copper gluconate was nephrotoxic as shown by the development of hyperkalemia, hypernatremia, uraemia and increased creatinine levels which were higher for the drug combination when compared to the single agent. These results are pointers to the development of kidney damage in the experimental animals. The researchers believe that the nephrotoxicity observed is achieved via a synergistic toxicological effect when disulfiram and copper gluconate are combined. These effects were observed at low, medium and high doses and should therefore be used with extreme caution.

Acknowledgements

The authors are grateful to Prof. O.A. Georgewill and Dr. Dawaye A. Georgewill for their useful contributions.

References

[1]   World Health Organization (2008) World Cancer Report 2008. International Agency for Research on Cancer, Lyon.

[2]   Chukwuma, M. (2006) Crude Oil Pollution Raises Cancer Risk among Nigerians. African Cancer Centre.

[3]   Duran-Frigola, M. and Aloy, P. (2012) Recycling Side Effects into Clinical Markers for Drug Repositioning. *Genome Medicine*, **4**, 3. http://dx.doi.org/10.1186/gm302

[4]   Li, Y.Y. and Jones, S.J. (2012). Drug Repositioning for Personalised Medicine. *Genome Medicine*, **4**, 27.

[5]   Blatt, J. and Corey, S.J. (2013) Drug Repositioning in Paediatrics and Pediatric Hematology Oncology. *Drug Discovery Today*, **18**, 4-10. http://dx.doi.org/10.1016/j.drudis.2012.07.009

[6]   Cvek, B. (2011) Targeting Malignancies with Disulfiram(antabuse); Multidrug Resistance, Angiogenesis, and Proteasome. *Current Cancer Drug Targets*, **11**, 332-337. http://dx.doi.org/10.2174/156800911794519806

[7]   Kast, R.E., Boockvar, J.A., Bruning, A., Capello, F., Chang, W.W., Cvek, B., Dou, Q.P., Duenas-Gonzalez, A., Efferth, T., Focosi, D., Ghaffari, S.H., Karpel-Massler, G., Ketola, K., Khoshnevisan, A., Keizman, D., Magne, N., Marosi, C., McDonald, K., Munoz, M., Paranjpe, A., Pourgholami, M.H., Sardi, I., Sella, A., Srivenugopal, K.S., Tucorri, M., Wang, W., Wirtz, C..R. and Halatsch, M.E. (2013) A Conceptually New Treatment Approach for Relapsed Glioblastoma; Coordinated Undermining of Survival Paths with Nine Repurposed Drugs (CUSP9) by the International Initiative for Accelerated Improvement of Glioblastoma Care. *Oncotarget*, **4**, 502-530.

[8]   Brar, S.S., Grigg, C., Wilson, K.S., Holder, W.D., Dreau, D., Austin, C., *et al.* (2010) Disulfiram Inhibits Activating Transcription Factor/Cyclic AMP Responsive Element Binding Protein and Human Melanoma Growth in a Metal-Dependent Manner *in Vitro*, in Mice and in a Patient with Cancer Cell Lines. *Cancer Letters*, **290**, 104-113.

[9]   Marikovsky, M., Nevo, N., Vadai, E. and Harris-Cerruti, C. (2002) Cu/Zn Superoxide Dismutase Plays a Role in Angiogenesis. *International Journal of Cancer*, **97**, 34-41. http://dx.doi.org/10.1002/ijc.1565

[10] Cen, D., Gonzalez, R.I., Buckmeier, J.A., Kahlon, R.S., Tohidian, N.B. and Meyskens Jr, F.L. (2002) Disulfiram Induces Apoptosis in Human Melanoma Cells: A Redox-Related Process. *Molecular Cancer Therapeutics*, **1**, 197-204.

[11] Chen, D., Cui, Q.C., Yang, H.J. and Dou, Q.P. (2006) Disulfiram, a Clinically Used Anti-Alcoholism Drug and Copper-Binding Agent, Induces Apoptotic Cell Death in Breast Cancer Cultures and Xenografts via Inhibition of the Proteasome Activity. *Cancer Research*, **66**, 10425-10433. http://dx.doi.org/10.1158/0008-5472.CAN-06-2126

[12] Johansson, B. (1992) A Review of the Pharmacokinetics and Pharmacodynamics of Disulfiram and Its Metabolites. *Acta Psychiatrica Scandinavica*, **86**, 15-26. http://dx.doi.org/10.1111/j.1600-0447.1992.tb03310.x

[13] Kristenson, H. (1995) How to Get the Best out of Antabuse. *Alcohol and Alcoholism*, **30**, 775-783.

[14] Skrott, Z. and Cvek, B. (2012) Diethyldithiocarbamate Complex with Copper: The Mechanism of Action in Cancer Cells. *Mini-Reviews in Medicinal Chemistry*, **12**, 1184-1192. http://dx.doi.org/10.2174/138955712802762068

[15] Papaioannou, M., Malonas, I., Kast, R.E. and Brüning, A. (2013) Disulfiram/Copper Causes Redox-Related Proteotoxicity and Concomitant Heat Shock Response in Ovarian Cancer Cells That Is Augmented by Auranofin-Mediated Thioredoxin Inhibition. *Oncoscience*, **1**, 21-29.

[16] Ries, F. and Klastersky, J. (1986) Nephrotoxicity Induced by Cancer Chemotherapy with Special Emphasis on Cisplatin Toxicity. *American Journal of Kidney Diseases*, **8**, 368-379. http://dx.doi.org/10.1016/S0272-6386(86)80112-3

[17] Barbier, O., Jacquillet, G., Tauc, M., Cougnon, M. and Poujeol, P. (2005) Effect of Heavy Metals on, and Handling by, the Kidney. *Nephron Physiology*, **99**, 105-110. http://dx.doi.org/10.1159/000083981

[18] Owunari, G.U., Minakiri, S.I. and Wolfe, O.A. (2015) Effect of Disulfiram/Copper Gluconate Combination on Haematological Indices in Rodents. *Pharmacology & Pharmacy*, **6**, 17-24. http://dx.doi.org/10.4236/pp.2015.61003

[19] Grossmann, K.F., Blankenship, M.B., Akerley, W., Terrazas, M.C., Kosak, K.M., Boucher, K.M., Buys, S.S., Jones, K., Werner, T.L., Agarwal, N., Weis, J., Sharma, S., Ward, J. and Shami, P.J. (2011) Abstract 1308: A Phase I Clinical Study Investigating Disulfiram and Copper Gluconate in Patients with Advanced Treatment-Refractory Solid Tumors Involving the Liver. *Cancer Research*, **71**, 1308. http://dx.doi.org/10.1158/1538-7445.AM2011-1308

[20] Olurishe, T.O., Kwanashie, H.O., Anukar, J.A., Muktar, H. and Sambo, J.S. (2013) Renal Impact of Subacute Lamivudine-Artesunate Treatment in Wistar Rats. *African Journal of Pharmacology and Therapeutics*, **2**, 48-53.

[21] Eaton, D.C. and Pooler, J.P. (2009) Vander's Renal Physiology. 7th Edition, Lange Medical Books/McGraw-Hill, Medical Pub. Division, New York.

[22] Traynor, J., Mactier, R., Geddes, C.C. and Fox, J.G. (2006) How to Measure Renal Function in Clinical Practice. *British Medical Journal*, **333**, 733-737. http://dx.doi.org/10.1136/bmj.38975.390370.7C

[23] Allen, P.J. (2012) Creatine Metabolism and Psychiatric Disorders: Does Creatine Supplementation Have Therapeutic Value? *Neuroscience & Biobehavioral Reviews*, **36**, 1442-1462. http://dx.doi.org/10.1016/j.neubiorev.2012.03.005

[24] Gross, J.L., de Azevedo, M.J., Silveiro, S.P., Canani, L.H., Caramori, M.L. and Zelmanovitz, T. (2005) Diabetic Nephropathy: Diagnosis, Prevention, and Treatment. *Diabetes Care*, **28**, 164-176. http://dx.doi.org/10.2337/diacare.28.1.164

6

Effect of Disulfiram/Copper Gluconate Combination on Haematological Indices in Rodents

Georgewill Udeme Owunari, Siminialayi Iyeopu Minakiri, Obianime Atuboyedia Wolfe

Department of Pharmacology, Faculty of Basic Medical Sciences, College of Health Sciences, University of Port Harcourt, Port Harcourt, Nigeria
Email: udgeorgewill@yahoo.com

Abstract

The chronic toxicological profile of disulfiram/copper gluconate (DSF/CG) combination was investigated in a 90 day time and dose dependent study. A total of 148 rats weighing 260 - 300 g were used for this study; 60 for the pilot study and 88 for the chronic toxicity test. 88 rats divided into eleven groups consisting of 8 rats each were used for the main experiment. Groups 1 and 2 served as control groups and received normal saline as placebo and 99.5% dimethyl sulfoxide (DMSO) (Solvent control), respectively. Drugs were administered orally via a 1 ml syringe. Animals were given three doses (1/5th, 1/10th and 1/20th) of the calculated LD_{50} of 373 mg/kg and 75 mg/kg for disulfiram and copper gluconate respectively. Dosing was done daily with that of the combination given 12 hours apart. Blood samples were obtained via cardiac puncture on days 30, 45, 60 and 90 for analysis. Haematological parameters showed a significant ($p < 0.05$) dose- and time-dependent decrease in the packed cell volume, red blood cell count, white blood cell count and platelet count respectively. The results indicate bone marrow depression evidenced by anemia, leucopenia and thrombocytopenia in the experimental animals. The DSF/CG combination appears to exhibit a synergistic dose-dependent haematotoxicity.

Keywords

Disulfiram, Copper gluconate, Haematological Indices

1. Introduction

Disulfiram (Antabuse) (**Figure 1**), a drug used for the aversive therapy of alcoholism and copper gluconate are being repurposed for cancer chemotherapy. Disulfiram, used for several decades in the treatment of alcoholism, now shows promise as an anticancer drug and radio sensitizer. Disulfiram-induced cytotoxicity has been reported to be mediated by oxidative stress [1] [2], and this may be enhanced by the presence of copper [1]. Many tumours contain elevated levels of copper which render them selectively susceptible to disulfiram-induced toxicity [3]. Copper binding drugs inhibit proteasome activity [3] and generate reactive oxygen species (ROS) [4]. Disulfiram chelates copper, and it has been suggested that the disulfiram-copper complex is the toxic form of the drug [5]. Researchers have observed that in the presence of copper, disulfiram exhibits cytotoxic effects on a number of cancer cell lines. It is postulated that disulfiram, chemically a bis-N, N-diethyldithiocarbamate forms a carbamato complex with copper II ions *in situ* which inhibits the proteasome activity, instigating apoptosis and eventual cell death [5]. This research work set out to study the chronic toxicological effect of the DSF/CG combination on haematological parameters in rodents.

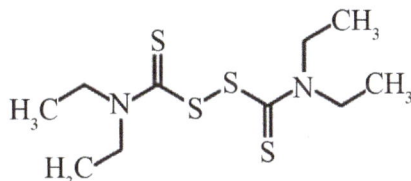

Figure 1. Chemical structure of Disulfiram (http://images.ddccdn.com/img/mol/DB00822.mol.t.jpg)

2. Methodology

148 Albino Swiss rats of both sexes weighing between 260 g - 300 g obtained from the Department of Pharmacology animal house were used for this study. 88 rats were used for the main experiment while 60 rats were used for the pilot study. The rats were bred and maintained under suitable conditions, allowed an acclimatization period of two (2) weeks, housed in hygienic cages in groups of four and allowed free access to feed obtained from vital feeds UAC PLC and water *ad libitum*. The beddings were changed and cages cleaned out on alternate days. Animals were handled according to Helsinki declaration on animal care. The animals were divided into 11 groups, each consisting of 8 rats each. The groups included those for treatment and the control groups. Drugs were administered orally via a 1ml syringe.

2.1. Pilot Study

Acute toxicity tests were done using the arithmetic method of Karber to determine the LD_{50} of disulfiram and copper gluconate. A total of 60 rats were used. This preliminary dose range finding test was done to determine the doses to be administered. Drugs were administered via the intra-peritoneal route. The Arithmetic method of Karber as adapted by (Patel, 2004) [6] was used as follows;

This method made use of the formula stated below:

$$LD_{50} = LD_{100} - \Sigma\{a \times b\}/n$$

where, LD_{50} = Median Lethal dose;
  LD_{100} = Dose that kills 100% of the test animals;
  a = Dose difference;
  b = Mean mortality;
  n = group population.

2.2. Chronic Toxicity Tests

This study spanned 3 months and was domiciled in the Department of Pharmacology, University of Port Harcourt, Animal house and Laboratory. A dose and time dependent toxicological evaluation of the effects of disulfiram, copper gluconate and disulfiram and copper gluconate combination on the haematological profiles of rodents was evaluated. A total of 88 rats obtained from the Department of Pharmacology animal house were divided into eleven groups consisting of 8 rats each. Groups 1 and 2 served as control groups and the rats received normal saline as placebo and 99.5% DMSO (Solvent control) respectively. Drugs were administered orally via a 1 ml syringe.

The test group rats were divided into groups 3, 4 and 5 consisting of 24 rats in each group. Drug administration was done orally for 90 days as follows:

Control group 1 rats received 1ml of normal saline orally daily for 90 days

Solvent control, group 2 received 0.5 ml of DMSO orally daily for 90 days

Group 3a rats received *15 mg/kg of copper gluconate daily orally

Group 3b rats received *7.5 mg/kg of copper gluconate daily orally

Group 3c rats received *3.75 mg/kg of copper gluconate daily orally

*doses were 1/5th, 1/10th and 1/20th of the LD_{50} of Copper gluconate

Group 4a rats received °74.6 mg/kg of DSF and *15 mg/kg of copper gluconate daily orally

Group 4b rats received °37.3 mg/kg of DSF and *7.5 mg/kg of copper gluconate daily orally

Group 4c rats received °18.65 mg/kg of DSF and *3.75 mg/kg of copper gluconate daily orally

°Doses were 1/5th, 1/10th and 1/20th of the LD_{50} of disulfiram (DSF)

*Doses were 1/5th, 1/10th and 1/20th of the LD_{50} of copper gluconate

N/B The drug combination was given following the protocol of Grossman et al., 2011 [7].

Group 5a rats received °74.6 mg/kg of DSF daily orally

Group 5b rats received °37.3 mg/kg of DSF daily orally

Group 5c rats received °18.65 mg/kg of DSF daily orally

°Doses were 1/5th, 1/10th and 1/20th of the LD_{50} of disulfiram (DSF)

2.3. Collection of Samples

Two animals per group were sacrificed under diethyl ether anaesthesia and blood samples were obtained with a 5 ml syringe on days 30, 45, 60 and 90 for analysis via cardiac puncture. The Packed cell volume, red blood cell count, white blood cell count and platelets were analyzed using the auto haematology analyzer (BC 2800) made in China.

2.4. Stock Solutions

These were prepared from 99.5% DMSO for disulfiram and distilled water for copper gluconate. Pure analytical grade samples, CAS No. 527-09-3 (98% min purity) and CAS No. 97-77-8 (98% min purity) obtained from Shijiazhuang Aopharm Import and Export Co. Limited China were used for the study.

2.5. Ethical Approval

This was obtained from the University of Port Harcourt Research Ethics Committee.

2.6. Statistical Analysis

This was done using graph pad prism 5 statistical package and ANOVA for comparison of the means of the various groups. Results are expressed as means ± SEM. Test group results were compared with that of the control groups. A p-value < 0.05 was considered significant.

3. Results

Table 1. LD_{50} determination of disulfiram (DSF).

DOSE (mg/kg)	NO. OF DEAD	MEAN DEAD (MD)	DOSE DIFF (DD)	MDXDD
200	0	0	0	0
300	1	0.5	100	50
350	2	1.5	50	60
400	3	2.5	50	125
450	4	3.5	50	175
500	5	4.5	50	225
TOTAL				635

LD_{50} = 373 mg/kg.

Table 2. LD$_{50}$ determination of copper gluconate (CG).

DOSE (mg/kg)	NO. OF DEAD	MEAN DEAD (MD)	DOSE DIFF (DD)	MD XDD
50	0	0	0	0
60	1	0.5	10	5
70	2	1.5	10	15
80	3	2.5	10	25
90	4	3.5	10	35
100	5	4.5	10	45
TOTAL				125

LD$_{50}$ = 75 mg/kg.

Table 3. Effect of low dose DSF (18.65 mg/kg), CG (3.75 mg/kg) and DSF/CG (18.65/3.75 mg/kg) combination on PCV (%).

	30 DAYS	45 DAYS	60 DAYS	90 DAYS
CONTROL 1	48.67 ± 1.856	50.00 ± 2.000	49.33 ± 1.333	52.67 ± 1.764
DSF	42.33 ± 1.453	42.67 ± 3.712	42.67 ± 3.712	44.33 ± 3.480
CG	40.00 ± 1.155*	39.33 ± 2.906*	39.33 ± 2.906*	39.33 ± 2.906*
DSF/CG	38.67 ± 1.333*	38.00 ± 3.786*	38.00 ± 3.786*	32.00 ± 4.619*

Results are expressed as mean ± SEM, the superscript (*) means significant difference with respect to control at $p < 0.05$ (ANOVA).

Table 4. Effect of medium dose DSF (37.3 mg/kg), CG (7.5 mg/kg), DSF/CG (37.3/7.5 mg/kg) combination on PCV (%).

	30 DAYS	45 DAYS	60 DAYS	90 DAYS
CONTROL 1	52.67 ± 0.667	52.67 ± 0.667	50.27 ± 0.176	50.07 ± 0.067
DSF	46.67 ± 1.764*	47.33 ± 1.764*	41.00 ± 2.646*	41.00 ± 2.646*
CG	47.33 ± 1.764*	44.00 ± 2.309*	42.00 ± 2.309*	42.00 ± 2.309*
DSF/CG	43.33 ± 2.404*	41.33 ± 2.906*	40.33 ± 3.283*	41.00 ± 2.646*

Results are expressed as mean ± SEM, the superscript (*) means significant difference with respect to control at $p < 0.05$ (ANOVA).

Table 5. Effect of high dose DSF (74.6 mg/kg), CG (15 mg/kg) and DSF/CG (74.6/15 mg/kg) combination on PCV (%).

	30 DAYS	45 DAYS	60 DAYS	90 DAYS
CONTROL 1	50.07 ± 1.097	52.67 ± 0.667	52.67 ± 0.667	52.00 ± 1.155
DSF	40.33 ± 3.283*	39.00 ± 4.583*	39.00 ± 4.583*	40.33 ± 3.283*
CG	38.67 ± 4.667*	40.67 ± 3.528*	40.67 ± 3.528*	44.33 ± 2.186*
DSF/CG	42.33 ± 3.180*	41.33 ± 3.712*	40.33 ± 4.177*	44.67 ± 1.764*

Results are expressed as mean ± SEM, the superscript (*) means significant difference with respect to control at $p < 0.05$ (ANOVA).

Table 6. Effect of low dose DSF (18.6 mg/kg), CG (3.75 mg/kg), DSF/CG (18.6/3.75 mg/kg) combination on RBC ($\times 10^{12}$).

	30 DAYS	45 DAYS	60 DAYS	90 DAYS
CONTROL 1	25.67 ± 0.667	26.67 ± 0.667	27.67 ± 1.202	31.00 ± 0.5774
DSF	20.33 ± 0.333*	22.00 ± 1.528*	22.00 ± 1.528*	22.00 ± 1.528*
CG	19.33 ± 0.667*	20.67 ± 1.333*	20.67 ± 1.333*	20.67 ± 1.333*
DSF/CG	19.07 ± 0.581*	19.40 ± 0.872*	19.40 ± 0.872*	19.40 ± 0.872*

Results are expressed as mean ± SEM, the superscript (*) means significant difference with respect to control at $p < 0.05$ (ANOVA).

Table 7. Effect of medium dose DSF (37.3 mg/kg), CG (7.5 mg/kg) and DSF/CG (37.3/7.5 mg/kg) combination on RBC ($\times 10^{12}$).

	30 DAYS	45 DAYS	60 DAYS	90 DAYS
CONTROL 1	32.00 ± 1.155	9.633 ± 0.067	9.633 ± 0.067	8.333 ± 0.167
DSF	$26.33 \pm 1.202^*$	$6.233 \pm 0.145^*$	$6.233 \pm 0.145^*$	$6.233 \pm 0.145^*$
CG	$24.00 \pm 2.309^*$	$6.167 \pm 0.203^*$	$6.167 \pm 0.203^*$	$6.167 \pm 0.203^*$
DSF/CG	$24.00 \pm 2.309^*$	$5.867 \pm 0.353^*$	$5.800 \pm 0.416^*$	$5.800 \pm 0.416^*$

Results are expressed as mean ± SEM, the superscript (*) means significant difference with respect to control at $p < 0.05$ (ANOVA).

Table 8. Effect of high dose DSF (74.6 mg/kg), CG (15 mg/kg) and DSF/CG (74.6/15 mg/kg) combination on RBC ($\times 10^{12}$).

	30 DAYS	45 DAYS	60 DAYS	90 DAYS
CONTROL 1	8.333 ± 0.167	9.640 ± 0.074	9.640 ± 0.074	9.833 ± 0.167
DSF	$6.167 \pm 0.203^*$	$6.167 \pm 0.203^*$	$6.100 \pm 0.265^*$	$5.833 \pm 0.524^*$
CG	$5.967 \pm 0.393^*$	$5.967 \pm 0.393^*$	$5.900 \pm 0.458^*$	$5.567 \pm 0.788^*$
DSF/CG	$5.800 \pm 0.416^*$	$5.800 \pm 0.416^*$	$5.733 \pm 0.481^*$	$5.467 \pm 0.742^*$

Results are expressed as mean ± SEM, the superscript (*) means significant difference with respect to control at $p < 0.05$ (ANOVA).

Table 9. Effect of low dose DSF (18.65 mg/kg), CG (3.75 mg/kg) and DSF/CG (18.65/3.75 mg/kg) combination on WBC ($\times 1000$).

	30 DAYS	45 DAYS	60 DAYS	90 DAYS
CONTROL 1	10.70 ± 0.520	10.70 ± 0.520	10.73 ± 0.536	11.63 ± 0.664
DSF	9.400 ± 0.208	9.000 ± 1.155	9.000 ± 1.155	9.000 ± 1.155
CG	$8.667 \pm 0.203^*$	$8.667 \pm 0.203^*$	$8.667 \pm 0.203^*$	$8.667 \pm 0.203^*$
DSF/CG	$7.433 \pm 0.449^*$	$7.100 \pm 0.737^*$	$7.100 \pm 0.737^*$	$7.100 \pm 0.737^*$

Results are expressed as mean ± SEM, the superscript (*) means significant difference with respect to control at $p < 0.05$ (ANOVA).

Table 10. Effect of medium dose DSF (37.3 mg/kg), CG (7.5 mg/kg) and DSF/CG (37.3/7.5 mg/kg) combination on WBC ($\times 1000$).

	30 DAYS	45 DAYS	60 DAYS	90 DAYS
CONTROL 1	14.67 ± 1.764	15.33 ± 0.667	11.97 ± 0.328	11.97 ± 0.328
DSF	9.000 ± 1.155	$9.000 \pm 1.155^*$	$5.533 \pm 0.291^*$	$5.533 \pm 0.291^*$
CG	$8.667 \pm 0.203^*$	$8.667 \pm 0.203^*$	$6.000 \pm 0.231^*$	$6.000 \pm 0.231^*$
DSF/CG	$7.100 \pm 0.737^*$	$7.100 \pm 0.737^*$	$5.200 \pm 0.603^*$	$5.200 \pm 0.603^*$

Results are expressed as mean ± SEM, the superscript (*) means significant difference with respect to control at $p < 0.05$ (ANOVA).

Table 11. Effect of high dose DSF (74.6 mg/kg), CG (15 mg/kg), DSF/CG (74.6/15 mg/kg) combination on WBC ($\times 1000$).

	30 DAYS	45 DAYS	60 DAYS	90 DAYS
CONTROL 1	11.97 ± 0.328	11.67 ± 0.167	11.50 ± 0.289	11.50 ± 0.289
DSF	$5.533 \pm 0.291^*$	$5.533 \pm 0.291^*$	$5.533 \pm 0.291^*$	$5.533 \pm 0.291^*$
CG	$5.933 \pm 0.291^*$	$5.933 \pm 0.291^*$	$5.800 \pm 0.416^*$	$5.533 \pm 0.677^*$
DSF/CG	$5.200 \pm 0.603^*$	$5.367 \pm 0.437^*$	$5.200 \pm 0.603^*$	$5.133 \pm 0.669^*$

Results are expressed as mean ± SEM, the superscript (*) means significant difference with respect to control at $p < 0.05$ (ANOVA).

Table 12. Effect of low dose DSF (18.65 mg/kg), CG (3.75 mg/kg) and DSF/CG (18.65/3.75 mg/kg) combination on PLT (×1000).

	30 DAYS	45 DAYS	60 DAYS	90 DAYS
CONTROL 1	471.3 ± 1.856	474.3 ± 2.603	480.0 ± 11.55	461.7 ± 1.667
DSF	433.3 ± 8.819*	440.0 ± 11.55*	413.3 ± 17.64*	420.0 ± 11.55*
CG	423.3 ± 12.02*	433.3 ± 13.33*	426.7 ±13.33*	388.3 ± 16.41*
DSF/CG	403.3 ± 8.819*	396.7 ± 26.03*	396.7 ± 26.03*	350.0 ± 28.87*

Results are expressed as mean ± SEM, the superscript (*) means significant difference with respect to control at p < 0.05 (ANOVA).

Table 13. Effect of medium dose DSF (37.3 mg/kg), CG (7.5 mg/kg) and DSF/CG (37.3/7.5 mg/kg) combination on PLT (×1000).

	30 DAYS	45 DAYS	60 DAYS	90 DAYS
CONTROL 1	512.0 ± 6.110	631.7 ± 9.280	543.3 ± 8.819	563.3 ± 18.56
DSF	420.0 ± 11.55*	420.0 ± 11.55*	446.7 ± 29.06*	460.0 ± 30.55*
CG	388.3 ± 16.41*	388.3 ± 16.41*	380.0 ± 11.55*	380.0 ± 11.55*
DSF/CG	350.0 ± 28.87*	350.0 ± 28.87*	350.0 ± 28.87*	350.0 ± 28.87*

Results are expressed as mean ± SEM, the superscript (*) means significant difference with respect to control at p < 0.05 (ANOVA).

Table 14. Effect of high dose DSF (74.6 mg/kg), CG (15 mg/kg) and DSF/CG (74.6/15 mg/kg) combination on PLT (×1000).

	30 DAYS	45 DAYS	60 DAYS	90 DAYS
CONTROL 1	563.3 ± 18.56	513.3 ± 6.667	511.7 ± 4.410	518.3 ± 7.265
DSF	460.0 ± 30.55*	416.7 ± 16.67*	416.7 ± 33.83*	416.7 ± 33.83*
CG	380.0 ± 12.00*	373.3 ± 17.64*	366.7 ± 24.04*	360.0 ± 30.55*
DSF/CG	350.0 ± 28.87*	346.7 ± 31.80*	343.3 ± 34.80*	333.3 ± 44.10*

Results are expressed as mean ± SEM, the superscript (*) means significant difference with respect to control at p < 0.05 (ANOVA).

4. Discussion

The median lethal dose (LD_{50}) of a drug is that dose that kills 50% of the study population and serves as a general indicator of a drug's acute toxicity. For disulfiram, our study revealed an LD_{50} of 373 mg/kg (**Table 1**) and for copper gluconate an LD_{50} of 75 mg/kg was obtained (**Table 2**).

Low dose disulfiram had no significant (p > 0.05) effect on the packed cell volume (PCV) compared to the control, but copper gluconate and disulfiram/copper gluconate combination produced reductions in PCV values that were significant at p < 0.05 when compared to the control (**Table 3**). The finding of the significant effect of the combination may not be unconnected with the synergistic actions of the two drugs when combined.

Disulfiram, copper gluconate and disulfiram/copper gluconate combination at medium and high doses produced reductions in packed cell volume (PCV) that were significant (p < 0.05) when compared to the control (**Table 4** and **Table 5**). The results were in agreement with the findings of Al Naimi et al. [8] whose work on $CuSo_4$ in rats revealed a significant decrease in PCV values.

The reductions produced in the red blood cell (RBC) fractions by disulfiram, copper gluconate and their combination at low, medium and high doses were all significant (p < 0.05) when compared to the control (**Tables 6-8**). The results were also in agreement with the findings of Al Naimi et al. [8] whose work on $CuSo_4$ in rats revealed a significant decrease in RBC counts and PCV values with marked decrease in haemoglobin concentration suggestive of chronic blood loss due to haemolytic anaemia. Adams et al. (1979) [9] in their research, reported marked reduction in the deformability of the RBCs as well as marked increases in membrane permeability and osmotic fragility. In 1977 Adam and Wasfi, [10] reported that Copper induced formation and subsequent degradation of peroxides from the membrane lipids of the RBCs which may be a critical factor in altering membrane integrity that leads to hemolysis. Other researchers assert that excess copper intake produces anaemia by interfering with iron transport and/or metabolism [11] [12]. These observations may explain the recorded findings of this current investigation

This study's findings, indicate that at low dose, copper gluconate and disulfiram/copper gluconate combination produced marked reductions in white blood count (WBC) values that were significant ($p < 0.05$) when compared with control (**Table 9**). Disulfiram at medium dose produced reductions in WBC values that were significant ($p < 0.05$) only on day 45, 60 and 90, while copper gluconate and disulfiram/copper gluconate combination produced WBC reductions that were significant ($p < 0.05$) throughout the test period (**Table 10**). However, at high dose, disulfiram, copper gluconate and disulfiram/copper gluconate combination produced marked reductions in white blood count (WBC) values that were significant ($p < 0.05$) when compared with the control (**Table 11**) throughout the duration of the study. These findings were not surprising as it is known that the effects of high-dose ingestion of heavy metals include degenerative changes in the liver and kidneys and that at very high doses these heavy metals can cause leukopenia and marked hypoplasia or aplasia of the bone marrow. The result of this current investigation on WBC value is however at variance with the findings of Beddard et al., 2000 [13] who found significant increase in WBC count of experimental animals given different doses of $CuSo_4 \cdot H_2O$ when compared with the control. A finding he described as unusual neutrophilia. Beddard and his co-investigators further explained that the neutrophilia could have been produced by inflammatory stimuli coming from the damaged liver cells.

Disulfiram, copper gluconate and disulfiram/copper gluconate combination produced marked reduction in platelet count that was significant ($p < 0.05$) at low, medium and high doses when compared with the control (**Tables 12-14**). This agrees with the findings of Beddard et al., 2000 [13] who also reported a significant decrease in platelet count in their study of effects of $CuSo_4$ in rats. It is believed that secondary thrombocytopenia resulting from poisoning with heavy metal causes interference with clotting and haemorrhage [13]. It has been reported by Turnlund et al., 2004 [14], that long-term high intake of copper can result in adverse effects on immune function. This perhaps explains the significant ($p < 0.05$) decrease recorded in the different haematological parameters studied. As the level of reduction obtained in this study on the different components of the blood would adversely reduce immunity.

5. Conclusion

This current investigation has clearly shown that, disulfiram/copper gluconate combination produced bone marrow depression as evidenced by anaemia (low PCV), leucocytopenia (low WBC count) and thrombocytopenia (low Platelet count) in the experimental animals following chronic use. The importance of the sequel effects of bone marrow depression on the overall health of an organism need not be overemphasized; therefore, we believe that there is a synergistic toxicological effect when disulfiram and copper gluconate are combined. While these effects appear mild at low and medium doses and can be advisedly used with caution, at high doses this combination is highly toxic and should therefore be used with extreme caution.

Acknowledgements

The authors are grateful to Prof. O. A. Georgewill and Dr. Dawaye A. Georgewill for their useful contributions.

References

[1]   Chen, S.H., Liu, S.H., Liang, Y.C., Lin, J.K. and Lin-Shiau, S.Y. (2001) Oxidative Stress and c-Junamino-Terminal Kinase Activation Involved in Apoptosis of Primary Astrocytes Induced by Disulfiram-Cu21 Complex. *European Journal of Pharmacology*, **414**, 177-188. http://dx.doi.org/10.1016/S0014-2999(01)00792-0

[2]   Cen, D., Gonzalez, R.I., Buckmeier, J.A., Kahlon, R.S., Tohidian, N.B. and Meyskens Jr., F.L. (2002) Disulfiram Induces Apoptosis in Human Melanoma Cells: A Redox-Related Process. *Molecular Cancer Therapeutics*, **1**, 197-204.

[3]   Daniel, K.G., Chen, D., Yan, B. and Dou, Q.P. (2007) Copper-Binding Compounds as Proteasome Inhibitors and Apoptosis Inducers in Human Cancer. *Frontiers in Bioscience*, **12**, 135-144.

[4]   Gupte, A. and Mumper, J. (2009) Elevated Copper and Oxidative Stress in Cancer Cells as a Target for Cancer Treatment. *Cancer Treatment Reviews*, **35**, 32-46. http://dx.doi.org/10.1016/j.ctrv.2008.07.004

[5]   Chen, D., Cui, Q.C., Yang, H. and Dou, Q.P. (2006) Disulfiram, a Clinically Used Anti-Alcoholism Drug and Copper-Binding Agent, Induces Apoptotic Cell Death in Breast Cancer Cultures and Xenograftsvia Inhibition of the Pro-

teasome Activity. *Cancer Research*, **66**, 10425-10433. http://dx.doi.org/10.1158/0008-5472.CAN-06-2126

[6]   Patel, S. (2004) Demonstration of Karber's Method of LD50 Determination. *Journal of Chemical Pharmaceutical Research*. http://m.authorstream.com/presentation/patelcharmi91-1826002-methods-determineLD50

[7]   Grossmann, K.F., Blankenship, M.B., Akerley, W., Terrazas, M.C., Kosak, K.M., Boucher, K.M., Buys, S.S., Jones, K., Werner, T.L., Agarwal, N., Weis, J., Sharma, S., Ward, J. and Shami, P.J. (2011) Abstract 1308: A Phase I Clinical Study Investigating Disulfiram and Copper Gluconate in Patients with Advanced Treatment-Refractory Solid Tumors Involving the Liver. *Cancer Research*, **71**. http://dx.doi.org/10.1158/1538-7445.AM2011-1308

[8]   Al-Naimi, R.A., Al-Tayar, N.H., Alsoufi, L.A.M. and Al-Taae, E.H.Y. (2013) Hematological and Biochemical Evaluation after Different Orally Doses of Copper Sulfate in Rats. *The Iraqi Journal of Veterinary Medicine*, **38**, 83-91.

[9]   Adams, K.F., Johnson, G., Hornowski, K.E. and Lineberger, T.H. (1979) The Effect of Copper on Erythrocytes Deformability: A Possible Mechanism of Hemolysis in Acute Copper Intoxication. 23. *Biochimica et Biophysica Acta*, **550**, 279-287.

[10] Adam, S.E.I. and Wasfi, I.A. (1977) Chronic Copper Toxicity in Nubain Goats. *Journal of Comparative Pathology*, **87**, 623-627.

[11] Ralph, A. and McArdle, H.J. (2001) Copper Metabolism and Requirements in the Pregnant Mother, Her Fetus, and Children. International Copper Association, New York.

[12] International Programme on Chemical Safety (1998) Environmental Health Criteria No. 200: Copper. World Health Organization, Geneva.

[13] Bedard, K., Fuentealba, I.C. and Cribb, A. (2000) The Long Evans Cinnamon (LEC) Rat Develops Hepatocellular Damage in the Absence of Antimicrosomal Antibodies. *Toxicology*, **146**, 101-109.

[14] Turnlund, J.R., Jacob, R.A., Keen, C.L., *et al.* (2004) Long-Term High Copper Intake: Effects on Indexes of Copper Status, Antioxidant Status, and Immune Function in Young Men. *The American Journal of Clinical Nutrition*, **79**, 1037-1044.

7

Development of the Japanese Medication Adherence Scale and Verification of Its Reliability and Validity in Hypertensive Patients

Rika Shimada[1], Yasuaki Dohi[2], Kazunori Kimura[3], Satoshi Fujii[4]

[1]Department of Critical Care Nursing, Graduate School of Nursing, Nagoya City University, Nagoya, Japan
[2]Department of Cardio-Renal Medicine and Hypertension, Graduate School of Medicine, Nagoya City University, Nagoya, Japan
[3]Pharmaceutical Department, Nagoya City University Hospital, Nagoya, Japan
[4]Department of Laboratory Medicine, Asahikawa Medical University, Asahikawa, Japan
Email: shimada@med.nagoya-cu.ac.jp

Abstract

A 32-Item Japanese Medication Adherence Scale had been developed as a tool for evaluating the medication-taking behavior of hypertensive patients and predicting therapeutic efficacy, and an Internet survey of 990 hypertensive patients throughout Japan was performed. As a result, factor 1 "Expectation of pharmacological efficacy" (9 items), factor 2 "Motivation to be self-controlled in taking medication" (6 items), and factor 3 "Negative feelings about taking medication" (4 items) were identified, comprising a total of 19 items. The scale was highly reliable. Because it proved capable of discriminating between the 2 groups with different medication-taking status and blood pressure, its validity had also been confirmed.

Keywords

Drug Therapy, Hypertension, Measure, Medication Adherence Scale

1. Introduction

Hypertension is a major risk factor for disorders such as coronary artery disease, heart failure, cerebral stroke, and renal failure, and it is important to keep high blood pressure under control. Essential hypertension, which accounts for 90% of cases of hypertension, may be caused by factors including obesity, stress, smoking, alcohol, and excessive salt intake, in addition to genetic factors [1]. It is standard medical practice to provide health education on these factors, as well as drug treatment. However, these factors are heavily dependent on patient self-care, and many hypertensive patients find it difficult to control their own blood pressure [2].

It is estimated that approximately 20 million men and approximately 17 million women in Japan suffer from hypertension. The increase in hypertensive patients has also influenced increase of medical expenses. The medical expenses used for the hypertensive disease in 2004 were 1900 billion yen [3]. If inadequately controlled blood pressure is left untreated and potential future secondary diseases are not prevented, this will be detrimental not only to individuals but also for society at large.

Recently, the concept of adherence has come into use as an outcome related to medication-taking behavior in an attempt to describe patient behavior in a holistic manner [4]. Adherence refers to whether patients are capable of implementing treatment with medication correctly. It is affected by a range of different factors, including the patient's own values regarding health, their capacity to understand the disease and its treatment, their attitude to medication and ability to take medication, and the state of control of their disease [5]. It is suggested that reducing the number of tablets and the frequency of medications are effective in improving adherence [6] [7]. Research on medication adherence is still in its infancy. In Japan, a scale has yet to be developed for the appropriate measurement of medication-taking behavior in hypertensive patients, while the factors associated with medication adherence have not yet been elucidated. Thus, the aim of this study was to develop a scale to evaluate adherence among hypertensive patients and confirm the validity and reliability of the new measure.

2. Methods

2.1. Development of the Medication Adherence Measure: Interview to Clarify Factors

After obtaining approval from the ethics committee of the Nagoya City University, patients aged ≥35 and <80 years who were attending the clinic of the Department of Cardiovascular Medicine as outpatients, were taking antihypertensive medication, and had consented to participate in this study were invited. Patients with serious liver or kidney damage, uncontrolled diabetes, or endocrine disorders were excluded. Semi-structured interview was undertaken to each participant. The contents of the interviews were capacity to take medication, awareness of medication, what sort of information was given, and his or her behavior toward to taking medication. The 59 subjects included 26 men and 33 women with a mean age of 68.1 ± 9.9 years. Blood pressure at the first survey was classified according to the Guidelines for the Management of Hypertension (Japanese Society of Hypertension), with 22 patients (37.3%) having normal blood pressure, 20 (33.9%) high normal blood pressure, 15 (25.4%) grade 1 hypertension, 1 (1.7%) grade 2 hypertension and 1 (1.7%) grade 3 hypertension. Six factors associated with medication-taking behavior were isolated by analysis of the results of the interviews: "Trust in doctors and medication," "Interest in pharmacological action," "Desire to acquire knowledge about medication," "Making an effort to take medication properly," "Values regarding health," and "Thoughts on prescribed medication."

2.2. Preparation of the Scale

2.2.1. The Japanese Medication Adherence Measure Version 1
Sixty questions were formulated with reference to the categories formed by these 6 factors, and the Japanese Medication Adherence Measure version 1 was prepared. Responses were requested on a 5-point scale from "Very applicable" to "Not applicable at all." A survey was carried out by an internet research company. All subjects were Japanese who were taking antihypertensive medication daily. The results of a survey of 441 male and female patients aged 50 - 69 years taking antihypertensive medication (271 men, 170 women, mean age 59.4 ± 5.3 years) carried out using this measure were then verified.

2.2.2. The Japanese Medication Adherence Measure Version 1
Based on the Japanese Medication Adherence Measure version 1, the Japanese Medication Adherence Measure version 2, which consisted of 4 factors comprising a total of 32 items scored on a 5-point scale from "Very applicable" to "Not applicable at all," was prepared. It was then used to carry out an Internet survey entitled "Questionnaire about how you take your medication" of 990 men and women from throughout Japan who were

taking medication to treat hypertension. Mean age was 59.5 ± 10.7 (40 - 79) (**Table 1**).

2.3. Statistical Analysis

Reliability was investigated in terms of internal consistency and the test-retest method, with retesting performed 2 weeks after the first survey. Discriminant validity was investigated by dividing patients into groups with blood pressure and number of times they forgot to take their medication as independent variables, and using the t-test to investigate the differences between the groups with subscale scores as dependent variables. The level of statistical significance was set at 5%.

3. Results

3.1. Verification of Results of a Survey Using the Japanese Medication Adherence Measure Version 1

The sum total of distribution reached to 45% by 4th factor. The scree plots of principal component analysis and a comparison of the factor content of each factor solution also suggested that a 4-factor solution was appropriate. Then, factor analysis was performed for a 4-factor solution using the principal factor method and promax rotation. Items for which factor loading were <0.40 and those for which loading was similar for multiple factors were excluded. Then, factor analysis was repeated and it was determined that 32 items were appropriate. These 32 items were categorized as follows.

Factor 1, "Motivation to be self-controlled in taking medication," comprised 12 items including "I sometimes can't take my medication when I'm tired" and "It is difficult to take my medication because of its size or shape."

Factor 2, "Expectation of pharmacological efficacy," comprised 10 items including "I believe medication is effective" and "I take it so my condition won't get worse."

Factor 3, "Concern about side effects," comprised 8 items including "I am worried about the possible side effects of medication" and "I would like to know how strong the medication I am taking is."

Table 1. Sample character.

Characteristics		Number (%)
Sex	Male	562 (56.8)
	Female	428 (43.2)
Frequency of checking blood pressure per day	Never	206 (20.8)
	Once	383 (38.7)
	2 times	270 (27.3)
	3 times	40 (4.0)
	4 times	7 (0.7)
	More than 5 times	8 (0.8)
	No answer	76 (7.7)
Classification of blood pressure	Optimum	58 (5.9)
	Normal	232 (23.4)
	High normal	374 (37.8)
	Grade 1	269 (27.2)
	Grade 2	53 (5.4)
	Grade 3	4 (0.4)
Frequency of taking medicine per day	Once	445 (44.9)
	2 times	315 (31.8)
	3 times	202 (20.4)
	4 times	21 (2.1)
	More than 5 times	7 (0.7)
Frequency of forgot to take medicine per week	None	755 (76.3)
	Once	170 (17.2)
	2 times	45 (4.5)
	3 times	10 (1.0)
	More than 4 times	10 (1.0)

Blood pressure was classified according to the guidelines for the management of hypertension (Japanese Society of Hypertension, 2014).

Factor 4, "Dealing with forgetting to take medication," comprised 2 items, "I do not think forgetting to take medication once or twice is a problem" and "I do not think forgetting to take medication can be helped."

Cronbach's α coefficient was calculated for each factor to confirm internal consistency, and it was 0.856 for factor 1, 0.810 for factor 2, 0.777 for factor 3, and 0.679 for factor 4.

3.2. Verification of the Reliability and Validity of the Japanese Medication Adherence Measure Version 2

Four of the 32 items, for which the ceiling effect was evident, had been excluded. The remaining 28 items were analyzed. From the results of scree plots of principal component analysis of scores and a comparison of the factor content of each factor solution, it was determined that a 3-factor solution was appropriate, and factor analysis was performed for a 3-factor solution using the principal factor method and promax rotation. Items for which factor loading were <0.40 and those for which loading was similar for multiple factors were excluded. Then, factor analysis was repeated. It was determined that 19 items were appropriate, and these were categorized as follows (**Table 2**).

Factor 1, "Expectation of pharmacological efficacy," comprised 9 items including "I believe medication is effective" and "I think medication is important."

Factor 2, "Motivation to be self-controlled in taking medication," comprised 6 items including "I make my own decision as to whether or not to take my medication" and "I choose for myself which medication I want to take."

Factor 3, "Negative feelings about taking medication" comprised 4 items, including "I want to stop taking medication" and "I am worried about the possible side effects of medication."

Cronbach's α coefficient was calculated for each factor to confirm internal consistency. Cronbach's α coefficient was 0.829 for factor 1, 0.743 for factor 2, and 0.616 for factor 3. The correlation coefficients for subscale scores measured during the first survey and by the retest method 2 weeks later (**Table 3**). The correlation coefficients between factors were (**Table 4**). The patients were divided according to self-measured blood pressure following the Guidelines for the Management of Hypertension (Japanese Society of Hypertension, 2009) into those with optimal or normal blood pressure and those with high normal blood pressure or hypertension. The statistical difference of 2 groups were determined by the t-test, scores for all subscales and total scores were significantly higher in the normal blood pressure group ($p < 0.05$) (**Table 5**). Then, they were divided into those

Table 2. Factor loading of adherence scale among hypertensive patients.

Items	Factor loading		
	F1	F2	F3
Factor 1: Expectation of pharmacological efficacy ($\alpha = 0.829$)			
I believe medication is effective.	**0.675**	0.067	−0.102
I trust the doctor who prescribes my medication.	**0.662**	0.027	−0.158
I am serious about taking medication.	**0.644**	−0.085	0.035
I think medication is important.	**0.642**	0.045	0.025
I take it so my condition won't get worse.	**0.606**	−0.068	0.171
I expect the medication to have an effect.	**0.590**	−0.028	0.187
I always try to take it when the time comes round.	**0.577**	0.249	0.010
I take it in the way the doctor told me to.	**0.546**	−0.153	0.009
I am accustomed to taking medication.	**0.535**	0.034	0.031
Factor 2: Motivation to be self-controlled in taking medication ($\alpha = 0.743$)			
I make my own decision as to whether or not to take my medication.	0.180	**0.675**	−0.116
I choose for myself which medication I want to take.	0.217	**0.671**	−0.131
Even if I ask medical professionals a question about medication, they won't answer me.	−0.118	**0.528**	0.128
I don't know why I'm taking medication.	−0.220	**0.523**	0.079
Even if you are unable to take medication properly, that's all right.	−0.174	**0.467**	0.044
I'm taking medication even though I don't know what effect it has.	−0.129	**0.442**	0.071
Factor 3: Negative feelings about taking medication ($\alpha = 0.689$)			
I want to stop taking medication.	−0.125	−0.067	**0.660**
If possible, I would prefer not to take medication.	0.087	−0.188	**0.607**
I am worried about the possible side effects of medication.	0.027	0.248	**0.457**
I am concerned about the efficacy of medication.	0.290	0.084	**0.434**

Table 3. Correlation between test and retest of the medication adherence scale.

		Retest		
		Factor 1	Factor 2	Factor 3
Test	Factor 1: Expectation of pharmacological efficacy	0.697**	−0.400**	0.046
	Factor 2: Motivation to be self-controlled in taking medication	−0.408**	0.663**	0.155**
	Factor 3: Negative feelings about taking medication More table copy[a]	0.021	0.159**	0.689**

**p < 0.01.

Table 4. Correlation between the domains of the medication adherence scale.

Factor	Factor 1	Factor 2	Factor 3
Factor 1: Expectation of pharmacological efficacy	1.000	−0.370**	0.126**
Factor 2: Motivation to be self-controlled in taking medication	−	1.000	0.242**
Factor 3: Negative feelings about taking medication copy	−	−	1.000

**p < 0.01.

Table 5. Sample *t-test* results from comparing variables according to blood pressure.

Total score	Normal (n = 290)		High (n = 700)		Significance
	Average	SD	Average	SD	
Factor 1	18.0	4.7	18.7	4.7	0.036
Factor 2	24.2	3.3	23.1	3.6	0.000
Factor 3	11.1	2.8	10.5	2.9	0.002
All	53.3	5.6	52.3	6.0	0.017

who had forgotten to take their medication at least once during the previous week and those who had not forgotten to take it. The 2 groups were compared using the t-test. All subscale scores were significantly higher for those who had not forgotten to take their medication (p < 0.01) (**Table 6**).

4. Discussion

The word "adhere" means "stick to" or "hold fast" [8]. The concept of "adherence" has become more widely accepted worldwide. "Adherence" is a patient-centered term that refers to patients actively participating in medical treatment of their own accord and sticking to the treatment method. Patients with high adherence can thus be expected to participate in the treatment of their own accord in the endeavor to increase its therapeutic efficacy. Adherence is affected by numerous factors, including the type of treatment, patient factors, and factors related to medical professionals. A prominent feature of this concept is that adherence is understood in terms of the mutual relationship between patients and medical professionals.

In the treatment of cardiovascular diseases, factors that affect adherence can be broadly divided into those concerning patients themselves and those concerning their relationships with other people [5]. Factors concerning patients themselves include the state of their disease, health risks (smoking, obesity, lack of exercise, blood lipids, diabetes, etc.), outlook on health and view of cardiovascular disease, the health education they have received, what targets have been set, motivation, desire for change, and belief in their own ability to achieve results [9]. Factors concerning their relationships with other people include patients' social backgrounds, whether or not they have a support framework and their relationships with medical professionals [10] [11]. These factors interact with each other to regulate patients' adherence.

Within the conceptual structure determining medication adherence by hypertensive patients in our study, "Expectation of pharmacological efficacy" and "Motivation to be self-controlled in taking medication" improve adherence, whereas "Negative feelings about taking medication" reduce it.

The state of taking medicine by hypertensive patients is also affected by adherence. In addition to generally identified factors, the method of administration of medication also contributes to adherence of hypertensive pa-

Table 6. Sample *t-test* results from comparing variables according to forget medication.

Total score	Normal (n = 290)		High (n = 700)		Significance
	Average	SD	Average	SD	
Factor 1	18.1	4.6	19.8	4.6	0.000
Factor 2	23.6	3.5	22.8	3.6	0.003
Factor 3	10.8	2.9	10.2	2.7	0.009
All	52.5	5.8	52.8	6.1	0.509

tients. Compound formulations, which combine several active ingredients in a single tablet, have been reported to have an increased rate of use compared with multidrug therapy in which several medications are taken at the same time [6]. Reducing the number of medications taken at once [12], the number of medications taken per day, and the number of doses per day has also been shown to be effective in improving adherence [7], suggesting that simpler methods of taking medication result in higher adherence. It has also been pointed out that providing sufficient information increases adherence and improves medication-taking behavior, resulting in improved blood pressure control [13]. We found that the expectation of pharmacological efficacy is an expression of the desire to keep blood pressure under good control, while the motivation to be self-controlled on the basis of an understanding of the medication involved overrides negative feelings about taking medication to improve adherence.

From previous studies, factors affecting adherence have been shown to include patient's socioeconomic status [14], patient knowledge, method of administration, anxiety about side effects, and the medical professional-patient relationship [6] [7] [9]-[12] [15]. In addition to practical patient intervention strategies, it will be necessary to obtain evidence on the outcomes of interventions in Japan. Scales for evaluating adherence by hypertensive patients have been developed overseas, including Self-reported Medication-taking Scaleby Morisky [16] from the 1980s and the 8-Item Medication Adherence Measure [17]. However, few studies using these scales have been carried out in Japan, and the reliability and validity of the Japanese versions have yet to be adequately verified.

The Japanese Medication Adherence Measure version 2 is the first adherence scale that demonstrates its reliability and validity. Reliability was investigated in terms of internal consistency and the retest method. Discriminated validity was investigated by dividing patients into groups with blood pressure and number of times they forgot to take their medication as independent variables, and using the t-test to investigate the differences between the groups with subscale scores as dependent variables. The Japanese Medication Adherence Measure version 2 proved to be a reliable, simple and valid method for assessing patients' medication-taking behavior in clinical practice. It will be a valuable tool for predicting therapeutic efficacy.

5. Conclusion

A 32-Item Japanese Medication Adherence Scale has been developed and evaluated. Identified factor contains 19 items, factor 1, "Expectation of pharmacological efficacy", factor 2, "Motivation to be self-controlled in taking medication", and factor 3, "Negative feelings about taking medication". The measure was highly reliable, and because it proved capable of discriminating between 2 groups with different medication-taking status and blood pressure, its validity has also been confirmed. This would enable the widespread assessment of medication-taking behavior in clinical practice in Japan and provide a valuable tool for predicting therapeutic efficacy. Adjustments between measure items, and differences between men and women and different age groups, are topics for further study.

Acknowledgements

This work was supported by the Grant in aid for Scientific Research (C) from the Japan Society for the Promotion of Science (grant numbers 22592451) and Grant-in-Aid for Research in Nagoya City University. The authors wish to thank sincerely all the patients who participated in this study.

Conflict of Interest

The authors have no financial conflicts of interest to disclose concerning the research.

References

[1]   The Japanese Society of Hypertension (2014) The Japanese Society of Hypertension Guidelines for the Management of Hypertension (JSH2014). Tokyo.

[2]   World Health Organization (2013) WHO: A Global Brief On Hypertension: Silent Killer, Global Public Health Crisis. http://www.who.int/features/2013/japan_blood_pressure/en/index.html#

[3]   The Ministry of Health (2006) Labor and Welfare: The National Medical Expenditures in the Heisei 16 Fiscal Year. http://www.mhlw.go.jp/toukei/saikin/hw/k-iryohi/04/kekka6.html

[4]   Mendis, S. and Salas, M. (2013) Hypertension, in World Health Organization, Adherence to Long-Term Therapies: Evidence for Action, 107-114. Geneva. http://www.who.int/chp/knowledge/publications/adherence_full_report.pdf

[5]   Cohen, S.M. (2009) Concept Analysis of Adherence in the Context of Cardiovascular Risk Reduction. *Nursing Forum*, **44**, 25-36. http://dx.doi.org/10.1111/j.1744-6198.2009.00124.x

[6]   Bangalore, S., Kamalakkannan, G., Parkar, S. and Messerli, F.H. (2007) Fixed-Dose Combinations Improve Medication Compliance: A Meta-Analysis. *American Journal of Medicine*, **120**, 713-719. http://dx.doi.org/10.1016/j.amjmed.2006.08.033

[7]   Schroeder, K., Fahey, T. and Ebrahim, S. (2004) How Can We Improve Adherence to Blood Pressure-Lowering Medication in Ambulatory Care? Systematic Review of Randomized Controlled Trials. *Archives of Internal Medicine*, **164**, 722-732. http://dx.doi.org/10.1001/archinte.164.7.722

[8]   Collins, U.K. (1999) Collins Concise Dictionary. 4th Edition, HarperCollins Publishers, Glasgow, 16.

[9]   Rajpura, J. and Nayak, R. (2014) Medication Adherence in a Sample of Elderly Suffering from Hypertension: Evaluating the Influence of Illness Perceptions, Treatment Beliefs, and Illness Burden. *Journal of Managed Care Pharmacy*, **19**, 58-65.

[10] Abel, W.M. and Efird, J.T. (2013) The Association between Trust in Health Care Providers and Medication Adherence among Black Women with Hypertension. *Front Public Health*, **1**, 66.

[11] Harmon, G., Lefante, J. and Krousel-Wood, M. (2006) Overcoming Barriers: The Role of Providers in Improving Patient Adherence to Antihypertensive Medications. *Current Opinion in Cardiology*, **21**, 310-315. http://dx.doi.org/10.1097/01.hco.0000231400.10104.e2

[12] Gerbino, P.P. and Shoheiber, O. (2007) Adherence Patterns among Patients Treated with Fixed-Dose Combination versus Separate Antihypertensive Agents. *American Journal of Health-System Pharmacy*, **64**, 1279-1283. http://dx.doi.org/10.2146/ajhp060434

[13] Lee, J.K., Grace, K.A. and Taylor, A.J. (2006) Effect of a Pharmacy Care Program on Medication Adherence and Persistence, Blood Pressure, and Low-Density Lipoprotein Cholesterol: A Randomized Controlled Trial. *The Journal of the American Medical Association*, **296**, 2563-2571. http://dx.doi.org/10.1001/jama.296.21.joc60162

[14] Wee, L.E. and Koh, G.C. (2012) Individual and Neighborhood Social Factors of Hypertension Management in a Low-Socioeconomic Status Population: A Community-Based Case-Control Study in Singapore. *Hypertension Research*, **35**, 295-303. http://dx.doi.org/10.1038/hr.2011.187

[15] Working Group on the Summit on Combination Therapy for CVD (2014) Combination Pharmacotherapy to Prevent Cardiovascular Disease: Present Status and Challenges. *European Heart Journal*, **35**, 353-364. http://dx.doi.org/10.1093/eurheartj/eht407

[16] Morisky, D.E., Green, L.W. and Levine, D.M. (1986) Concurrent and Predictive Validity of a Self-Reported Measure of Medication Adherence. *Medical Care*, **24**, 67-74. http://dx.doi.org/10.1097/00005650-198601000-00007

[17] Morisky, D.E., Ang, A., Krousel-Wood, M. and Ward, H.J. (2008) Predictive Validity of a Medication Adherence Measure in an Outpatient Setting. *Journal of Clinical Hypertension*, **10**, 348-354. http://dx.doi.org/10.1111/j.1751-7176.2008.07572.x

8

Overcoming the Bell-Shaped Dose-Response of Cannabidiol by Using *Cannabis* Extract Enriched in Cannabidiol

Ruth Gallily[1], Zhannah Yekhtin[1], Lumír Ondřej Hanuš[2]

[1]The Lautenberg Center for General and Tumor Immunology, The Hadassah Medical School, The Hebrew University of Jerusalem, Jerusalem, Israel
[2]Department of Medicinal and Natural Products, Institute for Drug Research, The Hadassah Medical School, The Hebrew University of Jerusalem, Jerusalem, Israel
Email: ruthg@ekmd.huji.ac.il

Abstract

Cannabidiol (CBD), a major constituent of *Cannabis*, has been shown to be a powerful anti-inflammatory and anti-anxiety drug, without exerting a psychotropic effect. However, when given either intraperitoneally or orally as a purified product, a bell-shaped dose-response was observed, which limits its clinical use. In the present study, we have studied in mice the anti-inflammatory and anti-nociceptive activities of standardized plant extracts derived from the *Cannabis sativa* L., clone 202, which is highly enriched in CBD and hardly contains any psychoactive ingredients. In stark contrast to purified CBD, the clone 202 extract, when given either intraperitoneally or orally, provided a clear correlation between the anti-inflammatory and anti-nociceptive responses and the dose, with increasing responses upon increasing doses, which makes this plant medicine ideal for clinical uses. The clone 202 extract reduced zymosan-induced paw swelling and pain in mice, and prevented TNFα production *in vivo*. It is likely that other components in the extract synergize with CBD to achieve the desired anti-inflammatory action that may contribute to overcoming the bell-shaped dose-response of purified CBD. We therefore propose that *Cannabis* clone 202 (Avidekel) extract is superior over CBD for the treatment of inflammatory conditions.

Keywords

Cannabis sativa L. Clone 202, Cannabidiol, Anti-Inflammation, Anti-Nociceptive, TNFα

1. Introduction

Inflammation and pain have accompanied human life for ages. Many anti-inflammation and anti-pain medications and various approaches have been employed through the centuries and in recent time. Many of used drugs, however, impose severe side effects. *Cannabis* from various origins and species has been employed in various forms as anti-pain agents for thousands of years [1]-[3]. One example is the legitimated drug Sativex® (Nabiximols) that is used in the treatment of severe spasticity in patients with multiple sclerosis [4]. Two other drugs, Marinol (Dronabinol) and Cesamet, have been approved for use in cancer-related anorexia-cachexia syndrome as well as for nausea and vomiting [3]. But a major disadvantage of *Cannabis* phytomedicine is its psychoactive effects due to the presence of Δ^9-Tetrahydrocannabinol (THC).

Recently, a science-based approach is being conducted to specify the benefits of *Cannabis* and its many constituents. A *Cannabis* plant contains hundreds of different chemicals with about 60 - 80 chemicals known as cannabinoids [5]. The major *Cannabis* psychoactive molecule is the Δ^9-tetrahydrocannabinol, known as THC, which binds with high affinity (K_i = 3 - 5 nM) [6] to both the cannabinoid CB1 receptor expressed in the brain and the CB2 receptor expressed on cells of the immune system [7]. Another major constituent is Cannabidiol (CBD) which is devoid of psychotropic effects and binds only with very low affinity (K_i > 10 μM) [6] to the CB1/CB2 receptors. The other cannabinoids are present in minute amounts. Stimulation of CB1 receptor is responsible for the *Cannabis* psychoactivity, while activation of the CB2 receptor leads to attenuated inflammation, decreased injury and accelerated regeneration in many disease states [7]. CBD has been shown to activate central nervous system's limbic and paralimbic regions, which can reduce autonomic arousal and feeling of anxiety [3]. This is in contrast to THC which can be anxiogenic [3]. CBD has also been shown to have anti-emetic, anti-inflammatory and anti-psychotic effects [3]. Studies are looking for potential benefits of phytocannabinoids in management of neuropathic pain, hypertension, post-stroke neuroprotection, multiple sclerosis, epilepsy and cancer [3]. Doses up to 1500 mg per day as well as chronic use of CBD have been reported as being well tolerated by humans [3].

During the last 10 - 15 years, many studies have focused on the anti-inflammatory effects of purified CBD in various animal models, including rheumatoid arthritis, diabetes type 1, inflammatory bowel disease and multiple sclerosis [8]-[13]. These studies showed that purified CBD gives a bell-shaped dose-response curve. Healing was only observed when CBD was given within a very limited dose range, whereas no beneficial effect was achieved at either lower or higher doses. This trait of purified CBD imposes serious obstacles in planning human and animal studies. The aim of the present study was to find a CBD source that could eliminate the bell-shaped dose-response of purified CBD. We found that by using standardized plant extracts from the *Cannabis* clone 202 obtained from Tikun Olam, Israel, which is highly enriched in CBD and barely contains THC, a correlative anti-inflammatory and anti-pain dose-response could be achieved when applied either intraperitoneally or orally in an inflammatory mouse model.

2. Material and Methods

2.1. CBD and *Cannabis* Clone 202 (Avidekel) Extract

Purified CBD was purchased from THC Pharm. GmbH, Frankfurt, Germany. *Cannabis sativa* L. flowers from the clone 202 (Avidekel) rich in CBD while low in any psychotropic constituents was supplied by Tikun Olam Company (a government-approved farm growing medicinal *Cannabis*), Israel. CBD-enriched extract was prepared from the flowers of *Cannabis* clone 202 grown under controlled temperature and light conditions. 100% ethanol (20 ml) was added to the chopped *Cannabis* dry flowers (200 mg) for 24 - 48 hrs, with occasional shaking at room temperature. Following filtration, samples were taken for analysis. Ethanol solutions of *Cannabis* clone 202 extracts (10 mg/ml - 20 mg/ml) were kept at −20°C in the dark. The extract was evaporated on Rotavapor (BÜCHI Labortechnik AG, Switzerland). For intraperitoneal injection, the dried *Cannabis* clone 202 extract was emulsified in a vehicle composed of ethanol:Cremophor:saline at a 1:1:18 ratio. Purified CBD was emulsified in the same vehicle. For oral administration, the dried *Cannabis* clone 202 extract and the purified CBD were dissolved in olive oil.

2.2. Analysis of the *Cannabis* Clone 202 Extract by Thin-Layer Chromatography (TLC)

Cannabis clone 202 extract (1 μl) was separated on TLC Silica Gel 60 F254 aluminium sheets (Merck, Darmstadt, Germany) using hexane:dioxane (4:1) as a solvent in a chamber of $13 \times 9 \times 12$ cm. The separated components were detected by spraying the plates with a freshly prepared solution of 0.5 g Fast Blue B (D9805, Sigma) in acetone/water (9:1; v/v). Cannabinoids in the dried plant material predominately appeared as cannabinoid acids. The TLC analysis shows two major spots corresponding to the acid and neutral form of CBD, respectively, with only a minor spot corresponding to the acid form of THC (**Figure 1(a)**).

2.3. Analysis of the *Cannabis* Clone 202 Extract by Gas Chromatography and Mass Spectrophotometry (GC/MS)

For analysis of the composition of the ethanol extracts of medicinal *Cannabis* clone 202, the ethanol was evaporated and the resin dissolved in 20 ml of methanol and filtered through cotton in a capillary. The concentration of the extract was adjusted to 1 mg/ml to which 50 μg internal standard (Tetracosane, Acros Organics, USA) was added. One μl of this sample was applied for the GC/MS analysis. The quantitative analysis of the samples by GC/MS was performed in a Hewlett Packard G 1800B GCD system with a HP-5971 gas chromatograph with electron ionization detector. The software used was GCD Plus ChemStation. The column used was SPB-5 (30 m $\times$ 0.25 mm $\times$ 0.25 μm film thickness). Experimental conditions were: inlet, 250°C; detector, 280°C; splitless injection/purge time, 1.0 min; initial temperature, 100°C; initial time, 2.0 min; rate, 10°C/min; final temperature, 280°C. The helium flow rate was 1 ml/min. Calibration curve was made from 25.0 to 100 μg/ml Cannabidiol (CBD), Δ^9-Tetetrahydrocannabinol (THC) or Cannabinol (CBN) together with 50.0 μg/ml tetracosane as internal standard. The cannabinoid composition of *Cannabis* clone 202 extract is presented in **Figure 1(b)**, **Figure 1(c)** and **Table 1**.

2.4. Commercial Anti-Nociceptive and Anti-Inflammatory Drugs

The non-steroid anti-inflammatory drug (NSAID) aspirin (acetylsalicylic acid) was purchased from Sigma and dissolved in olive oil. Fifty mg of aspirin was given per os per kg in a volume of 40 μl. The opioid anti-nociceptive Tramadol hydrochloride was obtained from Grunenthal and dissolved in saline. Five mg of Tramadol was given per os per kg.

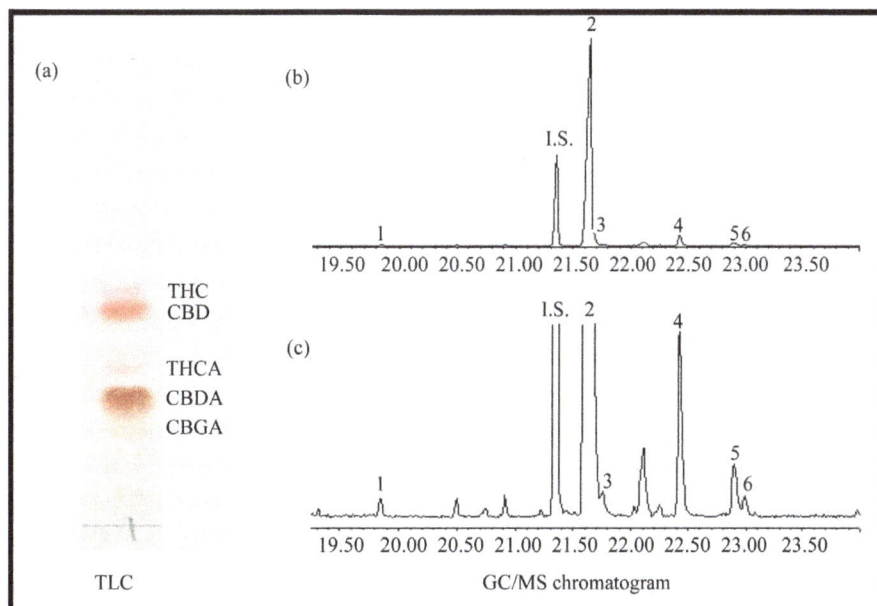

Figure 1. (a) TLC analysis of clone 202 extract. 1 μl of the extract was run on TLC as described in the Method section. CBD = Cannabidiol. CBDA = Cannabidiolic acid; (b) (c) GC/MS chromatograms of an extract from *Cannabis* clone 202. (b) The full chromatogram. (c) Magnification of weaker signals. Number keys: 1: Cannabidivarol (CBDV); 2: Cannabidiol (CBD); 3: Cannabichromene (CBC); 4: Δ^9-Tetrahydrocannabinol (Δ^9-THC); 5: Cannabigerol (CBG); 6: Cannabinol (CBN); I.S.-Internal Standard (Tetracosane).

Table 1. The percentage of main phytocannabinoids found in clone 202 extract according to GC/MS analysis (see **Figures 1(b)-(c)**).

Phytocannabinoid	Content
Cannabidiol (CBD)	17.9%
Δ^9-Tetrahydrocannabinol (Δ^9-THC)	1.1%
Cannabichromene (CBC)	1.1%
Cannabigerol (CBG)	0.2%
Cannabinol (CBN)	Traces
Cannabidivarol (CBDV)	Traces

As cannabinoid acids during injection to the GC/MS decarboxylate, the results are a total sum of neutral cannabinoids and cannabinoid acids that have decarboxylated into neutral cannabinoids. The content is the mass fraction (% w/w) of the given constituent in the extract.

2.5. Animals

Six to eight week old female Sabra mice (Israel) were maintained in the SPF unit of the Hebrew University-Hadassah Medical School, Jerusalem, Israel. The experimental protocols were approved by the Animal Care Ethical Committee of the Hebrew University-Hadassah Medical School, Jerusalem, Israel. The animals were maintained on standard pellet diet and water ad libitum. The animals were maintained at a constant temperature (20°C - 21°C) and a 12 h light/dark cycle.

2.6. Induction of Paw Inflammation in Mice and Treatment with Purified CBD or Clone 202 Extract

To induce inflammation, 40 µl of 1.5% (w/v) zymosan A (Sigma) suspended in 0.9% saline was injected into the sub-planter surface of the right hind paw of the mice. Immediately after zymosan injection, CBD or *Cannabis* clone 202 extract was injected intraperitoneally (i.p.) or given orally. For intraperitoneal injection, these agents were dissolved in 0.1 ml vehicle containing ethanol:Cremophore:saline at a ratio of 1:1:18. Control mice were injected with the vehicle only. For per os administration, the agents were dissolved in olive oil, each mouse receiving 40 µl. Control mice got 40 µl olive oil. After 2, 6 and 24 hrs, paw swelling and pain perception were measured. Serum TNFα titers were determined after 24 hrs. The effects of CBD and *Cannabis* clone 202 extract were compared to those of aspirin (50 mg/kg per os) and tramadol (5 mg/kg, i.p.).

2.7. Measurement of Oedema Formation

The paw swelling (thickness) was measured by calibrated calipers (0.01 mm), 2, 6 and 24 hrs following injections of zymosan alone or with CBD or *Cannabis* clone 202 extracts.

2.8. Pain Assay

The hyperalgesia was evaluated by the paw withdrawal von Frey test at 2, 6, and 24 hrs following injections of zymosan and/or the test compounds. In the von Frey nociceptive filament assay, von Frey calibrated monofilament hairs of logarithmically incremental stiffness (0.008 - 300 g corresponding to 1.65 - 6.65 log of force). In our study, only 1.4 - 60 g corresponding to 4.17 to 5.88 log of force was used, to test the mouse sensitivity to a mechanical stimulus on the swollen paw. The measurements were performed in a quiet room. Before paw pain measurements, the animals were held for 10 sec. The trained investigator applied the filament to the central area of the hind paw with gradual increasing size. The test consisted of poking the middle of the hind paw to provoke a flexion reflex followed by a clear flinch response after paw withdrawal. Each one of the von Frey filaments was applied for approximately 3 - 4 s to induce the end-point reflex. The first testing was done by using the force filament of 1.4 g. If there was no withdrawal response, the next higher stimulus was tried. The mechanical threshold force (in grams (g)) was defined as the lowest force imposed by two von Frey monofilaments of various sizes, required to produce a paw retraction. The untreated left hind paw served as a control.

2.9. Tumor Necrosis Factor α (TNFα) Plasma Levels

Plasma levels of TNFα were measured using a mouse TNFα ELISA kit (R&D System), according to the manufacturer's instructions.

2.10. Statistical Analysis

The results are presented as average ± standard error. Mice treated with CBD or *Cannabis* clone 202 extracts were compared with control mice receiving the vehicle only. Statistical significance was calculated using the ANOVA analysis of variance and Wilcoxon signed-rank test. Differences between the various doses of CBD and clone 202 extracts were analyzed for significance using the repeated measures ANOVA procedure with Post-Hoc test. All tests were 2-tailed and a p-value below 0.05 was considered statistically significant. A minimum of three to four animals was used in each treatment group for each experiment unless otherwise stated. Each experiment was performed at least three times. The graphs represent the average of all mice from the three different experiments. Thus, each bar corresponds to the average of 10 - 12 mice for each treatment group, for each time point, unless otherwise stated.

3. Results

3.1. Effect of CBD and CBD-Enriched Clone 202 Extract on Inflammation and Hyperalgesia (Pain Sensation)

In this study we have used the well-accepted mouse model of zymosan-induced inflammation [14] to investigate the anti-inflammatory and anti-nociceptive activities of *Cannabis* clone 202 extract versus purified CBD. The extent of hind paw swelling was determined 2, 6 and 24 hrs following paw injection of 60 µg zymosan together with either intraperitoneal injection or per os administration of various amounts of either purified CBD or *Cannabis* clone 202 extract, as indicated in the graphs (**Figure 2**, **Figure 3**). Following intraperitoneal injection of 1, 5, 25 and 50 mg/kg of purified CBD, a bell-shaped dose-response is observed (**Figure 2(a)**). The maximum inhibition of inflammation occurred after an injection of 5 mg/kg CBD with 50% and 57% inhibition after 6 and 24 hrs, respectively (p < 0.001), while a lower dose (1 mg/kg) being ineffective and higher doses (25 and 50 mg/kg) being less effective with 20% - 25% and 14% - 28% inhibition only, after 6 and 24 hrs, respectively (**Figure 2(a)**). In accordance with these findings, the anti-nociceptive effect, as determined by the von Frey monofilament assay, peaked at 5 mg/kg CBD (p < 0.001) (**Figure 2(c)**). The anti-nociceptive effect occurred prior (2 hrs) to inhibition of swelling (6 hrs), and peaked at 6 hrs. Higher concentrations of CBD had less anti-nociceptive effects (**Figure 2(c)**), again getting a bell-shaped dose-response. However, when clone 202 extract was used, a correlative dose-response was observed with increased inhibition of inflammation upon increased doses of the extract, reaching 43% and 64% inhibition at 25 mg and 50 mg, respectively, after 24 hrs (p < 0.001) (**Figure 2(b)**). These two dosages of clone 202 extract also showed strong anti-nociceptive effects after 6 and 24 hrs (p < 0.001) (**Figure 2(d)**). Although the anti-inflammatory effect of clone 202 extract was higher at 50 mg/kg than at 25 mg/kg with a p = 0.001, the anti-nociceptive effect was only slightly higher (p = 0.01), suggesting that a plateau has been reached. The clone 202 extract was more efficient for alleviating the pain than CBD (p = 0.01) (**Figure 2(d)** versus **Figure 2(c)**).

When CBD or *Cannabis* clone 202 extract was given orally, a similar response was observed. Namely, CBD gives a bell-shaped dose-response with an optimal inhibitory effect at 25 mg/kg (p < 0.001) (**Figure 3(a)** and **Figure 3(c)**), whereas *Cannabis* clone 202 extract provides a correlative dose-response curve with a maximum effect on swelling and pain relief at 50 and 150 mg/kg, respectively (p < 0.001) (**Figure 3(b)** and **Figure 3(d)**). Significant pain relief was already obtained with an oral clone 202 extract dose of 50 mg/kg (**Figure 3(d)**) that corresponds to about 10 mg/kg CBD (**Table 1**), while 25 mg/kg of purified CBD was needed to achieve the same effect (**Figure 3(c)**). This suggests for a better usage of clone 202 extract.

It should be noted that agents taken per os need to go through the enterohepatic route prior to exerting their effects, where the absorption rate and first-pass liver metabolism affect the blood drug level [15]. This may explain the higher doses required and the delayed response in comparison with the parenteral route, where the agents are immediately available for the blood circulation. The anti-inflammatory and anti-nociceptive effects peak at 6 hrs, which accords with the pharmacokinetics and pharmacodynamics of cannabinoids described by Grotenhermen [15].

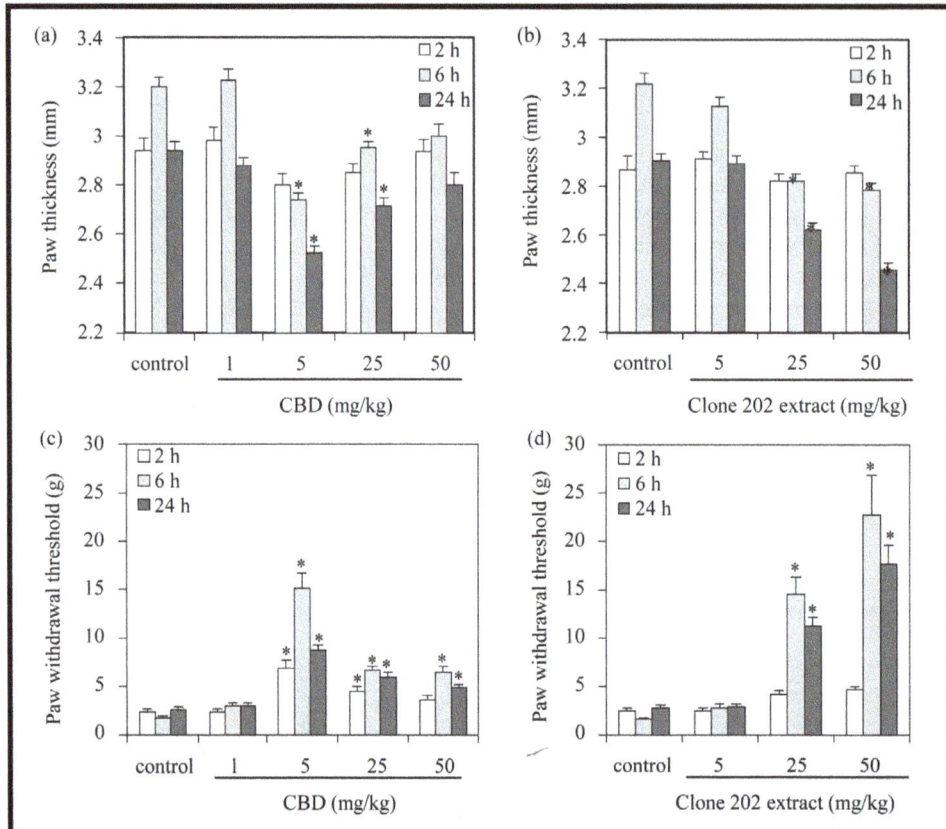

Figure 2. Anti-inflammatory and anti-nociceptive effects of intraperitoneally injected CBD and CBD-enriched clone 202 extract. (a) (b) Prevention of zymosan-induced swelling of hind paw. 1.5% zymosan in 40 μl was injected into the sub-planter surface of the right hind paw. Immediately thereafter, CBD (a) or *Cannabis* clone 202 extract (b) was injected intraperitoneally. The paw thickness indicative for paw swelling was measured 2, 6 and 24 hrs thereafter. The paw thickness of untreated mice was 2.0 - 2.2 mm, which made the baseline of the graph. N = 12 for each time point. $^*p < 0.001$ compared to control mice. $p < 0.001$ for 50 mg/kg vs 25 mg/kg of clone 202 extract at 24 hrs; (c) (d) Anti-pain effect of CBD (c) and *Cannabis* clone 202 extract (d). The hyperalgesia was measured by using the von Frey nociceptive filament assay. The higher the paw withdrawal threshold, the higher is the anti-nociceptive effect of the drug. The experiments were repeated three times, each experiment with 4 mice in each treatment group. The graphs presents the average of all mice in the three experiments, meaning that the N = 12 for each time point. The bars represent standard error. $^*p < 0.001$ compared to control mice. $p < 0.01$ for 50 mg/kg vs 25 mg/kg of clone 202 extract at 24 hrs. $p < 0.01$ for clone 202 extract vs CBD.

3.2. Suppression of TNFα Production by CBD and Clone 202 Extract

TNFα is a well-known pro-inflammatory cytokine secreted by activated macrophages upon inflammation that has been shown to be involved in initiation and amplification of inflammatory processes that ultimately leads to oedema [16]. Therefore, it was important to analyze the effect of CBD and clone 202 extracts on TNFα production. To this end, mice sera were analyzed for TNFα concentration by ELISA 24 hrs after treatment with zymosan in the absence or presence of CBD or clone 202 extract. When comparing the TNFα sera level in mice 24 hrs after injection of increasing doses of purified CBD, a bell-shaped dose-response curve of TNFα production was observed, with a maximum inhibitory effect (43%) achieved at 5 mg/kg (p < 0.001), while no inhibition was observed at either lower (1 mg/kg) or higher (25 and 50 mg/kg) doses (**Figure 4(a)**). In contrast, following injection of CBD-enriched clone 202 extract to mice, a clear dose dependent response was apparent. Increased inhibition of TNFα production (39%; 46% and 57%, respectively) was observed following injections with increasing amounts of extract (5 mg/kg, 25 mg/kg and 50 mg/ml, respectively) with a p value less than 0.001 (**Figure 4(b)**). Already at 5 mg/kg did clone 202 extract lead to a strong reduction in TNFα production (**Figure 4(b)**),

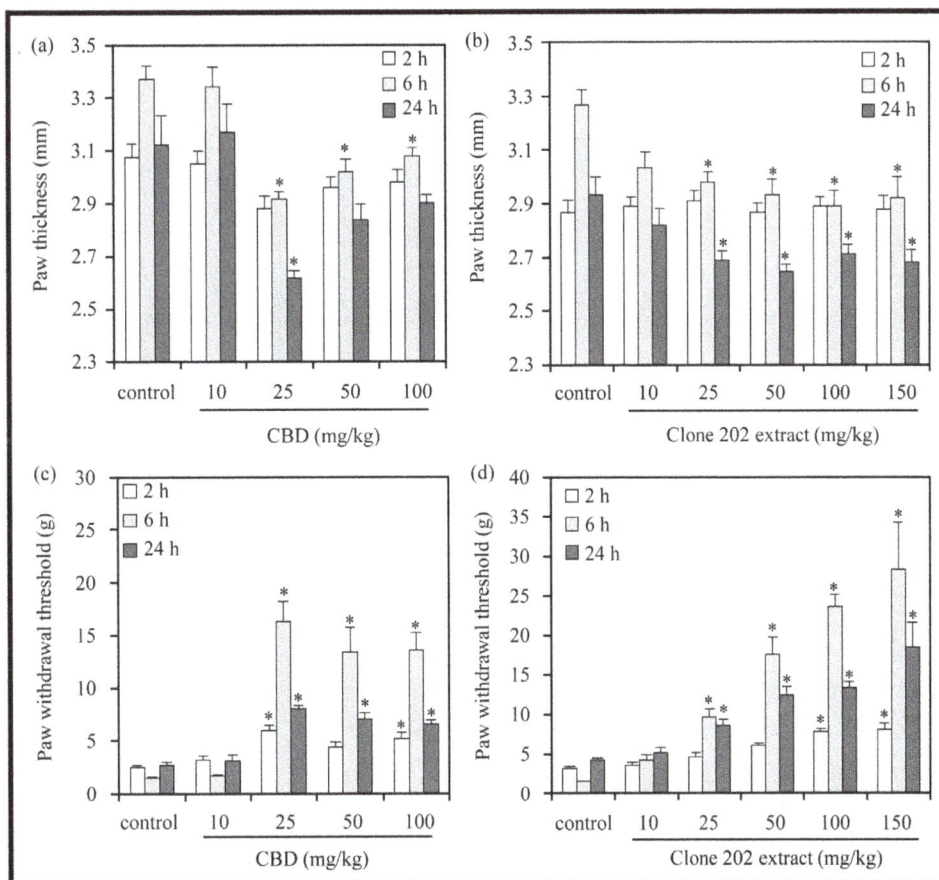

Figure 3. Anti-inflammatory and anti-nociceptive effects of CBD and CBD-enriched clone 202 extract administrated per os. (a) (b) Prevention of zymosan-induced swelling of hind paw. 1.5% zymosan in 40 μl was injected into the sub-planter surface of the right hind paw. Immediately thereafter, CBD (a) or *Cannabis* clone 202 extract (b) was given per os dissolved in olive oil (40 μl). The paw thickness indicative for paw swelling was measured 2, 6 and 24 hrs thereafter. The paw thickness of untreated mice was 2.0 - 2.2 mm, which made the baseline of the graph. N = 12 for each time point. *p < 0.001 in comparison to control mice. The anti-inflammatory effects of 25, 50, 100 and 150 mg/kg of clone 202 extract were similar; (c) (d) Anti-pain effect of CBD (c) and *Cannabis* clone 202 extract (d) when given orally. The hyperalgesia was measured by using the von Frey nociceptive filament assay. The higher the paw withdrawal threshold, the higher is the anti-nociceptive effect of the drug. The experiments were repeated three times, each experiment with 4 mice in each treatment group. The graphs presents the average of all mice in the three experiments, meaning that the N = 12 for each time point. The bars represent standard error. *p < 0.001 in comparison to control mice. p < 0.001 for 50 mg/kg clone 202 extract (containing 8.9 mg/kg CBD) vs 10 mg/kg purified CBD. p < 0.05 of 100 mg/kg and 150 mg/kg vs 50 mg/kg of clone 202 extract at 6 hrs, indicating a dose-dependent effect.

even though this dose was insufficient in reducing paw swelling (**Figure 2(b)**) or relieve pain (**Figure 2(d)**). At least 25 mg/kg extract, which corresponds to about 5 mg CBD, was required to achieve the anti-inflammatory effect. These data show that TNFα secretion is more sensitive to inhibition by clone 202 extract, than paw swelling and pain.

Similar to the results obtained with intraperitoneal injection, orally administrated CBD gave a bell-shape response, with an optimal response using 25 mg/kg (p < 0.001), while higher or lower doses had less effect (**Figure 4(c)**). In contrast, orally delivered clone 202 extract showed an increased inhibitory effect on TNFα production with increased doses (**Figure 4(d)**). Already at 25 mg/kg an inhibition of 48% was achieved that increased further to 66% when given 150 mg/kg clone 202 extract (**Figure 4(d)**). The inhibition of TNFα production was much stronger than the inhibitory effect on paw swelling of 27% - 35%.

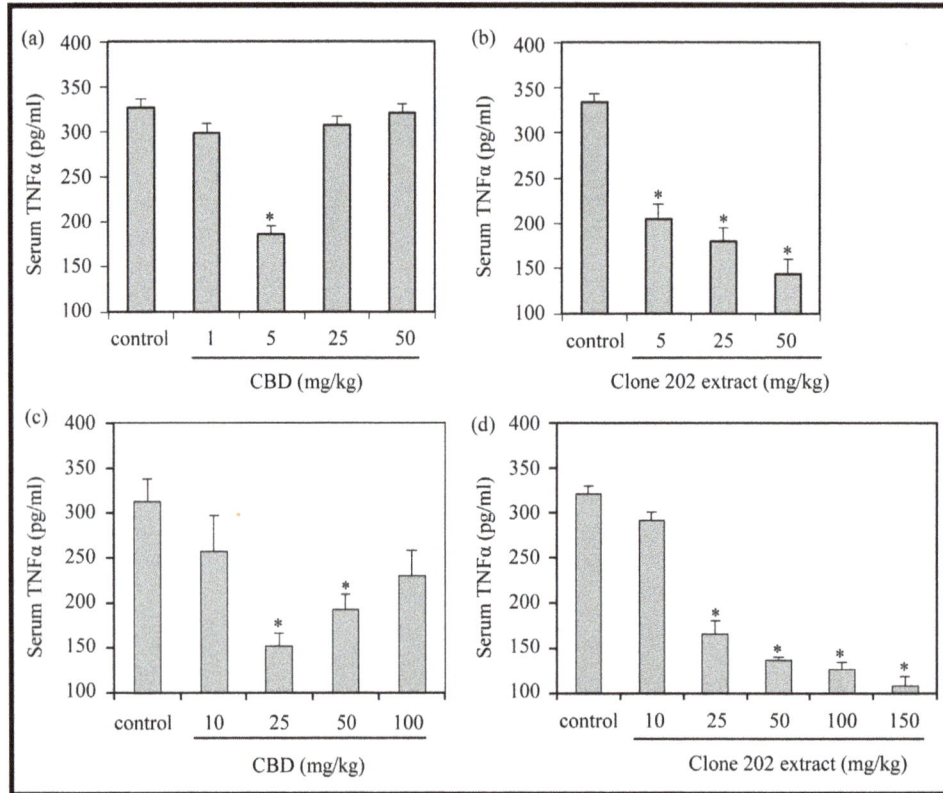

Figure 4. Prevention of zymosan-induced TNFα production by purified CBD and clone 202 extract. (a) (b) Twenty four hours after injecting zymosan and an intraperitoneal dose of CBD (a) or clone 202 extract (b), or a per os dose of CBD (c) or clone 202 extract (d), the TNFα concentration in the serum was determined by ELISA. The experiments were repeated three times, each experiment with 4 mice in each treatment group. The graphs presents the average of all mice in the three experiments, meaning an N = 12 for each treatment. TNFα serum level of untreated mice was 15 pg/ml. The bars represent standard error. *p < 0.001 in comparison to control mice. p < 0.01 when comparing clone 202 extract with purified CBD. p < 0.01 when comparing an increasing doses of clone 202 extract, emphasizing a dose-dependent effect.

3.3. Comparison of CBD and *Cannabis* Clone 202 Extract with Commercial Anti-Nociceptive and Anti-Inflammatory Drugs

Since *Cannabis* clone 202 extract has profound anti-inflammatory and anti-nociceptive effects as described above, it was important to compare its potency with commercial anti-nociceptive and anti-inflammatory drugs. We chose to use tramadol, a strong atypical opioid analgesic drug, and aspirin, a well-known non-steroid anti-inflammatory drug (NSAID) that is also a pain reliever. Immediately after zymosan injection, mice were treated with aspirin (50 mg/kg per os), tramadol (5 mg/kg i.p.), CBD (5 mg/kg i.p.) or clone 202 extract (50 mg/kg i.p.). While aspirin had a moderate effect on paw swelling (p < 0.001 at 6 h), tramadol barely had any effect (**Figure 5(a)**). Both CBD and clone 202 extract markedly prevented paw swelling to a much larger extent than aspirin (p < 0.005) (**Figure 5(a)**). As expected, aspirin and tramadol had a strong anti-nociceptive effect that exceeded that of CBD and clone 202 extract (p < 0.01) (**Figure 5(b)**). Aspirin, but not tramadol, showed a slight inhibitory effect on TNFα production, that was negligible in comparison to the strong inhibitory effect of CBD and clone 202 extract (p < 0.01) (**Figure 5(c)**). Thus, CBD and clone 202 extract are endowed with different traits than aspirin and tramadol, making them superior with respect to anti-inflammatory properties.

4. Discussion

In this manuscript we have observed different dose-response patterns when using purified CBD or plant extract

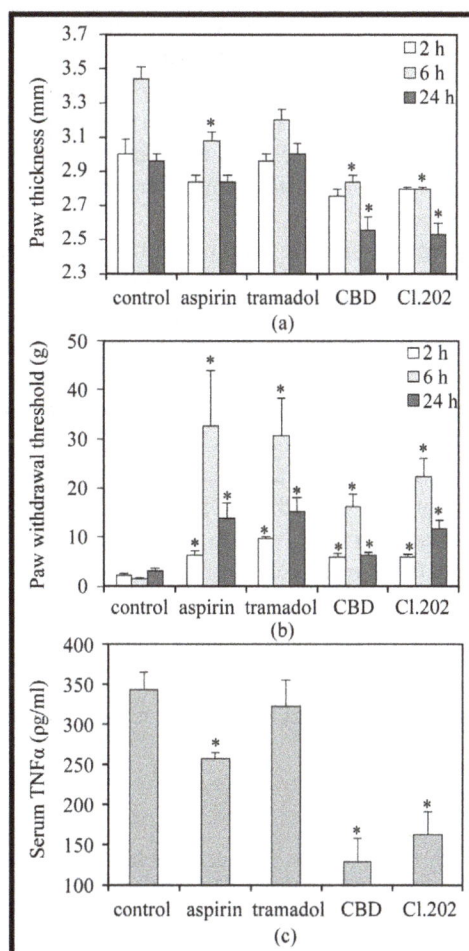

Figure 5. Comparison of anti-inflammatory and anti-nociceptive effects of CBD and *Cannabis* clone 202 extract with the commercial drugs aspirin and tramadol. (a) Prevention of zymosan-induced swelling of hind paw. 1.5% zymosan in 40 μl was injected into the sub-planter surface of the right hind paw. Immediately thereafter, aspirin (50 mg/kg per os), tramadol (5 mg/kg i.p.), CBD (5 mg/kg i.p.) or *Cannabis* clone 202 extract (50 mg/kg i.p.) was given. The paw thickness indicative for paw swelling was measured 2, 6 and 24 hrs later. The paw thickness of untreated mice was 2.0 - 2.2 mm, which made the baseline of the graph. N = 5 for each time point of each treatment group. $^*p < 0.001$ in comparison to control mice. $p < 0.005$ when comparing CBD and clone 202 extract with aspirin and tramadol; (b) Anti-pain effect of aspirin, tramadol, CBD and *Cannabis* clone 202 extract in mice treated as described in paragraph A. The hyperalgesia was measured by using the von Frey nociceptive filament assay. The higher the paw withdrawal threshold, the higher is the anti-nociceptive effect of the drug. N = 5 for each time point of each treatment group. The bars represent standard error. $^*p < 0.001$ in comparison to control mice. $p < 0.05$ when comparing CBD and clone 202 extract with aspirin and tramadol; (c) The TNFα serum concentration at 24 hrs in mice that were treated as described in paragraph A. N = 5 for each treatment. The bars represent standard error. $^*p < 0.001$ in comparison to control mice. $p < 0.01$ when comparing CBD and clone 202 extract with aspirin and tramadol.

of the *Cannabis sativa* L. clone 202, which is highly enriched in CBD. Purified CBD showed a bell-shaped dose-response, where a therapeutic response could only be achieved at a certain concentration. This narrow therapeutic window makes it difficult to use CBD in the clinics as a single agent. Therefore, we sought for a better preparation that can utilize the favorable therapeutic effects of CBD. We observed that plant extracts of the non-psychotropic clone 202 could fit this aim. A dose-dependent response was observed on all three parameters tested: namely, the extract prevented zymosan-induced paw oedema, zymosan-induced pain and zymosan-induced TNFα production in mice, with an improved therapeutic effect upon increased dosages. Thus, the limitation with purified CBD could be overcome when presented together with other natural components of the plant. Of note, TNFα secretion was more sensitive to clone 202 extract inhibition than paw swelling and pain.

Our finding that it is possible to get a correlative dose-response using *Cannabis* clone 202 extracts, makes it possible to use it in many pathological conditions. We suggest that clone 202 extracts may be a suitable substitute for the current used *Cannabis* strain in the clinics, especially taking into account that it does not have any psychotropic adverse effects. Following the clinical improvement by the clone 202 extracts, more tedious experiments with CBD might be planned.

Our findings that CBD in the presence of other plant constituents improve the dose-response are supported by some recent reports showing that CBD in a standardized *Cannabis sativa* extract is more potent or efficacious than pure CBD [17]-[19]. These research groups studied the anti-proliferative effect of CBD on tumor cells [17] [19] and the inhibitory effect of CBD on bladder contractility [18]. The higher efficiency of plant extract might be explained by additive or synergistic interactions between CBD and minor phytocannabinoids or non-cannabinoids presented in the extracts. Other phytocannabinoids, including Tetrahydrocannabivarin, Cannabigerol and Cannabichromene, exert additional effects of therapeutic interest [20]. A lot of research has been made to isolate and characterize isolated single constituents of traditional herbal medicine to find their rationale for therapeutic uses. However, our data together with those of others [21] provide legitimation to introduce a new generation of phytopharmaceuticals to treat diseases that have hitherto been treated using synthetic drugs alone. The therapeutic synergy observed with plant extracts results in the requirement for a lower amount of active components, with consequent reduced adverse effects.

5. Conclusion

In conclusion, we recommend standardized plant extract of the *Cannabis* clone 202 for treatment of various inflammatory conditions.

Acknowledgements

The authors would like to thank Dr. Ronit Sionov for her valuable editorial assistance.

Conflict of Interest

Prof. Ruth Gallily has been a consultant for Tikun Olam since 2013, and has received a research grant during the years 2012-2014 from Tikun Olam, Israel. There is no conflict of interest.

References

[1] Hazekamp, A., Ware, M.A., Muller-Vahl, K.R., Abrams, D. and Grotenhermen, F. (2013) The Medicinal Use of *Cannabis* and Cannabinoids—An International Cross-Sectional Survey on Administration Forms. *Journal of Psychoactive Drugs*, **45**, 199-210. http://dx.doi.org/10.1080/02791072.2013.805976

[2] Mechoulam, R. (2012) *Cannabis*—A Valuable Drug That Deserves Better Treatment. *Mayo Clinic Proceedings*, **87**, 107-109. http://dx.doi.org/10.1016/j.mayocp.2011.12.002

[3] Greydanus, D.E., Hawver, E.K., Greydanus, M.M. and Merrick, J. (2013) Marijuana: Current Concepts. *Frontiers in Public Health*, **1**, 42. http://dx.doi.org/10.3389/fpubh.2013.00042

[4] Syed, Y.Y., McKeage, K. and Scott, L.J. (2014) Delta-9-Tetrahydrocannabinol/Cannabidiol (Sativex®): A Review of Its Use in Patients with Moderate to Severe Spasticity Due to Multiple Sclerosis. *Drugs*, **74**, 563-578. http://dx.doi.org/10.1007/s40265-014-0197-5

[5] Brenneisen, R. (2007) Chemistry and Analysis of Phytocannabinoids and Other *Cannabis* Constituents. *Marijuana and the Cannabinoids*, **Chapter 2**, 17-49. http://dx.doi.org/10.1007/978-1-59259-947-9_2

[6] Pertwee, R.G. (2008) The Diverse CB1 and CB2 Receptor Pharmacology of Three Plant Cannabinoids: Delta9-Tetrahydrocannabinol, Cannabidiol and Delta9-Tetrahydrocannabivarin. *British Journal of Pharmacology*, **153**, 199-215. http://dx.doi.org/10.1038/sj.bjp.0707442

[7] Pacher, P. and Mechoulam, R. (2011) Is Lipid Signaling through Cannabinoid 2 Receptors Part of a Protective System? *Progress in Lipid Research*, **50**, 193-211. http://dx.doi.org/10.1016/j.plipres.2011.01.001

[8] Malfait, A.M., Gallily, R., Sumariwalla, P.F., Malik, A.S., Andreakos, E., Mechoulam, R. and Feldmann, M. (2000) The Nonpsychoactive *Cannabis* Constituent Cannabidiol Is an Oral Anti-Arthritic Therapeutic in Murine Collagen-Induced Arthritis. *Proceedings of the National Academy of Sciences USA*, **97**, 9561-9566.

http://dx.doi.org/10.1073/pnas.160105897

[9]　Mechoulam, R., Peters, M., Murillo-Rodriguez, E. and Hanus, L.O. (2007) Cannabidiol—Recent Advances. *Chemistry & Biodiversity*, **4**, 1678-1692. http://dx.doi.org/10.1002/cbdv.200790147

[10]　Weiss, L., Zeira, M., Reich, S., Slavin, S., Raz, I., Mechoulam, R. and Gallily, R. (2008) Cannabidiol Arrests Onset of Autoimmune Diabetes in NOD Mice. *Neuropharmacology*, **54**, 244-249. http://dx.doi.org/10.1016/j.neuropharm.2007.06.029

[11]　Kozela, E., Lev, N., Kaushansky, N., Eilam, R., Rimmerman, N., Levy, R., Ben-Nun, A., Juknat, A. and Vogel, Z. (2011) Cannabidiol Inhibits Pathogenic T Cells, Decreases Spinal Microglial Activation and Ameliorates Multiple Sclerosis-Like Disease in C57BL/6 Mice. *British Journal of Pharmacology*, **163**, 1507-1519. http://dx.doi.org/10.1111/j.1476-5381.2011.01379.x

[12]　Esposito, G., Filippis, D.D., Cirillo, C., Iuvone, T., Capoccia, E., Scuderi, C., Steardo, A., Cuomo, R. and Steardo, L. (2013) Cannabidiol in Inflammatory Bowel Diseases: A Brief Overview. *Phytotherapy Research*, **27**, 633-636. http://dx.doi.org/10.1002/ptr.4781

[13]　Jamontt, J.M., Molleman, A., Pertwee, R.G. and Parsons, M.E. (2010) The Effects of Delta-Tetrahydrocannabinol and Cannabidiol Alone and in Combination on Damage, Inflammation and *in Vitro* Motility Disturbances in Rat Colitis. *British Journal of Pharmacology*, **160**, 712-723. http://dx.doi.org/10.1111/j.1476-5381.2010.00791.x

[14]　Gadó, K. and Gigler, G. (1991) Zymosan Inflammation: A New Method Suitable for Evaluating New Anti-Inflammatory Drugs. *Agents and Actions*, **32**, 119-121. http://dx.doi.org/10.1007/BF01983335

[15]　Grotenhermen, F. (2003) Pharmacokinetics and Pharmacodynamics of Cannabinoids. *Clinical Pharmacokinetics*, **42**, 327-360. http://dx.doi.org/10.2165/00003088-200342040-00003

[16]　Rocha, A.C., Fernandes, E.S., Quintao, N.L., Campos, M.M. and Calixto, J.B. (2006) Relevance of Tumour Necrosis Factor-Alpha for the Inflammatory and Nociceptive Responses Evoked by Carrageenan in the Mouse Paw. *British Journal of Pharmacology*, **148**, 688-695. http://dx.doi.org/10.1038/sj.bjp.0706775

[17]　Romano, B., Borrelli, F., Pagano, E., Cascio, M.G., Pertwee, R.G. and Izzo, A.A. (2014) Inhibition of Colon Carcinogenesis by a Standardized *Cannabis Sativa* Extract with High Content of Cannabidiol. *Phytomedicine*, **21**, 631-639. http://dx.doi.org/10.1016/j.phymed.2013.11.006

[18]　Capasso, R., Aviello, G., Borrelli, F., Romano, B., Ferro, M., Castaldo, L., Montanaro, V., Altieri, V. and Izzo, A.A. (2011) Inhibitory Effect of Standardized *Cannabis Sativa* Extract and Its Ingredient Cannabidiol on Rat and Human Bladder Contractility. *Urology*, **77**, 1006.e9-1006e15. http://dx.doi.org/10.1016/j.urology.2010.12.006

[19]　De Petrocellis, L., Ligresti, A., Schiano Moriello, A., Iappelli, M., Verde, R., Stott, C.G., Cristino, L., Orlando, P. and Di Marzo, V. (2013) Non-THC Cannabinoids Inhibit Prostate Carcinoma Growth *in Vitro* and *in Vivo*: Pro-Apoptotic Effects and Underlying Mechanisms. *British Journal of Pharmacology*, **168**, 79-102. http://dx.doi.org/10.1111/j.1476-5381.2012.02027.x

[20]　Russo, E.B. (2011) Taming THC: Potential Cannabis Synergy and Phytocannabinoid-Terpenoid Entourage Effects. *British Journal of Pharmacology*, **163**, 1344-1364. http://dx.doi.org/10.1111/j.1476-5381.2011.01238.x

[21]　Wagner, H. and Ulrich-Merzenich, G. (2009) Synergy Research: Approaching a New Generation of Phytopharmaceuticals. *Phytomedicine*, **16**, 97-110. http://dx.doi.org/10.1016/j.phymed.2008.12.018

9

Formulation and *In-Vitro* Release Pattern Study of Gliclazide Matrix Tablet

Tanbir Ahammad[1], Marium Begum[2], A. F. M. Towheedur Rahman[3], Moynul Hasan[4], Saikat Ranjan Paul[5], Shaila Eamen[6], Md. Iftekhar Hussain[2], Md. Hazrat Ali[7], Md. Ashraful Islam[8], Mohammad Mizanur Rahman[2], Mamunur Rashid[9*]

[1]Department of Pharmacy, BRAC University, Dhaka, Bangladesh
[2]Department of Pharmacy, Primeasia University, Dhaka, Bangladesh
[3]Department of Pharmaceutical Sciences, North South University, Dhaka, Bangladesh
[4]Department of Pharmacy, Dhaka International University, Dhaka, Bangladesh
[5]Department of Pharmacy, Southeast University, Dhaka, Bangladesh
[6]Department of Pharmacy, Jahangirnagar University, Dhaka, Bangladesh
[7]Department of Pharmacy, International Islamic University of Chittagong, Chittagong, Bangladesh
[8]Department of Biomedical Imaging, Faculty of Bioscience, Abo Akademi University, Turku, Finland
[9]Department of Pharmacy, University of Rajshshi, Rajshahi, Bangladesh
Email: *mamun69jp@yahoo.com

Abstract

In current decade, pharmaceutical industries of Bangladesh are giving much emphasize on the formulation of time release preparation to treat various chronic diseases in order to decrease the frequency of administration and to improve patient compliance. Objectives: The objective of this investigation is to design and evaluate sustained release matrix tablet of Gliclazide by direct compression method employing polymers of hydroxypropylmethyl cellulose (HPMC) derivatives (K15M CR and K4M CR) and to select the optimized formulations and compression process by performing a comparative release kinetic study with a reference product, Diamicron MR (one of the worldwide brand of Gliclazide sustain released tablet manufactured by Servier one of the French pharmaceutical company) tablet. Methods: Release kinetics of Gliclazide matrix tablets were determined using USP paddle method at Phosphate buffer (pH 7.4). The release mechanism was explored and explained with zero order, first order, Higuchi and Korsmeyer model. Result: It is found that formulation with lower polymeric concentration follows Higuchi release kinetics and that the formulation with higher concentration best fits with zero order release kinetics. Among the formulations, F1 and F6 show almost similar dissolution profile with Diamicron MR Tablet, which can be suitable candidates for further *in-vivo* bioequivalence study. Conclusion: Findings of

---

*Corresponding author.

this investigation suggest that F1 and F6 formulations are potential candidates for further bioequivalence study among other formulations.

Keywords

Gliclazide, Sustained Release, Methocel K15M CR, Methocel K4M CR, *In-Vitro* Bioequivalence

1. Introduction

Matrix systems appear to be a very attractive approach from the economic as well as from the process development and scale-up points of view in modified-release system [1]. Methocel (HPMC) is used frequently as a rate-controlling polymer in matrix tablets and offers some advantages of being non-toxic and relatively inexpensive; it can be compressed directly into matrix and is available in different chemical substitution, hydration rates and viscosity grades [2]. In general, most of the sustain release matrix tablet manufactured by wet granulation process which is very tedious process and required organic granulation solvent because aqueous solvent make the process more tedious. But use of direct compression technique by using suitable excipients can give desired pharmaceutical and pharmacokinetic properties [3]. In the present study, direct compression method is used to produce matrix tablets.

Chemically Gliclazide is 1-(3-azabicyclo [3, 3, 0]oct-3-yl)-3-p-tolylsulphonylurea (**Figure 1**) which is a second-generation sulfonylurea, oral hypoglycemic drug and widely used in the treatment of non-insulin-dependent diabetes mellitus (NIDDM). However, the usage of the common formulation of gliclazide can be limited by some kinds of reasons, such as patient's age and renal impairment etc. [4].

Currently, both conventional and modified release preparation are available. But most of them are failed to give reproducible and desirable drug release profile and there is no evidence of bioavailability and bioequivalence study of such products in Bangladesh. So, a lot of researches are carried out to prepare modified release Gliclazide tablets with pharmacokinetic characteristics suited to the circadian glycemic profile of type II diabetes. This approach will minimize the complications associated with diabetes mellitus [4]. The development of a sustain release dosage form of Gliclazide will reduce the total requirement of API (In conventional tablet 80 mg per day is recommended where 30 mg/day in sustain release tablet are recommended [5] hence reduce the side effect and chance of hypoglycemic effect. Same time it reduces the price of drug and makes the drug more affordable to the patients. For those reasons, an attempt has been taken to develop a Giclazide sustained release matrix tablets and their dissolution profiles were compared by determining similarity and difference factor that are introduced by Moor and Flanner, 1996 [6]. This comparison will help the health professionals to find the best alternative. From the point of view of formulation scientist and commercial personnel, it is excellent tool to select one or two suitable formulation(s) for *in-vitro* bioequivalence study which will be more rational and cost effective instead of going for several formulations on the basis of random selection.

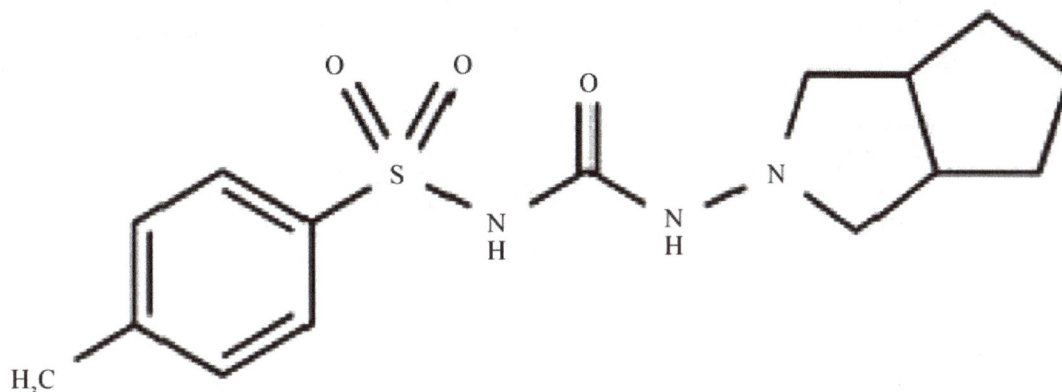

Figure 1. Chemical structure of Gliclazide.

2. Materials and Methods

2.1. Table Preparation by Direct Compression Technique

Individual ingredient was taken according to **Table 1** and was sieved through 30 mesh sieve. At first, Gliclazide and polymer (Methocel K15M CR or K4M CR) were mixed uniformly. Then lactose was added with this mixture and finally the powder mix was lubricated with magnesium stearate. Tablets were made by a compression machine (Erweka, TR 16, Germany) using a 5 × 10 mm caplet shaped punch and die set. Formulation code F1, F2, F3 represents the gliclazide matrix tablet prepared with Methocel K15M CR and Formulation code F4, F5, F6 represents the gliclazide matrix tablet prepared with Methocel K4M CR.

2.2. Study of Physical Properties of the Formulated Tablets

The weight variation was determined by taking 10 tablets using an electronic balance (AY120, Shimadzu, Japan). Friability was determined by testing 10 tablets in a friability tester (FTA-20, Campbell Electronics) for 4 minutes at 25 rpm. Tablet thickness, diameter and hardness were determined for 6 tablets using a Sotax HT10.

2.3. Dissolution Study of the Matrix Tablet

All dissolution studies were carried out for extended release Gliclazide formulations according to USP XII. Phosphate buffer at pH 7.4 was used as dissolution medium. The amount of Gliclazide was determined by employing UV spectrophotometer to measure the absorbance at the wavelength of maximum 226 nm and 290 nm. For this purpose absorbance of Standard solution against standard blank solution (0.6 ml methanol was diluted to 100 ml by Phosphate buffer (pH 7.4) and absorbance of sample solution against phosphate buffer (at pH 7.4) using 1 cm cell were measured. Differences between these two absorbances (at 226 and 290 nm) were calculated.

3. Result and Discussion

All of the studied physical properties were within the acceptable range with narrow variation and complied with the pharmacopoeial specifications for hardness, friability and weight variation. Range of hardness was 9.8 to 10.5 Kpa, friability was below 1.0% and rage was 0.34% to 0.40% and weight variation was 1.4% to 1.8% which is below 5%.

3.1. Effect of Methocel K15M CR on Release Pattern of Gliclazide from Matrix Tablet

Figure 2 is displaying the zero order release of Gliclazide from Methocel K15M CR (A) and Methocel K4M CR (B) and **Figure 3** is displaying Higuchi release of Gliclazide from Methocel K15M CR (A) and Methocel K4M CR (B).

The release profile of Gliclazide was monitored up to 10 hours. **Figure 2(a)** and **Figure 3(a)** represent the zero order and Higuchi release profile of Gliclazide matrix tablet compressed by direct compression. The total % of Gliclazide release from the formulation F1, F2 and F3 were 64.566%, 56.83% and 55.293% respectively. It has been observed that the drug release was extended with the increase of polymer % and with the decrease of lactose % which is due to a decrease in the total porosity *i.e.* release is extended to long period. Lactose causes a

Table 1. Composition of Gliclazide matrix tablets (mg/tablet; per tablet 180 mg).

Formulation	Gliclazide	% of Polymer	K15M CR	K4M CR	Lactose	Mg-Stearate
F1	30	20	36	-	113.1	0.9
F2	30	25	45	-	104.1	0.9
F3	30	30	54	-	95.1	0.9
F4	30	20	-	36	113.1	0.9
F5	30	25	-	45	104.1	0.9
F6	30	30	-	54	95.1	0.9

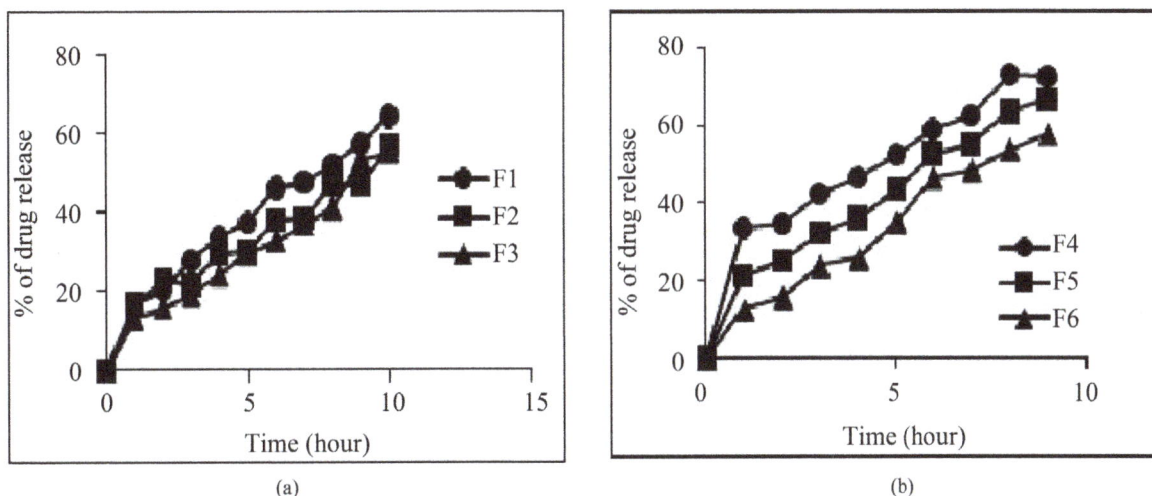

(a)

(b)

Figure 2. Zero order release of Gliclazide from Methocel K15M CR (a) and Methocel K4M CR (b).

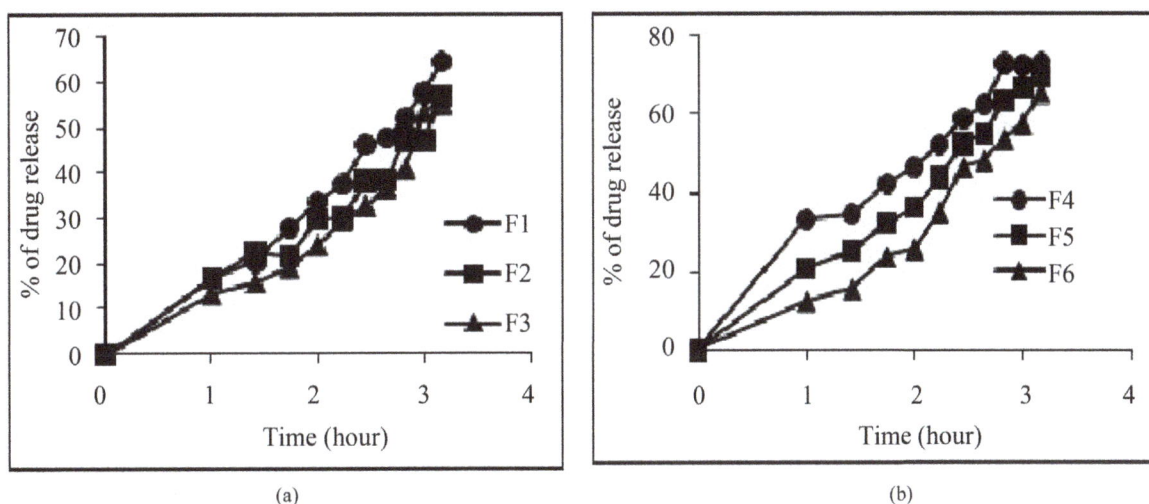

(a)

(b)

Figure 3. Higuchi release of Gliclazide from Methocel K15M CR (a) and Methocel K4M CR (b).

decreased tortuosity of the path of the drug due to its preferential solubility than Methocel K15 M CR, by its swelling effect; additionally weakened the integrity of the matrix [7]. The highest percent of drug release within 10 hours is obtained from formulation F1 where polymer content is 20% of total tablet weight. But in Formulation F3, the polymer content is 30% of total tablet weight and lactose content is 52.83%, the release of drug is controlled with 55.29% within 10 hours.

The kinetics data are presented in **Table 2** and it has been seen that all these formulations of this class show good linearity for Korsmeyer plot (r^2: 0.973 to 0.924) and follow Anomalous or non-Fickian transport (n: >0.45 and <0.89). From the table, it has been seen that all these formulations of this class follows zero order, first order and Higuchi release model. Formulation F1 best fits with first order release model followed by Higuchi and zero order where F2 best fit for Higuchi and F3 for zero order.

3.2. Effect of Methocel K4M CR on Release Pattern of Gliclazide Matrix Tablet

The release profile of Gliclazide from formulation F4, F5 and F6 were monitored up to 10 hours. **Figure 2(b)** and **Figure 3(b)** represent the zero order and Higuchi release profile of Gliclazide matrix tablet containing polymer Methocel K4M CR. The total % of Gliclazide release from the formulation F4, F5 and F6 were 73.076%, 69.259%, and 65.45% respectively.

The kinetics data are presented in **Table 3** and it has been seen that all the formulations of this class show

Table 2. Kinetic parameters of Gliclazide matrix tablets containing Methocel K15M CR.

Formulation code	Gliclazide release (%) after 10 hrs	Zero order		First order		Higuchi		Korsmeyer	
		r^2	K_0	r^2	K_1	r^2	K_H	r^2	n
F1	64.566	0.969	5.755	0.984	−0.040	0.976	20.06	0.924	0.517
F2	56.83	0.945	4.751	0.953	−0.030	0.953	16.58	0.978	0.603
F3	55.293	0.974	5.051	0.953	−0.032	0.922	17.07	0.938	0.645

Table 3. Kinetic parameters of Gliclazide matrix tablets containing Methocel K4M CR.

Formulation code	Gliclazide release (%) after 10 hrs	Zero order		First order		Higuchi		Korsmeyer	
		r^2	K_0	r^2	K_1	r^2	K_H	r^2	n
F4	73.07	0.885	6.266	0.958	−0.054	0.978	22.89	0.936	0. 395
F5	69.26	0.961	6.414	0.988	−0.049	0.979	22.50	0.970	0.565
F6	65.44	0.985	6.287	0.980	−0.043	0.936	21.31	0.966	0.769

good linearity for Korsmeyer plot (r^2: 0.991 to 0.936) where Formulation F4 follow Fickian (case I) diffusion (n: 0.395 < 0.45) and others follow Anomalous or non-Fickian transport (n > 0.45 but <0.89).

From **Table 3**, it has also been seen that formulation F5 best fits with first order release model follow by Higuchi and zero order where Formulation F4 best fit for Higuchi and F6 for zero order. Same trend was observed in formulations F1 to F3 where release kinetics shift from first order to zero order kinetics with the increase the % of polymer (20% to 30%).

3.3. Comparative Release Pattern Study between Diamicron MR Tablet and the Proposed Sustained Release Formulations

Figure 4 is showing Comparative *in vitro* Gliclazide release profile of Formulation F1 (A) & F6 (B) against Diamicron MR Tablet. The release rate of the proposed formulations were compared with the innovator's drug Diamicron MR Tablet in terms of Difference Factor (f_1) and Similarity Factor (f_2) [6]. For this purpose Diamicron MR (worldwide brand) of Servier was collected from local market and the dissolution of this product was studied for 10 hours in the same condition of the test sample. Similarity Factor (f_2) and Difference Factor (f_1) were determined by using the equation developed by Moor and Flanner (Equations (1) and (2)) and results are summarized in **Table 4**.

$$f_2 = 50\log \left[\left\{ 1 + 1/n \ (Rt - Tt)^2 \right\}^{-0.5} \times 100 \right] \tag{1}$$

$$f_1 = \left[\left\{ |Rt - Tt|/Rt \right\} \times 100 \right] \tag{2}$$

where Rt and Tt are the percent drug dissolved at each time point for the reference and test products, respectively; n is the number of dissolution sample times and t is the time points for collecting dissolution samples.

From the above study, it is seen that among the proposed formulations F1 and F6 are more likely to meet the specification with Diamicron MR in terms of Difference Factor (f_1) and Similarity Factor (f_2) and their release profile with Diamicron MR (**Figure 4**) are very identical. But others formulations don't showed desired dissolution pattern. Some are showing faster dissolution than Diamicron MR where others showing slower dissolution.

4. Conclusion

In the present study, Gliclazide matrix tablets have been prepared by employing polymers K15M CR and K4M CR with good tabletting properties like weight variation, thickness, diameter, hardness and friability (**Table 5**). Among the formulations, formulations F1 (containing 36 mg K15M CR) and F6 (containing 54 mg K15M CR) better meet the specification in terms of Difference Factor (f_1) and Similarity Factor (f_2) and exhibit similar release profile with Diamicron MR tablet. Both the Formulations F1 & F6 follow Anomalous or non-Fickian

Table 4. Summary of f_1 and f_2 test.

Formulation	Difference factor, (f_1) (0 to 15)	Similarity factor, (f_2) (50 to 100)
F1	5.6	72.3
F2	17.9	54.2
F3	21.6	50.7
F4	34.6	41.3
F5	14.2	59.0
F6	7.3	70.6

Table 5. Physical properties of the designed Gliclazide matrix tablets.

Formulation	Hardness (Kpa)	Thickness (mm)	Diameter (mm)	Friability (%)	Weight Variation
F1	09.9 ± 0.05	3.31	10.02	0.35	±1.8
F2	10.1 ± 0.08	3.32	10.01	0.37	±1.4
F3	10.5 ± 0.10	3.30	10.00	0.34	±1.6
F4	10.3 ± 0.50	3.33	10.00	0.38	±1.6
F5	10.3 ± 0.50	3.34	10.01	0.38	±1.4
F6	09.8 ± 0.10	3.33	09.99	0.40	±1.7

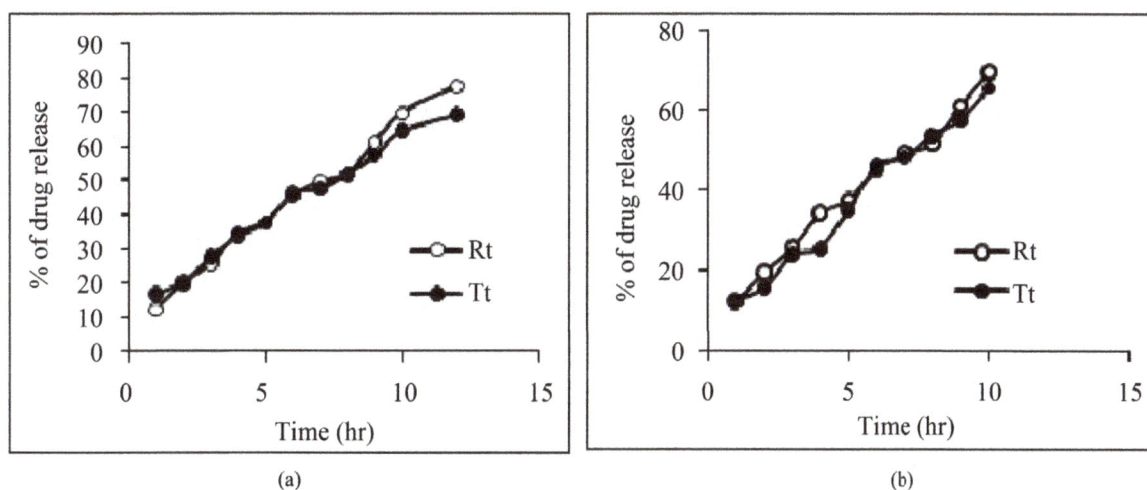

Figure 4. Comparative *in vitro* Gliclazide release profile of Formulations F1 (a) & F6 (b) against Diamicron MRTablet [Rt and Tt indicates the reference tablet and test tablet respectively].

transport. Formulation F1 best fits with first order release model indicating concentration dependent drug release where as Formulation F6 best fits with zero order release model indicating that the drug is released from the matrix tablet by both diffusion and erosion. For the further bioequivalence study, these two (F1 & F6) will be more prominent candidates than other formulations.

Acknowledgements

Authors are thankful to SQUARE Pharmaceuticals Ltd., Bangladesh for proving manufacturing facilities.

Conflict of Interest

The authors declare that they have no conflict of interest to disclose.

References

[1] Rekhi, G.S., Nellore, R.V. and Hussain, A.S. (1999) Identification of Critical Formulation and Processing Variables form Extended-Release (ER) Matrix Tablet. *Journal of Controlled Release*, **59**, 327-342. http://dx.doi.org/10.1016/S0168-3659(99)00004-8

[2] Perez-Marcos, B., Ford, J.L. and Amstrong, D.J. (1994) Release of Propranolol Hydrochloride from Matrix Tablets Containing Hydroxyl Propyl Methyl Cellulose K4M and Carbopol 974. *International Journal of Pharmaceutics*, **111**, 251-259. http://dx.doi.org/10.1016/0378-5173(94)90348-4

[3] Ahammad, T., Hasan, M., Ahamed, I. and Islam, M.A., (2011) Effect of Granulation Technique and Drug-Polymer Ratio on Release Kinetics of Gliclizade from Methocel K15M CR Matrix Tablet. *International Journal of Pharmaceutical Sciences and Research*, **2**, 1063-1068.

[4] British Pharmacopoeia (2009) The Stationery Office, London, Vol. I, 2761.

[5] McGavin, J.K., Perry, C.M. and Goa, K.L. (2002) Gliclazide Modified Release. *Drugs*, **62**, 1357-1364. http://dx.doi.org/10.2165/00003495-200262090-00010

[6] Moore, J.W. and Flanner, H.H. (1996) Mathematical Comparison of Curves with an Emphasis on *in Vitro* Dissolution Profiles. *Pharmaceutical Technology*, **20**, 64-74.

[7] Ju, R.T.C., Nixon, P.R., Patel, M.V. and Tong, D.M. (1995) A Mechanistic Model for Drug Release from Hydrophilic Matrixes Based on the Structure of Swollen Matrices. *Proceedings International Symposium on Control. Rel. Bioact. Mater*, **22**, 59-60.

10

Antiproliferative Activity of Acerogenin C, a Macrocyclicdiarylheptanoid, on PDGF-Induced Human Aortic Smooth Muscle Cells Proliferation

Byung-Yoon Cha[1], Wen Lei Shi[2], Kotaro Watanabe[3], Takayuki Yonezawa[1], Toshiaki Teruya[1], Kiyotake Suenaga[3], Yuichi Ishikawa[3], Shigeru Nishiyama[3], Kazuo Nagai[1,2], Je-Tae Woo[1,2]

[1]Research Institute for Biological Functions, Chubu University, Matsumoto, Japan
[2]Department of Biological Chemistry, Chubu University, Matsumoto, Japan
[3]Department of Chemistry, Faculty of Science and Technology, Keio University, Yokohama, Japan
Email: bycha@isc.chubu.ac.jp

Abstract

Platelet-derived growth factor (PDGF)-BB is one of the most potent factors in the development and progression of various vascular disorders, such as atherosclerosis and restenosis. PDGF is a major stimulant for vascular smooth muscle cells (VSMCs) proliferation via the mitogenesis signaling pathway. In the present study, we investigated the effect of acerogenin C, a macrocyclicdiarylheptanoid, on PDGF-BB-stimulated human aortic smooth muscle cells (HASMCs) proliferation. Acerogenin C significantly inhibited PDGF (20 ng/mL)-BB-induced [^{3}H]-thymidine incorporation into DNA at concentrations of 0.1, 1 and 10 μM without any cytotoxicity. Acerogenin C also blocked PDGF-BB-stimulated phosphorylation of PLCγ1 and Akt but had no effect on extracellular signal-regulated kinase 1/2 (ERK1/2) and PDGF beta-receptor (Rβ) activation. In addition, acerogenin C (0.1 - 10 μM) induced cell-cycle arrest in the G_1 phase, which was associated with the down-regulation of cyclins and the up-regulation of p27^{kip1}. These results suggest that acerogenin C blocks PDGF-BB-stimulated HASMCs proliferation via G_0/G_1 arrest in association with the induction of p27^{kip1} and the suppression of PLCγ1 and phosphatidylinositol 3-kinase (PI3-K)/Akt signaling pathways. Furthermore, acerogenin C may be used for prevention and treatment of atherosclerosis during restenosis after coronary angioplasty.

Keywords

HASMCs, Acerogenin C, PDGF-BB, p27^{kip1}, Cell Cycle

1. Introduction

Whereas PDGF is expressed at low levels in arteries in healthy adults, its expression is increased in conjunction with the inflammatory-fibroproliferative response that characterizes atherosclerosis [1]. Thus, studies of balloon catheter-injured arterial tissue [2]-[4], naturally occurring atherosclerosis [5]-[8], coronary arteries after percutaneous transluminal coronary angioplasty [9], and experimentally induced atherosclerosis [10] [11] revealed increased expression of PDGF and PDGF receptors in these lesions.

It is well-known that binding of signal transduction molecules to different phosphorylated tyrosine residues in PDGF-Rβ and PDGF-BB triggers the PI3-K/PKB (Akt) and PLCγ1 pathways in addition to the ERK pathway [12]. PI3-K mediates many different cellular responses, including actin reorganization, chemotaxis, cell growth and the serine/threonine kinase Akt/PKB for the antiapoptotic effect [13]-[15]. Interestingly, full activation of PLCγ is dependent on PI3-K; the PI(3,4,5)P3 formed by PI3-K binds the PH domain of PLCγ and may anchor the enzyme at the membrane [16]. Mitogenic growth factors such as PDGF-BB share a final common signaling pathway in the cell cycle. Quiescent (G_0) cells enter a gap period (G_1), during which the factors necessary for DNA replication in the subsequent synthetic (S) phase are assembled. After DNA replication is completed, the cells enter another gap phase (G_2) in preparation for mitosis (M). Restriction points at the G_1-S and G_2-M interphases ensure orderly cell cycle progression [17].

In the arterial media, VSMCs are normally quiescent, proliferate at low indices (<0.05%), and remain in the G_0/G_1 phases of the cell cycle [18]. After vessel injury, vascular smooth muscle cells migrate into the intimal layer of the arterial wall, where they leave their quiescent state and reenter the cell cycle [1]. In many cells, transit through G_1 of the cell cycle and entry into the S phase require the binding and activation of cyclin/CDK complexes, predominantly cyclin D1/CDK4 and cyclin E/CDK2 [19] [20]. The kinase activities of the cyclin/CDK complexes are negatively regulated by CDK inhibitors, such as p27[kip1] [21] [22].

Acerogenin is a diarylheptanoid whose characteristic structural feature is the presence of two hydroxylated aromatic rings tethered by a linear seven-carbon chain. Acerogenin C (**Figure 1**) was isolated from stems of *Boswellia ovalifoliolata* BAL. & HENRY (Burseraceae) [23], while acerogenin C has been synthesized by Gonzalez G. I. *et al.* [24]. This diarylheptanoid exhibits a broad range of potent biological activities that include anti-inflammatory, antihepatotoxic, antifungal, antibacterial and related effects [23] [25].

However, the mechanism by which acerogenin C affects VSMCs function is still largely unknown. The present study aimed to investigate, for the first time, the inhibitory effects of acerogenin C on PDGF-induced proliferation and signaling transduction pathways in HASMCs.

2. Materials and Methods

2.1. Materials and Reagents

PDGF-Rβ, Akt, PLCγ1, ERK1/2, cyclin D1, CDK4, cyclin E, CDK2, p27[kip1] and α-actin antibodies were purchased from Cell Signaling Technology Inc. (Beverly, MA, USA). Acerogenin C was a gift of Dr. Nishiyama (Department of Chemistry, Faculty of Science and Technology, Keio University; 3-14-1 Hiyoshi, Kohoku-ku, Yokohama 223-8522, Japan).

2.2. Cell Cultures

HASMCs were purchased from Cascade Biologics, Inc. (Portland, OR, USA). HASMCs were grown in Dulbecco's Modified Eagle Medium (DMEM) supplemented with 10% FBS, 100 IU/mL penicillin and 100 µg/mL

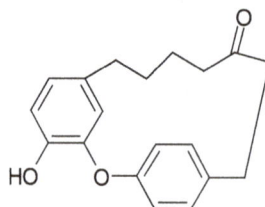

Figure 1. Chemical structures of acerogenin C.

streptomycin at 37°C in a humidified 95% air/5% CO_2 atmosphere. Cells were used at passages three through eight. For all experiments, HASMCs were grown to 80% - 90% confluence and quiescence was induced by starvation for at least 24 h.

2.3. [³H]-Thymidine Incorporation Assay

HASMCs proliferation was determined by [³H]-thymidine incorporation. HASMCs were incubated for 20 h with or without PDGF-BB (20 ng/mL) and various concentrations of acerogenins and then pulse-labeled with 1 µCi/mL of [³H]-thymidine for 4 h. Cells were harvested using a Universal Harvester (Perkin Elmer, Waltham, MA, USA) and then transferred to a GF/C filter (Perkin Elmer). The filter was dried and counted in scintillation fluid using a Microplate Scintillation and Luminescence Counter (Topcount NXT, Perkin Elmer).

2.4. Cell Viability

Cell viability was determined using the trypan blue dye exclusion method. Cells were incubated for 24 h with or without PDGF-BB (20 ng/mL) and various concentrations of acerogenin C and were then harvested from the dishes using a 0.1% w/v trypsin solution. Cell viability was examined by the trypan blue dye exclusion test. The number of viable cells was estimated by microscopic cell counting using a hemocytometer.

2.5. SDS-PAGE and Immunoblotting

Western blotting for protein analysis was performed as described previously [26]. Cells were harvested in lysis buffer containing 1 µM sodium vanadate, 1 µM phenylmethylsulfonyl fluoride, 5 µg/mL aprotinin and 5 µg/mL leupeptin. The protein concentration was determined by the Bradford assay (Bio-Rad, Hercules, CA, USA). Lysates corresponding to equal amounts of proteins were boiled in Laemmli sample buffer and the supernatants were loaded onto gels for SDS-PAGE. Proteins were transferred onto PVDF membranes and probed with the following primary antibodies: anti-phospho-PDGF-Rβ, anti-PDGF-Rβ, anti-phospho-PLCγ1 (Tyr783), anti-PLCγ1 anti-phospho-ERK1/2, anti-ERK, anti-phospho-Akt (Thr308) and anti-Akt. Appropriate horseradish peroxidase-coupled secondary antibodies were used at 1:10,000. Immunoreactive bands were visualized using enhanced chemiluminescence (ECL; Amersham Pharmacia Biotech, UK). The detected proteins were normalized to α-actin or the respective total protein, as appropriate. The intensities of bands were quantified using Sicon-Image for Windows (Scion Corporation, Frederick, MA, USA).

2.6. Cell Cycle Analysis

HASMCs were seeded in 6-well culture plates and grown in DMEM medium with growth supplement at 37°C in a humidified 95% air/5% CO_2 atmosphere. Cells were grown to 80% confluence and made quiescent by starvation for at least 24 h. Cells were incubated for 24 h with or without PDGF-BB (20 ng/mL) and various concentrations of acerogenin C. Cells were harvested, fixed in 70% ethanol for 12 h, and stored at -20°C. Cells were then washed twice with ice-cold PBS and incubated with 100 µg/mL RNase and 50 µg/mL propidium iodide and cell-cycle phase analysis was performed by flow cytometry using a Cytomics FC500 and CXP Software Ver. 2 software (Beckman Coulter, JAPAN).

2.7. Statistical Analysis

Experimental results are expressed as means ± S.E.M. One-way analysis of variance (ANOVA), followed by Dunnett's test, was used for multiple comparisons. P values of <0.05 and <0.01 were considered statistically significant.

3. Results

3.1. Effect of Acerogenins on PDGF-Induced HASMCs Proliferation and DNA Synthesis

In the [³H]-thymidine incorporation assay (**Figure 2(a)**), stimulation with PDGF-BB (20 ng/mL) increased cell proliferation by about 10-fold. Acerogenin C (0.1 to 10 µM) inhibited PDGF-induced cell proliferation in a concentration-dependent manner with about 90% inhibition observed at 10 µM. When quiescent cells were treated with acerogenin C (0.1 to 10 μM) for 24 h in the absence of PDGF-BB, no significant difference was observed in the extent of [^{3}H]-thymidine incorporation, suggesting that acerogenins are not cytotoxic at the concentrations tested. In particular, the lack of cytotoxicity of acerogenin C at the concentrations used in these experiments was confirmed by the trypan blue exclusion assay (**Figure 2(b)**). The number of cells was significantly increased after 20 ng/mL PDGF-BB stimulation (28.3 ± 0.3 × 10^4 cells/well) compared with the non-stimulated group (13.1 ± 0.1 × 10^4 cells/well) and the increased cells were significantly reduced to 21.2 ± 0.2, 15.3 ± 0.3 and 14.2 ± 0.2 × 10^4 cells/well at concentrations of 0.1, 1 and 10 μM, respectively (**Figure 2(b)**).

3.2. Effect of Acerogenin C on PDGF-Induced PDGF-Rβ, PCLγ1, Akt and ERK 1/2 Activation

The HASMCs were pre-incubated in the presence or absence of various concentrations of acerogenin C in a serum-free medium for 24 h and then stimulated for 10 min with 20 ng/mL PDGF-BB. As shown in **Figure 3**, PDGF-BB markedly increased phosphorylation levels on the PDGF-Rβ but acerogenin C treatment had no significant effect. To determine the effects of acerogenin C on the downstream intracellular signal transduction pathway of PDGF-BB, we determined the phosphorylation of PLCγ1, Akt and ERK1/2. PDGF-BB treatment clearly increased phosphorylation levels on the PLCγ1, Akt and ERK1/2. Acerogenin C blocked the phosphorylation of PLCγ1 and Akt in a concentration-dependent manner but had no effect on ERK 1/2 phosphorylation.

3.3. Effect of Acerogenin C on Cell Cycle Progression in HASMCs

Flow cytometric analysis was performed to determine whether acerogenin C-induced cell growth inhibition was due to an arrest in a specific point of the cell cycle. As shown in **Figure 4**, pre-incubation of HASMCs in a serum-free medium for 24 h resulted in approximately 91.8 ± 2.5% synchronization of the cell cycle in the G0/G1 phase. During cell cycle analysis, stimulation with PDGF-BB (20 ng/mL) increased the percentage of cells in the S phase from 5.6 ± 1.3% to 27.5 ± 2.1%. Acerogenin C (0.1 to 10 μM) significantly blocked cell cycle progression in a concentration-dependent manner. The percentage of cells in the S phase was significantly reduced to 12.6 ± 1.2% (P < 0.05, n = 3), 7.4 ± 1.4% (P < 0.05, n = 3) and 5.4 ± 1.4% (P < 0.05, n = 3) at concentrations of 0.1, 1 and 10 μM acerogenin C, respectively (**Figure 4**). These results suggest that acerogenin C may act against DNA synthesis in the early events of the cell cycle.

3.4. Effect of Acerogenin C on Cell Cycle Regulatory Protein Expression

Using immunoblot analysis, we analyzed the protein expressions of the cyclins and CDKs, which are known to

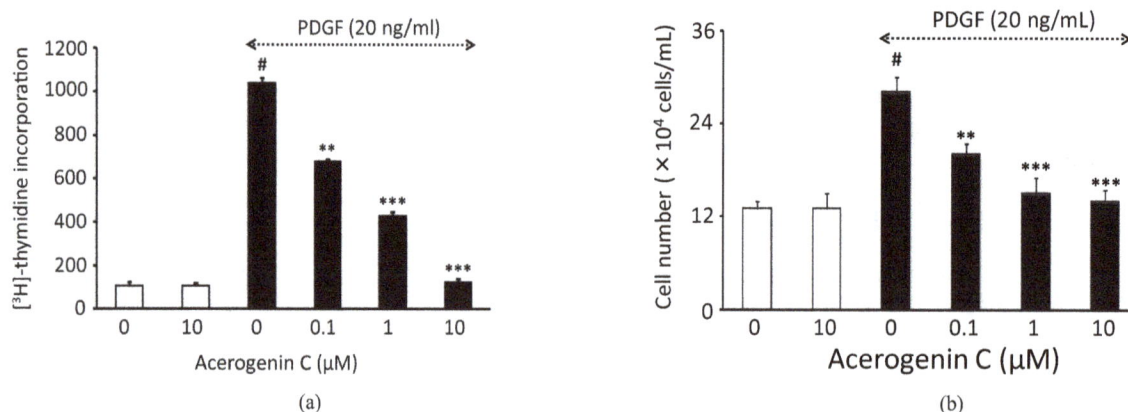

Figure 2. The effect of acerogenin on PDGF-BB-stimulated HASMCs proliferation. Cells were incubated for 20 h with or without PDGF-BB (20 ng/mL) and various concentrations of acerogenin C, and then pulse-labeled with [3H]-thymidine for 4 h (a). The cells were pre-incubated for 24 h with or without PDGF-BB and indicated concentrations of acerogenin C. The cells were trypsinized and then counted using a hemocytometer (b). Results are means ± S.E.M. from three independent experiments. #P < 0.005 compared with control; **P < 0.01 and ***P < 0.001 compared with PDGF-stimulation.

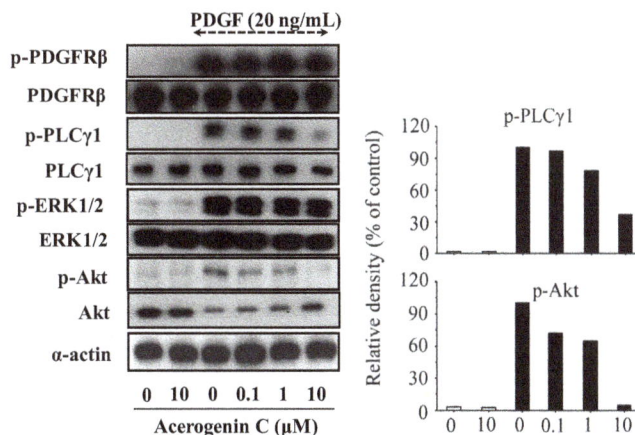

Figure 3. The effect of acerogenin C on PDGF-stimulated PDGF-Rβ, ERK 1/2, PLCγ1, and Akt phosphorylation in HASMCs. The cells were incubated for 10 min with or without PDGF-BB and various concentrations of acerogenin C in 6-well culture plates. Cells were lysed and lysates were immunoblotted with antibodies. Total protein was used for respective normalization. After densitometric quantification, data are representative of at least three independent experiments with similar results.

be regulated by p27^{kip1}, following treatment with acerogenin C. As shown in **Figure 5**, acerogenin C decreased the protein expression of cyclin E and CDK2, as well as cyclin D1 and CDK4, in a concentration-dependent manner. In addition, the expression of p27^{kip1}, one of the cyclin-dependent kinase inhibitors, was down regulated by PDGF-BB treatment. In contrast, the p27^{kip1} protein level was significantly increased by acerogenin C treatment in a concentration-dependent manner.

4. Discussion

In the present study, we found that acerogenin C inhibited DNA synthesis in response to PDGF-BB (**Figure 2(a)**). As a result, acerogeninC showed a concentration-dependent inhibition of the incorporation of [^{3}H]-thymidine into HASMCs. Furthermore, the antiproliferative effect of acerogenin C on HASMCs was not due to cellular cytotoxicity, as demonstrated by the cell counting (**Figure 2(b)**) and MTT assays (data not shown).

To understand the mechanism of down-regulation of PDGF-BB-stimulated HASMCs proliferation, we examined whether the effect of acerogenin C is mediated by down-regulation of the intracellular signaling pathways.

The PDGF-BB-stimulated mitogenesis signaling pathway has been well characterized. Binding of PDGF-BB to PDGF-Rβ can activate three major signal transduction pathways, PI3-K/Akt, PLCγ1 and ERK1/2, by activating Raf-1 [12]. As shown **Figure 3**, acerogenin C had no effect on the PDGF-BB-induced phosphorylation of PDGF-Rβ at various concentrations. This result suggests that the inhibition of acerogenin C on HASMCs proliferation does not occur at the receptor level. Thus, we did Western blotting to understand the effect of acerogenin C on the downstream signal transduction, such as the PI3-K/Akt, PLCγ1 and ERK1/2 signaling pathways. As shown in **Figure 3**, we observed that acerogenin C specifically inhibited PDGF-stimulated PLCγ1 and Akt activation but not PDGFR and ERK1/2 MAP kinase activation in HASMCs. These results are similar to a previous study, in which JM91 inhibited PDGF-induced PI3-K/Akt and ERK1/2 MAP kinase activation but not PDGF Rβ in HASMCs [12]. In the present study, PDGFRβ, PLCγ1, ERK1/2 and Akt were used as a control for protein loading. However, the total amount of Akt rapidly decreased upon its activation. PDGF caused a rapid decrease in the Akt protein levels, concomitant with Akt activation. PDGF causes the regulated proteolytic down-regulation of Akt, which is dependent on PI3-K and proteasome activities. The proteasome-dependent down- regulation of Akt might be a fundamental mechanism that regulates the activity and function of Akt in VSMCs [27]. Interestingly, full activation of PLCγ is dependent on PI3-K; the PI(3,4,5)P3 formed by PI3-K binds the PH domain of PLCγ and may anchor the enzyme at the membrane [16]. PLCγ appears not to be of primary impor-

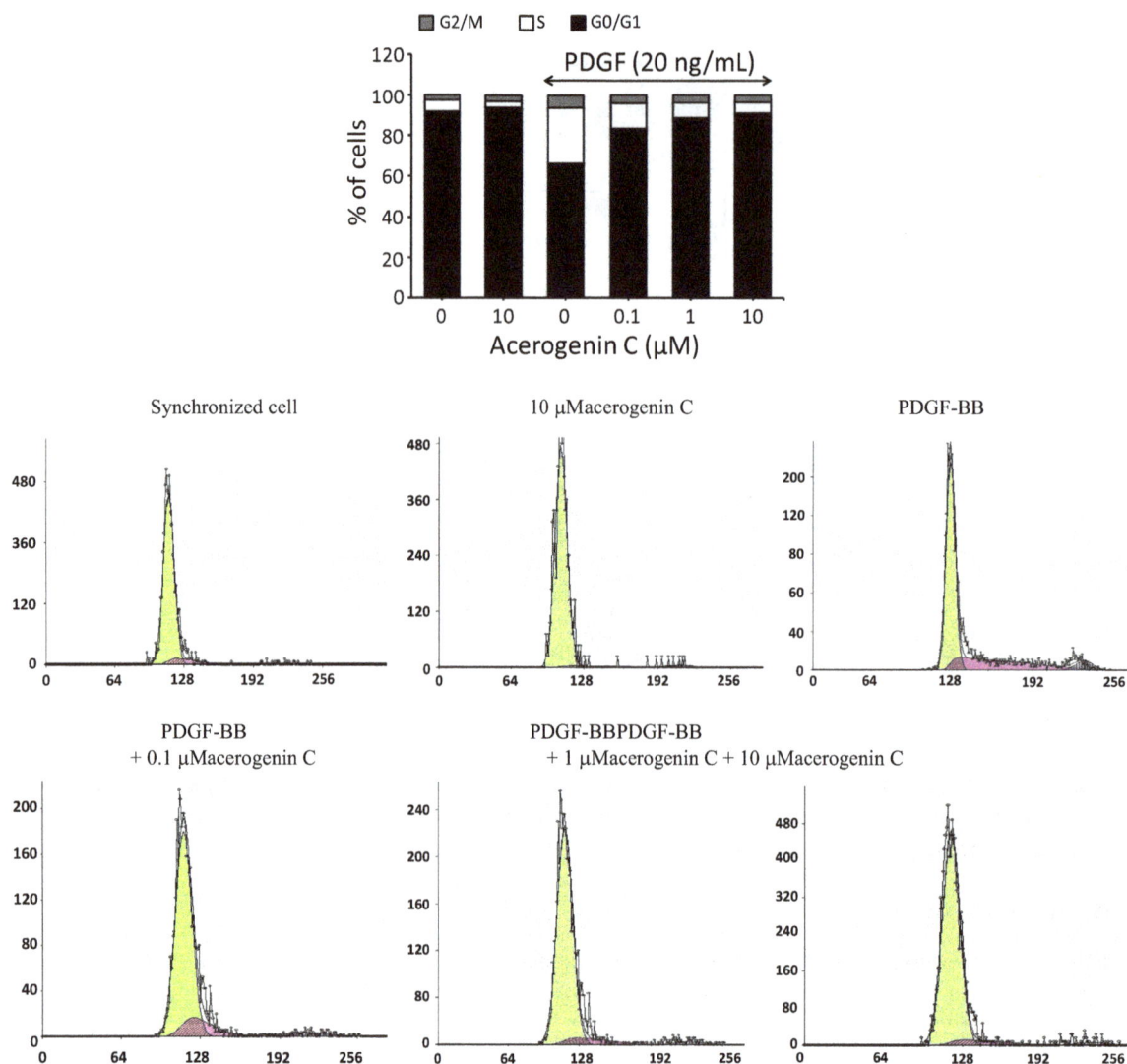

Figure 4. The effect of acerogenin C on PDGF-BB-stimulated cell cycle progression in HASMCs. The cells were incubated for 24 h with or without PDGF-BB and various concentrations of acerogenin C in 6-well culture plates. The cells were trypsinized and then analyzed by flow cytometry. Each item is derived from a representative experiment where data from at least 10,000 events were obtained. Data are representative of at least three independent experiments with similar results.

tance for the stimulation of cell growth and motility in most cell types. However, in certain cell types, PLCγ affects these responses [28]. Members of the PI3-K family that bind to and are activated by tyrosine kinase receptors consist of a regulatory subunit, p85, and a catalytic subunit, p110. Their preferred substrate is phosphatidylinositol 4,5-bisphosphate [PI(4,5)P2], which is phosphorylated to phosphatidylinositol 3,4,5-trisphosphate [PI(3,4,5)P3]. Phosphatidylinositol 39-kinase plays a central role in intracellular signal transduction; it can be activated by several different signals, it has a number of downstream effector molecules, and it mediates many different cellular responses, including actin reorganization, chemotaxis, cell growth and antiapoptosis [15].

In addition, cell cycle analysis was performed to investigate the antiproliferative effect of acerogenin C. As shown in **Figure 4**, acerogenin C inhibits PDGF-BB-stimulated HASMCs proliferation via G_0/G_1 arrest. Several reports suggest that the G_1 phase is a major point of control for cell proliferation in mammalian cells [29]. Many studies have attributed the regulation of G_1 cell-cycle arrest to a number of cellular proteins, including the CDK inhibitor, p27^{kip1} [22]. Our data demonstrates a significant up-regulation of p27^{kip1}. However, under similar experimental conditions, the expression levels of another cyclin-dependent kinase inhibitor, p21^{waf1} protein, was not changed (data not shown), suggesting that p21^{waf1} is unlikely to be involved in the cell-cycle arrest induced

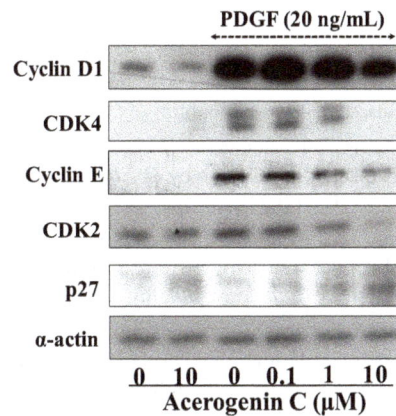

Figure 5. The effect of acerogenin C on PDGF-stimulated expression of cell cycle regulatory proteins in HASMCs. The cells were incubated for 24 h with or without PDGF-BB and various concentrations of acerogenin C in 6-well culture plates. The cells were lysed and proteins were analyzed by SDS-PAGE and immunoblotting. α-actin was used for normalization. Data are representative of at least three independent experiments with similar results.

by acerogenin C. We assessed the effect of acerogenin C treatment on the cyclins and CDKs operative in the G_1-phase of the cell cycle, such as cyclin D1, CDK4, cyclin E and CDK2. Acerogenin C inhibited the expression of cyclin D1, CDK4, cyclin E and CDK2 in a concentration-dependent manner. Our results indicate that cell cycle arrest in the G_1-phase might be due to the down-regulation of CDKs/cyclins complex expression.

5. Conclusion

We showed that acerogenin C inhibited PDGF-BB-induced HASMCs proliferation via G_0/G_1 arrest, in association with the down-regulation of the expression of cyclin D1, CDK4, cyclin E and CDK2 and the up-regulation of $p27^{kip1}$. Therefore, acerogenin C may be useful for prevention and treatment of vascular diseases, such as restenosis after coronary angioplasty.

Acknowledgements

This study was performed at a laboratory supported by an endowment from Erina Co., Inc.

References

[1] Ross, R. (1993) The Pathogenesis of Atherosclerosis: A Perspective for the 1990s. *Nature*, **362**, 801-809. http://dx.doi.org/10.1038/362801a0

[2] Kanzaki, T., Shinomiya, M., Ueda, S., Morisaki, N., Saito, Y. and Yoshida, S. (1994) Enhanced Arterial Intimal Thickening after Balloon Catheter Injury in Diabetic Animals Accompanied by PDGF Beta-Receptor Overexpression of Aortic Media. *European Journal of Clinical Investigation*, **24**, 377-381. http://dx.doi.org/10.1111/j.1365-2362.1994.tb02179.x

[3] Majesky, M.W., Reidy, M.A., Bowen-Pope, D.F., Hart, C.E., Wilcox, J.N. and Schwartz, S.M. (1990) PDGF Ligand and Receptor Gene Expression during Repair of Arterial Injury. *Journal of Cell Biology*, **111**, 2149-2158. http://dx.doi.org/10.1083/jcb.111.5.2149

[4] Uchida, K., Sasahara, M., Morigami, N., Hazama, F. and Kinoshita, M. (1996) Expression of Platelet-Derived Growth Factor B-Chain in Neointimal Smooth Muscle Cells of Balloon Injured Rabbit Femoral Arteries. *Atherosclerosis*, **124**, 9-23. http://dx.doi.org/10.1016/0021-9150(95)05742-0

[5] Libby, P., Salomon, R.N., Payne, D.D., Schoen, F.J. and Pober, J.S. (1989) Functions of Vascular Wall Cells Related to Development of Transplantation-Associated Coronary Arteriosclerosis. *Transplantation Proceedings*, **21**, 3677-3684.

[6] Libby, P., Warner, S.J., Salomon, R.N. and Birinyi, L.K. (1988) Production of Platelet-Derived Growth Factor-Like Mitogen by Smooth-Muscle Cells from Human Atheroma. *New England Journal of Medicine*, **318**, 1493-1498.

http://dx.doi.org/10.1056/NEJM198806093182303

[7]   Rubin, K., Tingström, A., Hansson, G.K., Larsson, E., Rönnstrand, L., Klareskog, L., *et al.* (1988) Induction of B-Type Receptors for Platelet-Derived Growth Factor in Vascular Inflammation: Possible Implications for Development of Vascular Proliferative Lesions. *Lancet*, **1**, 1353-1356. http://dx.doi.org/10.1016/S0140-6736(88)92177-0

[8]   Wilcox, J.N., Smith, K.M., Williams, L.T., Schwartz, S.M. and Gordon, D. (1988) Platelet-Derived Growth Factor mRNA Detection in Human Atherosclerotic Plaques by *in Situ* Hybridization. *Journal of Clinical Investigation*, **82**, 1134-1143. http://dx.doi.org/10.1172/JCI113671

[9]   Ueda, M., Becker, A.E., Kasayuki, N., Kojima, A., Morita, Y. and Tanaka, S. (1996) *In Situ* Detection of Platelet-Derived Growth Factor-A and -B Chain mRNA in Human Coronary Arteries after Percutaneous Transluminal Coronary Angioplasty. *American Journal of Pathology*, **149**, 831-843.

[10] Golden, M.A., Au, Y.P., Kirkman, T.R., Wilcox, J.N., Raines, E.W., Ross, R., *et al.* (1991) Platelet-Derived Growth Factor Activity and mRNA Expression in Healing Vascular Grafts in Baboons. Association *in Vivo* of Platelet-Derived Growth Factor mRNA and Protein with Cellular Proliferation. *Journal of Clinical Investigation*, **87**, 406-414. http://dx.doi.org/10.1172/JCI115011

[11] Ross, R., Masuda, J., Raines, E.W., Gown, A.M., Katsuda, S., Sasahara, M., *et al.* (1990) Localization of PDGF-B Protein in Macrophages in All Phases of Atherogenesis. *Science*, **248**, 1009-1012. http://dx.doi.org/10.1126/science.2343305

[12] Seo, J.M., Jin, Y.R., Ryu, C.K., Kim, T.J., Han, X.H., Hong, J.T., *et al.* (2008) JM91, a Newly Synthesized Indoledione Derivative, Inhibits Rat Aortic Vascular Smooth Muscle Cells Proliferation and Cell Cycle Progression through Inhibition of ERK1/2 and Akt Activations. *Biochemical Pharmacology*, **75**, 1331-1340. http://dx.doi.org/10.1016/j.bcp.2007.11.013

[13] Dudek, H., Datta, S.R., Franke, T.F., Birnbaum, M.J., Yao, R., Cooper, G.M., *et al.* (1997) Regulation of Neuronal Survival by the Serine-Threonine Protein Kinase Akt. *Science*, **275**, 661-665. http://dx.doi.org/10.1126/science.275.5300.661

[14] Kauffmann-Zeh, A., Rodriguez-Viciana, P., Ulrich, E., Gilbert, C., Coffer, P., Downward, J., *et al.* (1997) Suppression of c-Myc-Induced Apoptosis by Ras Signalling through PI(3)K and PKB. *Nature*, **385**, 544-548. http://dx.doi.org/10.1038/385544a0

[15] Vanhaesebroeck, B., Leevers, S.J., Panayotou, G. and Waterfield, M.D. (1997) Phosphoinositide 3-Kinases: A Conserved Family of Signal Transducers. *Trends in Biochemical Sciences*, **22**, 267-272. http://dx.doi.org/10.1016/S0968-0004(97)01061-X

[16] Falasca, M., Logan, S.K., Lehto, V.P., Baccante, G., Lemmon, M.A. and Schlessinger, J. (1998) Activation of Phospholipase Cγ by PI 3-Kinase-Induced PH Domain-Mediated Membrane Targeting. *EMBO Journal*, **17**, 414-422. http://dx.doi.org/10.1093/emboj/17.2.414

[17] Elledge, S.J. (1996) Cell Cycle Checkpoints: Preventing an Identity Crisis. *Science*, **274**, 1664-1672. http://dx.doi.org/10.1126/science.274.5293.1664

[18] Gordon, D., Reidy, M.A., Benditt, E.P. and Schwartz, S.M. (1990) Cell Proliferation in Human Coronary Arteries. *Proceedings of the National Academy of Sciences of the United States of America*, **87**, 4600-4604. http://dx.doi.org/10.1073/pnas.87.12.4600

[19] Sherr, C.J. (1994) G1 Phase Progression: Cycling on Cue. *Cell*, **79**, 551-555. http://dx.doi.org/10.1016/0092-8674(94)90540-1

[20] Sherr, C.J. (1996) Cancer Cell Cycles. *Science*, **274**, 1672-1677. http://dx.doi.org/10.1126/science.274.5293.1672

[21] Xiong, Y., Hannon, G.J., Zhang, H., Casso, D., Kobayashi, R. and Beach, D. (1993) p21 Is a Universal Inhibitor of Cyclin Kinases. *Nature*, **366**, 701-704. http://dx.doi.org/10.1038/366701a0

[22] Toyoshima, H. and Hunter, T. (1994) p27, a Novel Inhibitor of G1 Cyclin-Cdk Protein Kinase Activity, Is Related to p21. *Cell*, **78**, 67-74. http://dx.doi.org/10.1016/0092-8674(94)90573-8

[23] Akihisa, T., Taguchi, Y., Yasukawa, K., Tokuda, H., Akazawa, H., Suzuki, T., *et al.* (2006) Acerogenin M, a Cyclic Diarylheptanoid, and Other Phenolic Compounds from *Acer nikoense* and Their Anti-Inflammatory and Anti-Tumor-Promoting Effects. *Chemical and Pharmaceutical Bulletin*, **54**, 735-739. http://dx.doi.org/10.1248/cpb.54.735

[24] Gonzalez, G.I. and Zhu, J. (1997) First Total Synthesis of Acerogenin C and Aceroside IV. *Journal of Organic Chemistry*, **62**, 7544-7545. http://dx.doi.org/10.1021/jo9714324

[25] Keseru, G.M. and Nogradi, M. (1995) The Chemistry of Natural Diarylheptanoids. In: Rahman, A.U., Ed., *Studies in Natural Products Chemistry*, Vol. 17, Elsevier, Amsterdam, 357-394.

[26] Cha, B.Y., Shi, W.L., Yonezawa, T., Teruya, T., Nagai, K. and Woo, J.T. (2009) An Inhibitory Effect of Chrysoeriol on Platelet-Derived Growth Factor (PDGF)-Induced Proliferation and PDGF Receptor Signaling in Human Aortic Smooth Muscle Cells. *Journal of Pharmacological Sciences*, **110**, 105-110. http://dx.doi.org/10.1254/jphs.08282FP

[27] Adachi, M., Katsumura, K.R., Fujii, K., Kobayashi, S., Aoki, H. and Matsuzaki, M. (2003) Proteasome-Dependent Decrease in Akt by Growth Factors in Vascular Smooth Muscle Cells. *FEBS Letters*, **554**, 77-80. http://dx.doi.org/10.1016/S0014-5793(03)01109-8

[28] Heldin, C.H. and Westermark, B. (1999) Mechanism of Action and *in Vivo* Role of Platelet-Derived Growth Factor. *Physiological Reviews*, **79**, 1283-1316.

[29] Fang, F. and Newport, J.W. (1991) Evidence That the G1-S and G2-M Transitions Are Controlled by Different cdc2 Proteins in Higher Eukaryotes. *Cell*, **66**, 731-742. http://dx.doi.org/10.1016/0092-8674(91)90117-H

11

Trends of Pediatric Outpatients Prescribing in Umm Al Quwain, United Arab Emirates

Suleiman I. Sharif*, Aseel H. Nassar, Fatima K. Al-Hamami, Maha M. Hassanein, Ashkur H. Elmi, Rubian S. Sharif

Department of Pharmacy Practice & Pharmacotherapeutics, College of Pharmacy, University of Sharjah, Sharjah, United Arab Emirates
Email: *sharifsi@sharjah.ac.ae

Abstract

Background: Data with regard to local drug prescribing in pediatric population is scarce. This study was carried out to investigate the patterns of drug prescribing for pediatric outpatient in a general hospital in the United Arab Emirates. Methods: A total of 707 prescriptions were collected from a governmental hospital in Umm Al Quwain, United Arab Emirates covering the months of June and July, 2014. Encounters issued for patients older than 12 years were rejected. A total of 520 prescriptions for age groups ranging from 1 week to 12 years were studied. Prescriptions were analyzed using WHO drug use indicators. Results: All prescriptions were electronic and head lettered by the name of the hospital. Average number of drugs per prescriptions was 2.6 and all drugs were generics. Name of patient, age and gender and prescriber's name and E-signature were present in 100%. Patient's address, allergy and diagnosis were present in 21.15%, 83.26% and 64.42% of prescriptions respectively. Complete dosage regimen was present in all encounters. Patients were prescribed one, two, three, four or more than four drugs per prescription in 23.84%, 27.88%, 26.53%, 12.69%, and 8.65% respectively. The most commonly prescribed therapeutic classes of drugs were antibiotics (44.60%), antihistamines (43.65%), and analgesics/antipyretics (32.30%). The most commonly prescribed drugs among each class were amoxicillin (40%), xylometazoline (61.23%), and paracetamol (87.5%). Conclusion: Present results indicate that prescribing trends for pediatric population seems to be rational. However, there is over use of antibiotics and there are some areas that warrant further attention by the prescribers for a more significantly rational prescribing.

Keywords

Prescriptions, Trends, Pediatrics, Outpatients, Drug Use Indicators

---

*Corresponding author.

1. Introduction

Irrational drug use increases the cost of treatment, incidence of adverse drug reactions and hospitalization. On the other hand, rational prescribing can be evaluated through prescription analysis to study the patterns of prescribing among physicians. Periodical evaluation of trends of prescribing is essential to point out areas for improvement and increase the awareness of prescribers to possible errors in their daily practice. In studying prescribing patterns, focus is mainly on errors which may be in the form of incomplete prescription or incorrect content [1]. It has been suggested that as community pharmacists have no access to patient's information, their use of scientific knowledge is not possible in cases of prescriptions with errors or incomplete information [2]. On the other hand, the situation in hospital practice is different. However, it is still possible to demonstrate encounters with errors or incomplete information.

The World Health Organization (WHO) [3] has formulated a set of core drug use indicators (**Table 1**), which measure the performance of prescribers, patients experience at health facilities and whether the health personnel can function effectively. The assessment of drug use indicators according to WHO guidelines on how to investigate drug use in health facilities is prescribing indicators, patient care indicators, facility indicators and complementary indicators [4].

Studies that investigated the prescribing trends in adults [5]-[20] are far in excess of those in pediatric patients [21]-[28]. It has been pointed out that drugs marketed for adult use, may possibly, be used in an off-label manner in children [2]. It has been shown that 80% - 93% of medications used in European and Australian neonatal wards are off-label or unlicensed [29].

Moreover, harmful medication errors are three times more common in pediatric than adult patients [30]. It must be remembered that most of the drugs prescribed for children have not been tested in the pediatric population due to the difficulties in carrying out clinical studies in children and ethical issues due to children not being able to make their own decisions to participate in a clinical trial. Therefore, many medications have not been approved by the Food and Drug Administration for children [31]. An essential component in rational drug prescribing is the availability of an approved guideline such as a list of essential drugs. For prescribing for children, the first guideline was issued by the WHO in October, 2007 [32].

Children are among the most vulnerable groups to possible harmful adverse effects of drugs and studies on drug use in children in UAE are lacking. The present study was undertaken to evaluate patterns of prescribing in paediatric population.

Table 1. Core drug use indicators in pediatric outpatients of a general hospital.

Prescribing indicators	
Average number of drugs per encounter.	2.6
Percentage of drugs prescribed by generic name.	100%
Percentage of antibiotics prescribed.	44.6%
Percentage of injections prescribed.	0.38%
Percentage of drugs prescribed from essential drug list or formulary.	100%
Patient care indicators	
Average consultation time.	20 Minutes
Average dispensing time.	12 Minutes
Percentage of drugs actually dispensed.	98%
Percentage of drugs adequately labeled.	100%
Patient's knowledge of correct dosage.	Not assessed
Facility indicators	
Availability of essential drugs list or formulary.	BNF
Availability of key drugs.	85%

2. Methods

A hospital base cross sectional study was carried out on prescriptions issued to pediatric outpatients. The study was approved by the Ethics Committee of the Medical Campus of the University of Sharjah and hospital approval was obtained prior to collecting prescriptions. A total of 707 prescriptions were collected from a governmental general hospital in the Emirate of Umm Al Quwain, United Arab Emirates. All prescription were issued during the months of June and July, 2014. All collected encounters were electronic prescriptions issued to outpatient aged one week to 19 years. A total of 187 prescriptions issued to patients older than 12 years of age were rejected and not included in the study. The rest (520) of prescription were subjected to the study. These prescriptions were subjected to analysis according to WHO core indicators for drug use in health facilities [3]. Indicators (**Table 1**) addressed include prescribing indicators such as average number of drugs per encounter, % of drugs prescribed by generic name, % of encounters with an antibiotic prescribed, % of encounters with an injection prescribed and % of drugs prescribed from essential drugs list or formulary. Under patient care indicators, we determined average consultation and dispensing times, % of drugs actually dispensed and those adequately labeled. For facility indicators, availability of key drugs and a copy of essential drugs list or formulary were determined. Collected prescriptions were also analyzed for the presence of information with regard to prescriber, patient and prescribed drugs. These include patient's name, age, sex, and address, and the physician's name, address, signature, and license number. The number of drugs per prescription, dosage, frequency of administration, duration of treatment, duplicate drugs of the same therapeutic class, possible drug-drug interactions and whether prescription is clear and illegible were also considered. We also studied the most commonly prescribed therapeutic classes and the most frequently prescribed drug of each common class were counted. Documentation of history of allergy and brief diagnosis of the condition were observed. We also determined the % of prescriptions with increasing number of drugs and the most common pathological conditions for which drugs were prescribed

3. Results

3.1. Prescribing Indicators

As shown in **Table 1** the number of prescriptions studied was 520 with a total number of 1,336 drugs prescribed and an average number of 2.6 drugs per prescription. The percentages of encounters with an antibiotic and those with an injection were 44.6% and 0.38% respectively. All prescribed drugs were from a formulary namely embedded in the electronic prescribing system used in the hospital.

3.2. Patient Care Indicators

Average consultation and dispensing times were 20 and 12 minutes respectively. All prescribed drugs were adequately labeled using the electronic system, and almost all (98%) of the prescribed drugs were actually dispensed. Parent's knowledge of correct dosage was not assessed in the present study (**Table 1**).

3.3. Facility Indicators

The electronic system of the hospital relies on an electronic drug formulary. In addition, the British National Formulary (BNF) was also available (**Table 1**).

Patients were distributed into males (56.34%) and females (43.65%). The majority (53.46%) of patients were 13 months - 6 years of age. Neonates comprised (1.15%), infants (5 weeks - 1 year, 13.65%) and the rest (31.73%) were 6 - 12 years of age (**Table 2**).

All prescriptions were electronic and were head lettered by the name of the hospital. As shown in **Table 3**, patient's name, age and gender were present in 100% of the prescriptions. Patients address, history of allergy and brief diagnosis of the condition were present in 21.15%, 83.26% and 64.42% of the prescriptions respectively. Regarding the prescriber information, the name was present in 100 % of the prescriptions while signature of the prescriber was an electronic one.

Table 3, also shows that the dose, route of administration, frequency of administration and the duration of treatment were present in all prescriptions. All drugs were prescribed by generic name. As shown in **Table 4**, patients were prescribed one, two, three, four or more than four drugs per prescription in 24%, 28%, 26.53%, 12.69% and 8.65% respectively.

Table 2. Distribution of pediatric outpatients according to age and gender.

	Parameter	Number of patients (%) (n = 520)
Age	Neonates (up to 4 weeks)	6 (1.15%)
	Infants (5 weeks - 1 year)	71 (13.65%)
	Children (13 months - 6 years)	278 (53.46%)
	Children (7 - 12 years)	165 (31.73%)
Sex	Females	227 (43.65%)
	Males	293 (56.34%)

Table 3. Percentages of prescriptions containing prescriber's, patient's and prescribed drug's information.

	Information	% (n = 520)
Prescriber's	Name	100%
	Address	100%
	Signature	E-signature
Patient's	Name	100%
	Address	100%
	Gender	100%
	Address	21.15%
	Allergy	83.26%
	Diagnosis	64.42%
Drug	Dose	100%
	Route of administration	100%
	Frequency of administration	100%
	Duration of treatment	100%

Table 4. Number of drugs per prescription.

Number of drugs/prescription	Number (%) of prescriptions (n = 520)
One drug	125 (24%)
Two drugs	146 (28%)
Three drugs	138 (26.53%)
Four drugs	66 (12.69%)
More than four drugs	45 (8.65%)

Antibiotics were the most commonly (44.6%) prescribed drugs with amoxicillin being the most frequently (40%) given drug. Second in ranking were antihistmaines (43.65%) with xylometazoline (61.23%) and third are the analgesic/antipyretic drugs (32.30%) with paracetamol (87.5%) as number one of this class (**Table 5**). The most frequent diagnosis encountered were in the order of; dermatological disorders, tonsillitis, rhinitis, otitis media, gastroenteritis, upper respiratory tract infection, bronchial asthma, acute bronchitis, fever, iron deficiency anemia, mouth ulceration, urinary tract infection, conjunctivitis, cerebral palsy, cough, enuresis, cerumen impaction, and seizures (**Table 6**).

4. Discussion

Several tools have been introduced to evaluate the quality of prescribing. The aim of this study was to determine

Table 5. Most commonly prescribed therapeutic classes and drugs of each class.

Therapeutic class	Number (%)	Drug (s) (n = 520)	Number (%)
Antibiotics 232(44.6%)		Amoxicillin	93(40.0%)
		Cefuroxime axetil	54 (23.3%)
		Fusidic acid	48 (20.7%)
Antihistamines 227 (43.7%)		Xylometazoline	139 (61.2%)
		Cetirizine HCl	104 (45.8%)
		Loratidine	57 (25.1%)
Analgesics/antipyretics 168(32.3%)		Paracetamol	147 (87.5%)
		Ibuprofen	11 (6.5%)
		Diclofenac	5 (3%)

Table 6. Number and percentage of diagnosed conditions for which drugs were prescribed.

Condition	Number of cases (%) (n = 520)
Dermatological disorders	30 (5.77%)
Tonsillitis	23 (4.42%)
Rhinitis	16 (3.08%)
Otitis media	14 (2.69%)
Gastroentiritis	13 (2.50%)
Upper respiratory tract infection	10 (1.92%)
Bronchial asthma	6 (1.15%)
Acute bronchitis	5 (0.96%)
Fever	5 (0.96%)
Iron deficiency anaemia	4 (0.77%)
Mouth ulceration	3 (0.58%)
Urinary tract infection	3 (0.58%)
Conjunctivitis	2 (0.38%)
Cerebral palsy	2 (0.38%)
Cough	2 (0.38%)
Enuresis	2 (0.38%)
Cerumen impaction Seizures	2 (0.38%)
Seizures	1 (0.19%)

the quality of prescribing in paediatric outpatients in a general hospital in one of the Emirates of United Arab Emirates using the WHO core indicators for drug use. In the present study, the average number of drugs per encounter was 2.6. This is higher than the recommended figure of 2, however, it is similar to 2.5 in India [2], more than that in Ethiopia [21] but less than that in KSA [22]. Prescribing large number of drugs to a child increases the risk of adverse effects, drug interactions, dispensing errors and leads to less understanding of parents of dosages regimens [23] [26]. It has been suggested that the optimal indicator values for the average number of drugs per encounter, and prescribing antibiotics and injections largely depend on disease patterns, policies and treatment guidelines and therefore may vary from country to country and over time [33].

Our results indicate that there is a tendency for polypharmacy as almost 47.87% of prescriptions contain three drugs and more. However, since all prescriptions were electronic, the possible risks of interaction is reduced as the electronic system reminds the prescriber of such possible interactions. Again the electronic system must have had an influence on prescribing as in all encounters only generic drugs were prescribed. Increasing generic prescribing would rationalize the use and reduce the cost of drugs [34]. It has been reported that usually poor generic prescribing is due to non-availability of the pediatric formulations in the hospital pharmacy [27] [35]. In the present study, almost all (98%) of the prescribed drugs were dispensed.

Drug doses, dosing interval, and duration of dosing were present in all encounters. Selection of drugs to be prescribed from an electronic drug database verifies prescriptions and ensures the consideration of all drug related parameters, such as dose, route, and duration of treatment [5].

In the present study, the information on patient's name, age, and gender were present in all encounters. However, address of patient was missing from about 80% of prescriptions. This may not be a problem if the prescriber or pharmacist need to correct an error of prescribing or dispensing or to follow up with the patient because the hospital have the address of the patient in his file. Not mentioning the patient's address constitutes a problem only if the patient has to seek medications outside the hospital and a dispensing error need to be corrected by the community pharmacist who dispensed the medication.

Allergy was not documented in 17% of the prescriptions. This is important particularly in paediatric population and when one consider the high % of encounters (44.6%) with antibiotics. Such use of antibiotics is similar to 43.19% in India [36], much higher than (21%) reported for Omani pediatric population [37] and less than (53.42%) reported in Ethiopia [21]. It is a fact that antibiotics are routinely used for the treatment of pediatric illnesses and still irrationally used for inappropriate indications such as upper respiratory tract infections, acute otitis media and acute gastroenteritis. These three condition were among the most frequently diagnosed in the present study. The irrational use of antibiotics calls for more efforts and effective interventions to promote rational antibiotic use particularly in pediatric population. It is important to stress on the importance of continuous monitoring of drug use in pediatrics as part of evaluation of risk/benefit of therapeutics in children [38].

Results of our study indicate that about one third of encounters did not mention the diagnosis. A brief diagnosis of the condition is also helpful to the pharmacist to ensure that the drugs prescribed are appropriate for the patient's condition [5] and also can be helpful to the pharmacist in correcting, in consultation with the prescriber, any possible medication error. With regard to the prescriber's information, all encounters were letter headed in the name and address of hospital, name of prescriber was mentioned and each encounter carried an electronic signature of the prescriber.

The most commonly prescribed therapeutic class was antibiotics These were encountered in (44.6%) of all prescriptions studied, and amoxicillin (40.0%) was the most commonly prescribed of this class. Antihistamines were the second most commonly (43.65%) prescribed class and xylometazoline (61.23%) was the most common antihistamine used. Third on the list were analgesic antipyretic drugs (32.30%) with paracetamol (87.5%) being the most common drug of the class. Studies from Sweden, the Netherlands, and Denmark showed that anti-infective drugs, respiratory drugs, and dermatological drugs were the most commonly prescribed drugs in pediatric patients [39]-[41]. On the other hand, the most frequently diagnosed conditions were; dermatological disorders, tonsillitis, rhinitis, otitis media, gastroenteritis, upper respiratory tract infection, bronchial asthma, acute bronchitis, fever, iron deficiency anemia. This may have bearing on the most commonly prescribed drug classes.

5. Conclusion

In conclusion, the present study provides baseline data useful for comparison with results of future local pediatric drug utilization studies. Results of the present study indicate that there is, in general, a trend for rational prescribing practice in pediatrics ward of the hospital, especially with regard to information concerning prescriber, patient and prescribed drugs. Attention must be made to document the diagnosed condition and history of allergy. Irrational use of antibiotic for inappropriate indications such as upper respiratory tract infections and acute Otitis media should be discouraged through proper and effective interventions. This could be achieved by stressing on rational drug use, evidence-based medicine and the hazards of irrational antibiotic use in medical curriculum, and continuing medical education and healthcare professional development programs.

Acknowledgements

We are grateful to the administration of Umm Al Qwuain Hospital and Umm Al Qwuain Medical District for their kind cooperation during data collection process.

References

[1]   Rupp, M.T., Schondelmeyer, S.W., Wilson, G.T. and Krause, J.E. (1988) Documenting Prescribing Errors and Pharmacist Interventions in Community Pharmacy Practice. *American Pharmacy*, **28**, 30-37.

[2]   Pandey, A.A., Prakash, S.B. and Bhatkule, R. (2010) Prescription Analysis of Pediatric Outpatient Practice in Nagpur City. *Indian Journal of Community Medicine*, **35**, 70-73. http://dx.doi.org/10.4103/0970-0218.62564

[3]   World Health Organization (1993) How to Investigate Drug Use in Health Facilities: Selected Drug Use Indicators. WHO/DAP/93.1. World Health Organization, Geneva, 1-87.

[4]   Akhtar, M.S., Divya, V., Pillai, K., Kiran, D., Roy, M.S., Najmi, A.K., *et al.* (2012) Drug Prescribing Practices in Paediatric Department of a North Indian University Teaching Hospital. *Asian Journal of Pharmaceutical and Clinical Research*, **5**, 146-149.

[5]   Sharif, S.I., AlShaqra, M., Hajar, H., Shamout, A. and Weis, L. (2008) Patterns of Drug Prescribing in a Hospital in Dubai-UAE. *Libyan Journal of Medicine*, **3**, 10-12.

[6]   Sharif, S.I., Alabdouli, A.H. and Sharif, R.S. (2013) Drug Prescribing Trends in a General Hospital in Sharjah, United Arab Emirates. American. *Journal of Pharmacological Sciences*, **1**, 6-9.

[7]   Guyon, A.B., Barman, A., Ahrned, J.U., Ahmed, A.U. and Alam, M.S. (1994) A Baseline Survey on Use of Drugs at the Primary Health Care Level in Bangladesh. *Bull WHO*, **72**, 265-271.

[8]   Krause, G., Borchert, M., Benzler, J., *et al.* (1999) Rationality of Drug Prescriptions in Rural Health Centres in Burkina Faso. *Health Policy and Planning*, **14**, 291-298. http://dx.doi.org/10.1093/heapol/14.3.291

[9]   Chareonkul, C., Khun, V.L. and Boonshuyar, C. (2002) Rational Drug Use in Cambodia: Study of Three Pilot Health Centers in Kampong Thorn Province. *Southeast Asian Journal of Tropical Medicine and Public Health*, **33**, 418-424.

[10] Desta, Z., Abula, T., Beyene, L., Fantahun, M., Yohannes, A.G. and Ayalew, S. (1997) Assessment of Rational Drug Use and Prescribing in Primary Health Care Facilities in North West Ethiopia. *East African Medical Journal*, **74**, 758-763.

[11] Bosu, W.K. and Ofori-Adjei, D. (2000) An Audit of Prescribing Practices in Health Care Facilities of the Wassa West District of Ghana. *West African Journal of Medicine*, **19**, 298-303.

[12] Hamadeh, G.N., Dickerson, L.M., Saab, B.R. and Major, S.C. (2001) Common Prescriptions in Ambulatory Care in Lebanon. *Annals of Pharmacotherapy*, **35**, 636-640. http://dx.doi.org/10.1345/aph.10175

[13] Simon, N., Hakkou, F., Minani, M., Jasson, M. and Diquet, B. (1998) Drug Prescription and Utilization in Morocco. *Therapie*, **53**, 113-120.

[14] Ravi Shankar, P., Partha, P. and Nagesh, S. (2002) Prescribing Patterns in Medical Outpatients. *International Journal of Clinical Practice*, **56**, 549-551.

[15] Chukwuani, C.M., Onifade, M. and Sumonu, K. (2002) Survey of Drug Use Practices and Antibiotic Prescribing Pattern at a General Hospital in Nigeria. *Pharmacy World and Science*, **24**, 188-195. http://dx.doi.org/10.1023/A:1020570930844

[16] Najmi, M.H., Hafiz, R.A., Khan, I. and Fazli, F.R. (1998) Prescribing Practices: An Overview of Three Teaching Hospitals in Pakistan. *Journal of Pakistan Medical Association*, **48**, 73-77.

[17] Massele, A.Y., Nsimba, S.E. and Rimoy, G. (2001) Prescribing Habits in Church-Owned Primary Health Care Facilities in Dar Es Salaam and Other Tanzanian Coast Regions. *East African Medical Journal*, **78**, 510-514. http://dx.doi.org/10.4314/eamj.v78i10.8958

[18] Trap, B., Hansen, E.H. and Hogerzeil, H.V. (2002) Prescription Habits of Dispensing and Non-Dispensing Doctors in Zimbabwe. *Health Policy and Planning*, **17**, 288-295. http://dx.doi.org/10.1093/heapol/17.3.288

[19] Biswas, N.R., Biswas, R.S., Pal, P.S., *et al.* (2000) Patterns of Prescriptions and Drug Use in Two Tertiary Hospitals in Delhi. *Indian Journal of Physiology and Pharmacology*, **44**, 109-112.

[20] Rehan, H.S. and Lal, P. (2002) Drug Prescribing Pattern of Interns at a Government Healthcare Centre in Northern India. *Tropical Doctor*, **32**, 4-7.

[21] Bergicho, M., Mohammed, M.A. and Wabe, N.T. (2012) Assessment of the Pattern of Drug Prescribing in Pediatrics Ward in Tertiary Setting Hospital in Addis Ababa, Ethiopia. *Gaziantep Medical Journal*, **18**, 61-65.

[22] Gupta, N., Safhi, M.M., Sumaily, J.M.Y. and Agarwal, M. (2013) Drug Prescribing Patterns in Children Registered in the Department of Pediatrics of Jizan General Hospital of Jizan, KSA. *International Journal of Pharmacy and Pharmaceutical Sciences*, **5**, 397-399.

[23] Karande, S., Sankhe, P. and Kulkarni, M. (2005) Patterns of Prescription and Drug Dispensing. *The Indian Journal of Pediatrics*, **72**, 117-121. http://dx.doi.org/10.1007/BF02760693

[24] Ghaleb, M.A. and Wong, I.C. (2006) Medication Errors in Paediatric Patients. *Archives of Disease in Childhood—Education and Practice*, **91**, 20. http://dx.doi.org/10.1136/adc.2005.073379

[25] Thiruthopu, N.S., Mateti, U.V., Bairi, R., Sivva, D. and Martha, S. (2014) Drug Utilization Pattern in South Indian Pediatric Population: A Prospective Study. *Perspectives in Clinical Research*, **5**, 178-183. http://dx.doi.org/10.4103/2229-3485.140558

[26] Dinesh, K.G., Padmasani, L., Vasantha, J., Veera, R.B., Sudhakar, P. and Uma, M.R. (2011) Drug Prescribing Pattern among Pediatricians in an Out-Patient Department of Tertiary Care Teaching Hospital. *Indian Journal of Pharmacy Practice*, **4**, 64-68.

[27] Nazima, Y.M., Sagun, D. and Barna, G. (2009) Prescribing Pattern in a Pediatric Out-Patient Department in Gujarat. *Bangladesh Journal of Pharmacology*, **4**, 39-42.

[28] Shamshy, K., Mufidabegum, I. and Perumal, P. (2011) Drug Utilization of Antimicrobial Drug in Pediatrics Population in a Tertiary Care Hospital in Erode, Tamilnadu, India. *International Journal of PharmTech Research*, **3**, 1530-1536.

[29] Lindell-Osuagwu, L., Korhonen, M.J., Saano, S., Helin-Tanninen, M., Naaranlahti, T. and Kokki, H. (2009) Off-Label and Unlicensed Drug Prescribing in Three Pediatric Wards in Finland and Review of the International Literature. *Journal of Clinical Pharmacology & Therapeutics*, **34**, 277-287. http://dx.doi.org/10.1111/j.1365-2710.2008.01005.x

[30] Kaushal, R., Bates, D.W., Landrigan, C., McKenna, K.J., Clapp, M.D., Federico, F. and Goldmann, D.A. (2001) Medication Errors and Adverse Drug Events in Pediatric Inpatients. *The Journal of the American Medical Association*, **285**, 2114-2120. http://dx.doi.org/10.1001/jama.285.16.2114

[31] You, M.L., Chun, Y., Yung, T.K., Man, Y.H. and Hsiang, Y.C. (2010) Outcomes of Pharmacy Interventions on Pediatric Medication Prescribing Patterns in Taiwan. *International Journal of Clinical and Experimental Medicine*, **2**, 173-180. http://dx.doi.org/10.1016/S1878-3317(10)60027-7

[32] WHO (2007) WHO Model List of Essential Medicines for Children. First List. http://www.who.int/medicines/publications/essentialmedicines/en/index.html

[33] Mahmoud, R.K., Kheder, S.I. and Ali, H.M. (2014) Prescribing Rationality in Khartoum State, Sudan: An update. *Sudan Medical Monitor*, **9**, 61-66. http://dx.doi.org/10.4103/1858-5000.146575

[34] Quick, J.D., Hogerzeil, H.V., Velasquez, G. and Rago, L. (2002) Twenty-Five Years of Essential Medicines. *Bulletin of the World Health Organization*, **80**, 913-914.

[35] Pramil, T., Rajiv, A. and Gaurav, G. (2012) Pattern of Prescribing at a Pediatric Outpatient Setting in Northern India. *Indian Journal of Pharmacy Practice*, **5**, 40-44.

[36] Ashraf, H., Handa, S. and Khan, N.A. (2010) Prescribing Pattern of Drugs in Outpatient Department of Child Care Centre in Moradabad City. *International Journal of Pharmaceutical Sciences Review and Research*, **3**, Article 001.

[37] Al-Balushi, K.A., Al-Ghafri, F., Al-Zakwani, I. and Al-Sawafi, F. (2013) Drug Utilization Pattern in an Omani Pediatric Population. *Journal of Basic and Clinical Pharmacy*, **4**, 68-72.

[38] Chai, G., Governale, L., McMahon, A.W., Trinidad, J.P., Staffa, J. and Murphy, D. (2012) Trends of Outpatient Prescription Drug Utilization in US Children, 2002-2010. *Pediatrics*, **130**, 23-31.

[39] Madsen, H., Andersen, M. and Hallas, J. (2001) Drug Prescribing among Danish Children: A Population-Based Study. *European Journal of Clinical Pharmacology*, **57**, 159-165. http://dx.doi.org/10.1007/s002280100279

[40] Schirm, E., Tobi, H. and de Jong-van den Berg, L.T. (2002) Unlicensed and off Label Drug Use by Children in the Community: Cross Sectional Study. *British Medical Journal*, **324**, 1312-1313. http://dx.doi.org/10.1136/bmj.324.7349.1312

[41] Silwer, L. and Lundborg, C.S. (2005) Patterns of Drug Use during a 15 Year Period: Data from a Swedish County, 1988-2002. *Pharmacoepidemiology and Drug Safety*, **14**, 813-820. http://dx.doi.org/10.1002/pds.1124

12

Evaluation of Cisplatin-Loaded Polymeric Micelles and Hybrid Nanoparticles Containing Poly(Ethylene Oxide)-Block-Poly(Methacrylic Acid) on Tumor Delivery

Andang Miatmoko[1], Kumi Kawano[1], Etsuo Yonemochi[2], Yoshiyuki Hattori[1]*

[1]Department of Drug Delivery Research, Hoshi University, Shinagawa, Japan
[2]Department of Physical Chemistry, Hoshi University, Shinagawa, Japan
Email: *yhattori@hoshi.ac.jp

Abstract

Particulate carriers such as polymeric micelles (PMs) and liposomes have been investigated to increase drug accumulation in tumors and reduce distribution to healthy tissues. In this study, we prepared PM and hybrid nanoparticles (HNPs) with poly(ethylene oxide)-block-poly(methacrylic acid) (PEO-b-PMAA) for loading cisplatin, and evaluated cisplatin release, cytotoxicity, and biodistribution in mice. PM composed of PEO-b-PMAA and HNPs composed of egg phosphatidylcholine (EPC)/PEO-b-PMAA at molar ratios of 50/2.8 (HNP-P5) and 50/50 (HNP-P50), respectively, were prepared by a nanoprecipitation method. The sizes of PM, HNP-P5, and HNP-P50 after inclusion of cisplatin were approximately 200, 100, and 55 nm, respectively, and their entrapment efficiencies were approximately 44% - 66%. In the drug-release study, HNP-P5 and HNP-P50 showed reduced release of cisplatin compared with PM. Regarding the cytotoxic assay, HNP-P5 exhibited lower cytotoxicity for mouse Lewis lung carcinoma (LLC) and mouse colon carcinoma Colon 26 cells than PM and HNP-P50. In terms of biodistribution, PM could significantly improve blood circulation and tumor accumulation after intravenous injection into Colon 26 tumor-bearing mice compared with free cisplatin, but HNP-P5 and HNP-P50 did not. EPC in HNPs might be destabilized in the circulation, although it could reduce release of cisplatin in *in vitro* experiments. This study suggested that polymeric micelles composed of PEO-b-PMAA are a better carrier for cisplatin than hybrid nanoparticles composed of PEO-b-PMAA and EPC.

Keywords

Polymeric Micelles, Hybrid Nanoparticles, Cisplatin, PEO-b-PMAA

---

*Corresponding author.

1. Introduction

Cisplatin is a platinum (Pt) complex classified as an alkylating agent that has been widely used as monochemo-therapy for cancers including lung, testicular, ovarian, bladder, head, neck, and esophageal cancer, or in combination with other drugs such as taxanes, gemcitabines, befuximab, bleomycin, etoposide, and vinca alkaloids [1]-[3]. Despite its clear benefits in clinical therapy, severe side-effects such as nephrotoxicity and distal neuropathy [4] [5], nausea, vomiting, anorexia, hearing loss [6] [7], and liver toxicities [8] have been reported. To overcome the problems of toxicities caused by cisplatin, particulate carriers such as polymeric micelles (PMs) and liposomes have been investigated to obtain high drug accumulation in tumors and reduce distribution to healthy tissues. Liposomal cisplatin, such as PEGylated liposomes e.g. Lipoplatin TM and SPI-077 [9] [10], or pH-sensitive PEGylated liposomes [11], could have high efficacy for the treatment of cancer and reduce the toxicity of cisplatin. However, the low solubility of cisplatin in water causes inefficient entrapment efficiency (7% - 19%) of cisplatin into liposomes [12].

Cisplatin can interact with carboxylic acid in an aqueous environment [13]. Therefore, it can be loaded into PMs composed of a biodegradable block ionomers containing carboxylic acid such as poly(ethylene oxide)-block-poly(methacrylic acid) (PEO-b-PMAA). The polymer has two different functional block segments, called a diblock polymer that can produce PM. Poly(ethylene oxide) (PEO) is a water soluble non-ionic polymer that is relatively non-toxic. It has the ability to reduce the recognition of PM by the immune system, resulting longer retention in plasma in the circulation [14]. In addition, poly(methacrylic acid) (PMAA) can form the inner core of PM by interaction with Pt [15]. Therefore, PM composed of PEO-b-PMAA might be a suitable carrier for cisplatin. However, an excess dilution upon systemic administration often causes the disintegration of PMs [16].

Hybrid nanoparticles (HNPs) consist of polymer and lipid components and have the properties of both lipid vesicles and polymeric micelles [17]. Thus, an additional lipid layer at the surface of hydrophobic block segment, such as with egg phosphatidylcholine (EPC) may be useful to protect the inner core and enhance particle stability. Therefore, in this study, to examine the possibility that incorporating cisplatin into HNPs could improve tumor accumulation of cisplatin *via* stabilization in the circulation, we prepared the PM composed of PEO-b-PMAA and HNPs composed of PEO-b-PMAA and EPC for cisplatin-loading, and compared cisplatin release, cytotoxicity, and biodistribution in mice.

2. Materials and Methods

2.1. Materials

Cisplatin was purchased from Wako Pure Chemical Industries Co., Ltd. (Tokyo, Japan). EPC (Coatsome NC-50) was obtained from NOF Corporation (Tokyo, Japan). PEO-b-PMAA (Mw of PEO = 7,500, Mn of PMAA = 11,000) was purchased from Polymer Source, Inc. (Quebec, Canada). All other reagents used in this study were the finest grade.

2.2. Preparation of Polymeric Micelles and Hybrid Nanoparticles

For preparation of PM, PEO-b-PMAA was dissolved in acetone. For preparation of HNP, the PEO-b-PMAA solution was added into EPC solution dissolved in methanol at a molar ratio of EPC/PEO-b-PMAA of 50/2.8 or 50/50 (HNP-P5 and HNP-P50, respectively). The solution of PEO-b-PMAA or mixture of EPC and PEO-b-PMAA was added dropwise into water and stirred continuously for 30 min at room temperature. In order to remove the organic solvents, these mixtures were dialyzed against water using Spectra Por®7 dialysis membrane with molecular weight cut-off (MWCO) 2,000 (Spectrum Laboratories, Inc., CA, USA).

Cisplatin was incorporated into PM, HNP-P5 and HNP-P50 by direct mixing of cisplatin solution at pH 9 adjusted with ammonia solution at a molar ratio of carboxylic acid of PEO-b-PMAA/cisplatin of 1/2, and then incubated with shaking at 37°C for 48 h. The concentration of carboxylic acid was determined by an acid-base titration method. Finally, free cisplatin was removed from the cisplatin-loaded PM, HNP-P5 and HNP-P50 by centrifugation at 2500 g for 20 min using an Amicon® Ultra filter (MWCO 30,000, Merck Millipore Ltd, Carrigtwohill, Ireland).

2.3. Measurement of Particle Size, ζ-Potential, and Entrapment Efficiency

The particle sizes of PM, HNP-P5 and HNP-P50 were measured by the cumulant method using a light-scattering photometer (ELS-Z2, Otsuka Electronics Co, Ltd., Osaka, Japan) at 25°C after diluting the dispersion to an appropriate volume with water. The ζ-potentials were measured by electrophoresis light-scattering methods using ELS-Z2 at 25°C after diluting the dispersion to an appropriate volume with water. For calculating the entrapment efficiency of cisplatin, cisplatin was extracted from PM, HNP-P5, and HNP-P50 by solubilizing lipid layer using the Bligh and Dyer method [18]. Briefly, 20 μL of PM, HNP-P5, or HNP-P50 solution was mixed with 180 μL 0.1 N HCl solution. A 750 μL aliquot of a solution of methanol: chloroform (1:2), 250 μL chloroform and 250 μL 0.1 N HCl was added and then centrifuged to separate the aqueous (upper) and organic solvent (lower) phases. The cisplatin content of the upper phase was measured with a high-performance liquid chromatography (HPLC) system (Shimadzu Co. Kyoto, Japan) composed of an LC-10 ATVP pump, an SIL-10 AF autoinjector, and an SPD-10 AVP UV detector at an absorbance at 306 nm. The upper phase was applied to an anion exchange column Inertsil AX® (250 mm × 4.6 mm, GL Sciences, Tokyo, Japan) equilibrated in a mixture of 8:40:10:20 (v/v) of ethyl acetate, methanol, water and N, N-dimethylformamide at a flow rate of 1 mL/min. The entrapment efficiency (EE%) of cisplatin in PM, HNP-P5 and HNP-P50 was calculated using the following equation.

EE% = (Amount of drug entrapped)/(Amount of drug added) × 100.

2.4. Drug Release Study

The release studies of cisplatin were performed by placing 200 μL of PM, HNP-P5, or HNP-P50 solution into Spectra Por®7 dialysis tubing with MWCO 3500 (Spectrum Laboratories, Inc.). The PM and HNPs were then immersed in 50 mL of phosphate-buffered saline (PBS; pH 5.5 or 7.4) with continuous stirring in a water bath at 37°C. At various time points, 200 μL aliquots were withdrawn from the outer aqueous solution and replaced with 200 μL of PBS. The Pt concentration was measured by a graphite furnace atomic absorption spectrophotometry (GF-AAS) method after diluting with 0.1 N HCl to an appropriate volume. The analysis program of the GF-AAS involved three steps: 1) a drying stage at 80°C - 100°C for 40 s, 2) an ashing stage at 800°C for 30 s, 3) an atomization stage by heating at 3000°C for 7 s, and then cooling down. The concentration of Pt was measured at 265.9 nm with a slit bandwidth of 0.4 nm, and then converted into cisplatin concentration. Wurster correction was used for calculating the cumulative amount of cisplatin released.

2.5. *In Vitro* Cytotoxic Assay

Murine Lewis lung carcinoma (LLC) and colon carcinoma Colon 26 cells were obtained from the Cell Resource Center for Biomedical Research, Tohoku University (Miyagi, Japan). The cells were cultured in RPMI-1640 medium with 10% heat-inactivated fetal bovine serum and kanamycin (100 μg/mL) in a humidified atmosphere containing 5% CO_2 at 37°C. For the *in vitro* cytotoxic assay, LLC and Colon 26 cells were seeded separately at a density of 1×10^4 cells per well in 96-well plates, respectively, and maintained in the medium for 24 h before treatment.

To examine the cytotoxicity of cisplatin, the cells were treated with medium containing various concentrations of cisplatin in PM, HNP-P5, and HNP-P50, and they were then incubated for 48 h. After treatment, the cell number was determined using a Cell Counting Kit-8 (Dojindo Laboratories, Kumamoto, Japan). Cell viability (%) was expressed relative to the absorbance of untreated cells at 450 nm.

2.6. *In Vivo* Biodistribution Study

All animal experiments were performed with approval from the Institutional Animal Care and Use Committee of Hoshi University. To generate Colon 26 tumors, 1×10^6 cells were inoculated subcutaneously into the flank of female BALB/c mice (female, 6 weeks old, Sankyo Lab. Service Corp., Tokyo, Japan). After the tumor size had reached 100 mm³, PM, HNP-P5, and HNP-P50 were administered intravenously *via* the tail vein at a dose equivalent to 4 mg cisplatin per kg. Twenty-four hours after injection, blood was collected in heparinized tubes by decapitation to obtain plasma, and the tumor and kidneys were excised.

For analysis of Pt levels, plasma, tumor, and kidneys were digested with concentrated HNO_3, and then heated at 70°C for 1 h followed by heating at 120°C overnight. The concentration of Pt was measured by GF-AAS method after diluting with 0.1 N HCl in appropriate volume as described above section, and calculated as μg·Pt/mL plasma or μg·Pt/g tissue.

2.7. Statistical Analysis

All data were produced in replicates and presented as the mean ± SD. To evaluate the significance of differences, data were analyzed by one-way ANOVA, followed by Tukey's HSD post-hoc test, with P values less than 0.05 considered as statistically significant.

3. Results and Discussion

3.1. Characterizations of Hybrid Nanoparticles

PM, HNP-P5, and HNP-P50 were prepared by the nanoprecipitation method. PM consisted of 100% PEO-b-PMAA, and HNP-P5 and HNP-P50 contained at 5.3 and 50 mol% PEO-b-PMAA with EPC, respectively. EPC comprises a polar head of choline, with fatty acid forming the double tail chains [19]. These lipophilic chains are expected to associate with the hydrophobic segment of PEO-b-PMAA to form an additional protective layer of the micelle and avoid micelle breakage during the excessive dilution in body fluids.

The sizes of PM, HNP-P5, and HNP-P50 before inclusion of cisplatin were approximately 220 nm, 110 nm, and 65 nm, respectively, and their ζ-potentials were approximately −21 mV, −13 mV, and −17 mV, respectively (**Table 1**). Generally, the size of PM was smaller than the vesicles of liposomes [20]. However, the size of PM was large compared with HNP-P5 and HNP-P50. It has been reported previously that divalent cation metal is needed to form self-assembly ionomer complexes with PEO-b-PMAA [21]. The large size of PM may relate to the hydration of PEO-b-PMAA by water without divalent cation metals. In contrast, in HNPs, the hydrophobicity of EPC might change the amphiphatic balance of PEO-b-PMAA.

After cisplatin loading, the particle sizes of PM, HNP-P5, and HNP-P50 were not significantly changed, but their ζ-potentials were increased (**Table 1**), indicating that the negatively charged carboxylic acid of PMAA interacted electrostatically with cisplatin. In contrast, increasing the EPC content in HNP slightly reduced entrapment efficiency (**Table 1**), suggesting that the high content of PEO-b-PMAA in PM and HNP-P50 could interact well with cisplatin.

3.2. *In Vitro* Drug-Release Study of Hybrid Nanoparticles

The *in vitro* profiles of cisplatin release from PM, HNP-P5, and HNP-P50 were evaluated by immersing nanoparticles in PBS (pH 5.5 and 7.4). Decreasing the pH from 7.4 to 5.5 increased the release of cisplatin from PM, HNP-P5, and HNP-P50 (**Figure 1(a)**, **Figure 1(b)**). It has been reported that dissociation of cisplatin from PMAA depended on the pH and ionic strength of the environment [15]. HNP-P5 and HNP-P50 showed low release of cisplatin at approximately 40% and 67%, respectively, of the cumulative dose over 120 h in PBS pH 5.5, whereas PM exhibited the highest release of up to 90% (**Figure 1(b)**). HNP-P5 exhibited reduced cisplatin release compared with HNP-P50, indicated that increasing EPC content in HNPs reduced cisplatin release. The presence of the lipid layer could limit water diffusion into the inner part of particles [22]; therefore, the barrier of EPC in HNPs might reduce cisplatin release.

3.3. *In Vitro* Cytotoxicity Assay

Next, we evaluated the cytotoxicity of PM, HNP-P5, and HNP-P50 on Colon 26 and LLC cells by 48 h exposure. PM and HNP-P50 had similar cytotoxic effects on Colon 26 (IC_{50} = 1.79 and 1.71 µg/mL, respectively) (**Figure 2(a)**) and LLC cells (IC50 = 0.42 and 0.87 µg/mL, respectively) (**Figure 2(b)**) compared with cisplatin solution

Table 1. Characterization of polymeric micelle (PM) and hybrid nanoparticles (HNPs) before and after inclusion of cisplatin.

Formulation	Particle size (nm)[a]		ζ-potential (mV)[a]		Entrapment efficiency (%)[a]
	Before	After	Before	After	
PM	221.7 ± 186.4	203.7 ± 194.3	−21.3 ± 4.5	0.5 ± 1.7	66.1 ± 4.0
HNP-P5	107.7 ± 9.4	103.3 ± 7.7	−13.4 ± 0.7	2.2 ± 3.4	44.5 ± 2.4
HNP-P50	65.4 ± 5.5	54.6 ± 4.7	−16.9 ± 1.3	2.5 ± 2.3	56.2 ± 14.3

[a]Each value represents the mean ± SD (n = 3). HNP-P5 and HNP-P50, hybrid nanoparticles (HNPs) composed of egg phosphatidylcholine/poly(ethylene oxide)-block-poly(methacrylic acid) at molar ratios of 50/2.8 and 50/50, respectively.

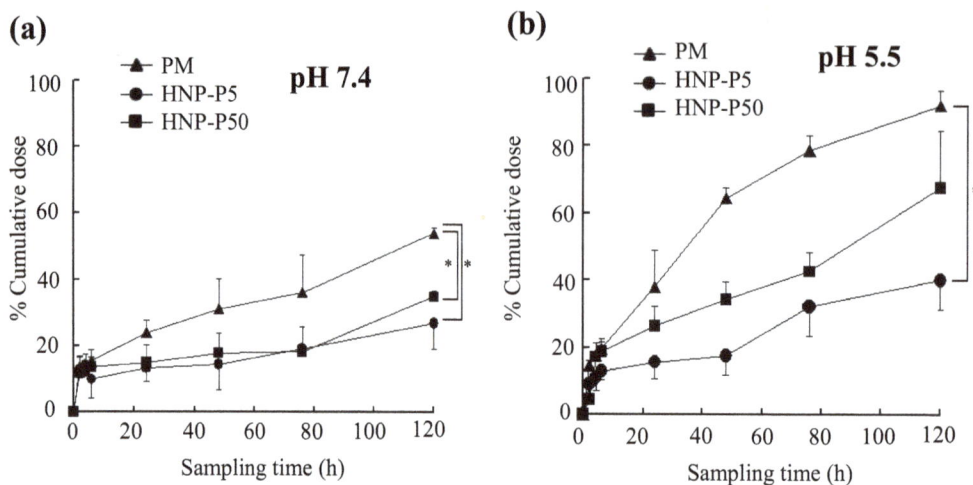

Figure 1. Profiles of cisplatin release from polymeric micelle (PM) and hybrid nanoparticles (HNPs) composed of egg phos phatidylcholine/poly(ethylene oxide)-block-poly(methacrylic acid) at molar ratios of 50/2.8 (HNP-P5) and 50/50 (HNP-P50) in phosphate-buffered saline (PBS), pH 7.4 (a) and pH 5.5 (b) at 37°C. Each value represents mean ± SD (n = 3). *$P < 0.05$.

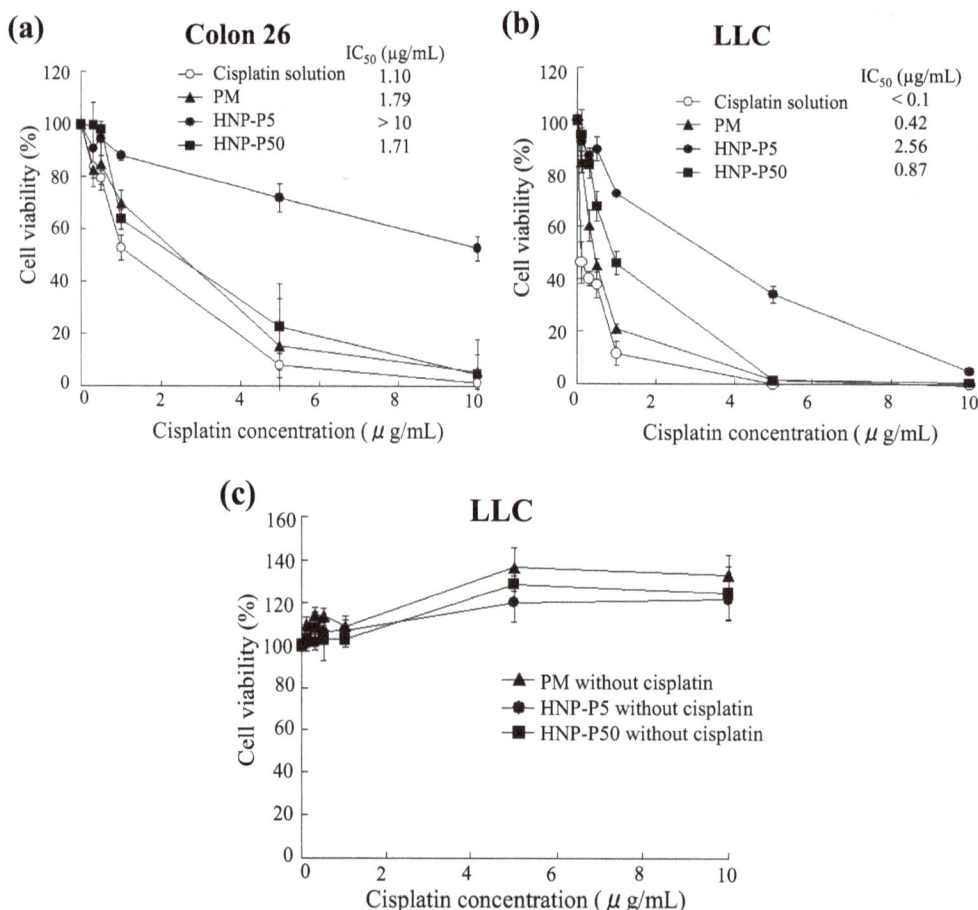

Figure 2. *In vitro* cytotoxicity of polymeric micelle (PM) and hybrid nanoparticles (HNPs) composed of egg phosphatidyl-choline/poly(ethylene oxide)-block-poly(methacrylic acid) at molar ratios of 50/2.8 (HNP-P5) and 50/50 (HNP-P50) with Colon 26 cells (a) and Lewis lung carcinoma (LLC) cells ((b), (c)). Cisplatin-loaded PM, HNP-P5, and HNP-P50 were incu-bated at various concentrations of cisplatin ((a) and (b)) for 48 h. In (c), PM, HNP-P5, and HNP-P50 without cisplatin were incubated with LLC cells. The concentration of cisplatin indicates the same amount of PM or HNPs with cisplatin-loaded PM or HNPs. Each value represents mean ± SD (n = 3).

(IC_{50} = 1.10 µg/mL for Colon 26 and <0.1 µg/mL for LLC cells). In contrast, HNP-P5 decreased cytotoxic effects ($IC_{50} \geq$ 10 µg/mL for Colon 26 and 2.56 µg/mL for LLC) compared with PM and HNP-P50. These results correlated well with the slow release of cisplatin from HNPs. Furthermore, to confirm the effect of carriers on the cell viability, LLC cells were exposed to PM, HNP-P5, and HNP-P50 without cisplatin, and no effects were observed on the cell viability (**Figure 2(c)**).

3.4. *In Vivo* Biodistribution after Intravenous Injection

Finally, we evaluated the biodistribution 24 h after injection of cisplatin-loaded PM, HNP-P5, and HNP-P50 on Colon 26 tumor-bearing mice. Compared with cisplatin solution (0.1 µg·Pt/mL plasma), which was almost cleared from the systemic circulation, the concentration of Pt in plasma after injection of PM remained at 5.3 µg·Pt/mL at 24 h (**Figure 3(a)**). Higher tumor accumulation of cisplatin was also observed with PM (1.7 µg·Pt/g tumor) than HNP-P5 or HNP-P50 (0.5 and 0.9 µg·Pt/g tumor, respectively) (**Figure 3(b)**). This suggested that PM could significantly improve tumor accumulation of cisplatin by prolonged circulation in the bloodstream (EPR effect), compared with cisplatin solution. Although HNP-P5 and HNP-P5 did not significantly increase cisplatin levels in plasma and tumors compared with cisplatin solution, they were still better than cisplatin solution. We speculated that EPC in HNPs might be destabilized in the circulation by interaction with blood components, although it could reduce the release of cisplatin in the *in vitro* experiments (**Figure 1** and **Figure 2**). In contrast, the accumulation of cisplatin in the kidneys after injection of PM, HNP-P5, and HNP-P50 was low and did not show significant differences (**Figure 3(c)**). We also prepared other types of HNPs composed of EPC/ PEO-b-PMAA/sodium deoxycholate or EPC/PEO-b-PMAA/Tween 80 at a molar ratio of 50/2.8/5, and evaluated their biodistribution at 24 h after intravenous injection into mice; however, their cisplatin levels in plasma (1.1 and 0.8 µg·Pt/mL, respectively) and tumor (0.3 and 0.3 µg·Pt/g tumor, respectively) were low compared with PM (data not shown). In HNPs, further improvement might be required to obtain better stability *in vivo*. Using lipids with higher phase transition temperature such as HSPC for the formulation of HNPs may be able to improve *in vivo* tumor delivery.

4. Conclusion

In the present study, we found that hybrid nanoparticles composed of PEO-b-PMAA and EPC showed improved *in vitro* stability; however, they did not increase circulatory concentration or tumor accumulation of cisplatin after intravenous injection compared with PM composed of PEO-b-PMAA. The present work suggested that further improvement of the formulation of hybrid nanoparticles might be required to obtain better stability *in vivo*.

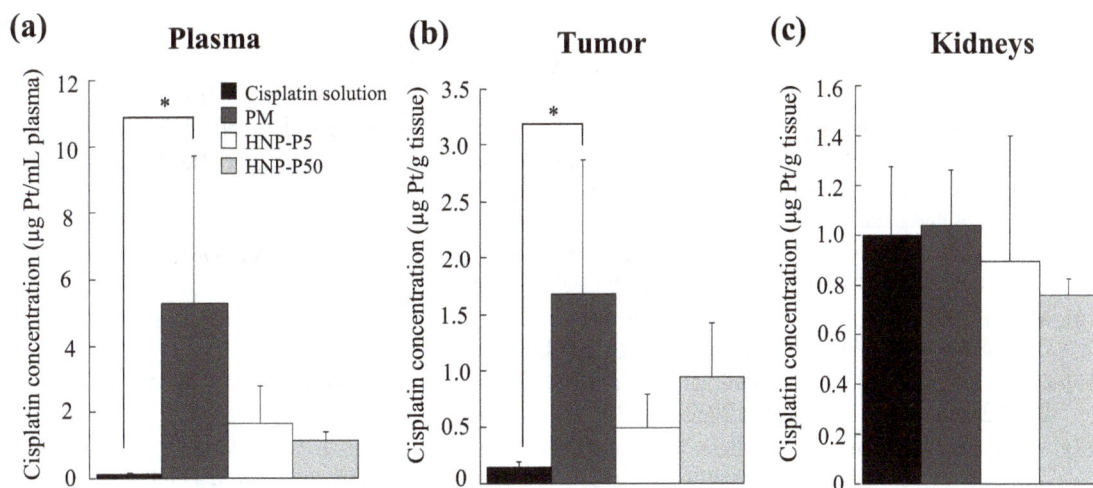

Figure 3. Biodistribution of cisplatin in Colon 26 tumor-bearing mice at 24 h after a single intravenous injection of polymeric micelle (PM) or hybrid nanoparticles (HNPs) composed of egg phosphatidylcholine/poly(ethylene oxide)-block-poly(methacrylic acid) at molar ratios of 50/2.8 (HNP-P5) and 50/50 (HNP-P50) at doses equal to 4 mg cisplatin per kg. Each value represents mean ± SD (n = 4). *P < 0.05.

Conflicts of Interest

The authors declare that they have no potential conflict of interests by any means to any institution, organization while publishing this study.

References

[1]   Kelland, L. (2007) The Resurgence of Platinum-Based Cancer Chemotherapy. *Nature Reviews Cancer*, **7**, 573-584. http://dx.doi.org/10.1038/nrc2167

[2]   Homesley, H.D., Bundy, B.N., Hurteau, J.A. and Roth, L.M. (1999) Bleomycin, Etoposide, and Cisplatin Combination Therapy of Ovarian Granulosa Cell Tumors and Other Stromal Malignancies: A Gynecologic Oncology Group Study. *Gynecologic Oncology*, **72**, 131-137. http://dx.doi.org/10.1006/gyno.1998.5304

[3]   Ray-Coquard, I., Biron, P., Bachelot, T., Guastalla, J.P., Catimel, G., Merrouche, Y., Droz, J.P., Chauvin, F. and Blay, J.Y. (1998) Vinorelbine and Cisplatin (CIVIC Regimen) for the Treatment of Metastatic Breast Carcinoma after Failure of Anthracycline- and/or Paclitaxel-Containing Regimens. *Cancer*, **82**, 134-140. http://dx.doi.org/10.1002/(SICI)1097-0142(19980101)82:1<134::AID-CNCR16>3.0.CO;2-3

[4]   Miller, R.P., Tadagavadi, R.K., Ramesh, G. and Reeves, W.B. (2010) Mechanisms of Cisplatin Nephrotoxicity. *Toxins (Basel)*, **2**, 2490-2518. http://dx.doi.org/10.3390/toxins2112490

[5]   Quasthoff, S. and Hartung, H.P. (2002) Chemotherapy-Induced Peripheral Neuropathy. *Journal of Neurology*, **249**, 9-17. http://dx.doi.org/10.1007/PL00007853

[6]   Kurihara, N., Kubota, T., Hoshiya, Y., Otani, Y., Ando, N., Kumai, K. and Kitajima, M. (1996) Pharmacokinetics of Cis-Diamminedichloroplatinum (II) Given as Low-Dose and High-Dose Infusions. *Journal of Surgical Oncology*, **62**, 135-138. http://dx.doi.org/10.1002/(SICI)1096-9098(199606)62:2<135::AID-JSO10>3.0.CO;2-7

[7]   Simon, T., Hero, B., Dupuis, W., Selle, B. and Berthold, F. (2002) The Incidence of Hearing Impairment after Successful Treatment of Neuroblastoma. *Klinische Padiatrie*, **214**, 149-152. http://dx.doi.org/10.1055/s-2002-33179

[8]   El-Sayyad, H., Ismail, M.F., Shalaby, F.M., Abou-El-Magd, R.F., Gaur, R.L., Fernando, A., Raj, M.H. and Ouhtit, A. (2009) Histopathological Effects of Cisplatin, Doxorubicin and 5-Flurouracil (5-FU) on the Liver of Male Albino Rats. *International Journal of Biological Sciences*, **5**, 466-473. http://dx.doi.org/10.7150/ijbs.5.466

[9]   Newman, M.S., Colbern, G.T., Working, P.K., Engbers, C. and Amantea, M.A. (1999) Comparative Pharmacokinetics, Tissue Distribution, and Therapeutic Effectiveness of Cisplatin Encapsulated in Long-Circulating, Pegylated Liposomes (SPI-077) in Tumor-Bearing Mice. *Cancer Chemotherapy and Pharmacology*, **43**, 1-7. http://dx.doi.org/10.1007/s002800050855

[10] Slingerland, M., Guchelaar, H.J. and Gelderblom, H. (2012) Liposomal Drug Formulations in Cancer Therapy: 15 Years along the Road. *Drug Discovery Today*, **17**, 160-166. http://dx.doi.org/10.1016/j.drudis.2011.09.015

[11] Leite, E.A., Giuberti Cdos, S., Wainstein, A.J., Wainstein, A.P., Coelho, L.G., Lana, A.M., Savassi-Rocha, P.R. and De Oliveira, M.C. (2009) Acute Toxicity of Long-Circulating and pH-Sensitive Liposomes Containing Cisplatin in Mice after Intraperitoneal Administration. *Life Sciences*, **84**, 641-649. http://dx.doi.org/10.1016/j.lfs.2009.02.002

[12] Carvalho Jr., A.D., Vieira, F.P., Melo, V.J., Lopes, M.T., Silveira, J.N., Ramaldes, G.A., Garnier-Suillerot, A., Pereira-Maia, E.C. and Oliveira, M.C. (2007) Preparation and Cytotoxicity of Cisplatin-Containing Liposomes. *Brazilian Journal of Medical and Biological Research*, **40**, 1149-1157. http://dx.doi.org/10.1590/S0100-879X2006005000125

[13] Cepeda, V., Fuertes, M.A., Castilla, J., Alonso, C., Quevedo, C. and Perez, J.M. (2007) Biochemical Mechanisms of Cisplatin Cytotoxicity. *Anti-Cancer Agents in Medicinal Chemistry*, **7**, 3-18. http://dx.doi.org/10.2174/187152007779314044

[14] Kwon, G.G. and Katoka, K. (2012) Block Copolymer Micelles as Long-Circulating Vehicles. *Advanced Drug Delivery Reviews*, **64**, 237-245. http://dx.doi.org/10.1016/j.addr.2012.09.016

[15] Mori, H. and Muller, A.H.E. (2003) New Polymeric Architectures with (Meth)acrylic Acid Segments. *Progress in Polymer Science*, **28**, 1403-1439. http://dx.doi.org/10.1016/S0079-6700(03)00076-5

[16] Owen, S.C., Chan, D.P.Y. and Shoichet, M.S. (2012) Polymeric Micelle Stability. *Nano Today*, **7**, 53-65. http://dx.doi.org/10.1016/j.nantod.2012.01.002

[17] Mandal, B., Bhattacharjee, H., Mittal, N., Sah, H., Balabathula, P., Thoma, L.A. and Wood, G.C. (2013) Core-Shell-Type Lipid-Polymer Hybrid Nanoparticles as a Drug Delivery Platform. *Nanomedicine*, **9**, 474-491. http://dx.doi.org/10.1016/j.nano.2012.11.010

[18] Bligh, E.G. and Dyer, W.J. (1959) A Rapid Method of Total Lipid Extraction and Purification. *Canadian Journal of Biochemistry and Physiology*, **37**, 911-917. http://dx.doi.org/10.1139/o59-099

[19] Walker, R.A., Gruetzmacher, J.A. and Richmond, G.L. (1998) Phosphatidylcholine Monolayer Structure at a Liq-

uid-Liquid Interface. *Journal of the American Chemical Society*, **120**, 6991-7003. http://dx.doi.org/10.1021/ja980736k

[20] Nishiyama, N. and Kataoka, K. (2006) Current State, Achievements, and Future Prospects of Polymeric Micelles as Nanocarriers for Drug and Gene Delivery. *Pharmacology & Therapeutics*, **112**, 630-648. http://dx.doi.org/10.1016/j.pharmthera.2006.05.006

[21] Kim, J.O., Nukolova, N.V., Oberoi, H.S., Kabanov, A.V. and Bronich, T.K. (2009) Block Ionomer Complex Micelles with Cross-Linked Cores for Drug Delivery. *Polymer Science Series A*: *Polymer Physics*, **51**, 708-718. http://dx.doi.org/10.1134/S0965545X09060169

[22] Hadinoto, K., Sundaresan, A. and Cheow, W.S. (2013) Lipid-Polymer Hybrid Nanoparticles as a New Generation Therapeutic Delivery Platform: A Review. *European Journal of Pharmaceutics and Biopharmaceutics*, **85**, 427-443. http://dx.doi.org/10.1016/j.ejpb.2013.07.002

Preparation of Microcapsules Containing Grape Polyphenol with the Spray Drying Method Followed by the Layer-by-Layer Method

Yoshinari Taguchi, Shinji Arakawa, Natsukaze Saito, Masato Tanaka*

Graduate School of Science and Technology, Niigata University, Niigata, Japan
Email: *tanaka@eng.niigata-u.ac.jp

Abstract

It was tried to prepare the microcapsules containing grape polyphenol with the spray drying method followed by the layer-by-layer method. As grape polyphenol was water soluble, the spray drying method was adopted to obtain the higher content. As the shell material of the first microcapsules prepared by the spray drying method, palmitic acid with the melting point of 60°C was adopted in order to prevent grape polyphenol from dissolution into water. As the shell material of the second microcapsules prepared by the layer-by-layer method, chitosan was used to coat the first microcapsules and to give the microcapsules alcohol resistance. In the experiment, the spray drying conditions such as the inlet temperature and the spraying pressure, the oil soluble surfactant species and the chitosan concentration were changed. The mean diameters of microcapsules could be controlled in the range from 5 μm to 35 μm by changing the spraying pressure and the inlet temperature. The yield of microcapsules and the microencapsulation efficiency over 50% could be obtained under the conditions of P = 1.0 kgf/cm^2 and T_{in} = 100°C. Furthermore, the microencapsulation efficiency could be increased by adding the oil soluble surfactant with the larger HLB value. Coating with chitosan could considerably increase alcohol resistance.

Keywords

Grape Polyphenol Containing Microcapsules, Palmitic Acid Shell, Chitosan Shell, Spray Drying Method, Layer-by-Layer Method

---

*Corresponding author.

1. Introduction

Many kinds of microcapsules have been prepared with the chemical and the physicochemical method and applied in various fields such as latent heat storage, cosmetics, foods, drugs, paintings, adhesives, textile, electric materials and so on [1]-[3].

The main functions of microcapsules are to protect the core materials from environment for the desired time, to optionally release the core materials according to appropriate stimuli and to modify the surface of core materials [1]-[3]. The microcapsules with these functions can be prepared by selecting the core and the shell materials with the desired chemical and physicochemical properties and by developing the microencapsulation procedure.

In these microencapsulation methods, the spray drying method has been generally utilized to prepare various powdery composite particles and microcapsules, because the products with stable quality can be continuously manufactured in large quantities [4]-[6]. Furthermore, the spray drying method has a strong point that the various shell materials can be used to prepare the microcapsules [7] [8].

It is well known that grape polyphenol is water-soluble and has a few physiological effects such as anti-aging effect and anti-oxidation effect, but has a few defects such as a bitter taste and reaction activity [9]. Accordingly, if grape polyphenol could be microencapsulated with some edible shell materials and released by appropriate stimulus, it should be expected that the application fields of grape polyphenol will be considerably extended.

Various stimuli-responsive microcapsules for optionally releasing the core material have been applied in many fields such as drug delivery systems (DDS), painting, self-healing agent, cosmetics, foods, and agriculture [2] [3].

As stimuli, mechanical pressure, temperature, water, pH, specified enzyme and ultra violet ray have been utilized according to the physical properties of shell materials.

Among these stimuli, temperature was frequently utilized for controlled release of the core material. As the temperature-responsive shell materials, fatty acids, paraffin wax, fatty acid ester and polymers (poly-N-isopropylacryl-amid) have been applied to form the microcapsule shell. Furthermore, if the thermal responsible shell microcapsules could be coated by another shell material, the microcapsules could be applied in the extensive fields, because the microcapsules could be given another stimuli responsibility.

In this study, it was tried to microencapsulate grape polyphenol with palmitic acid as a hydrophobic shell material by using the spray drying method followed by the layer-by-layer method in order to give alcohol resistance with chitosan shell. The purposes of this study are to prepare the microcapsules containing grape polyphenol with the spray drying method, to coat the microcapsules with chitosan by the layer-by-layer method and to characterize the microcapsules.

2. Experimental

2.1. Materials

Materials used to prepare the microcapsules containing grape polyphenol were as follows.

Grape polyphenol (GP) (Sunprite Ind. Co., Ltd., Tokyo, Japan) was used as the core material and palmitic acid (PA) (Wako Pure Chemical Ind. Co., Ltd., Tokyo, Japan) was used as the shell material of first microcapsules. Homologue of polyoxyethylene lauryl ether (POEL) with the different HLB values was added as the oil soluble surfactant. The HLB values of POEL were 6.3, 9.6, 11.3. Hereafter, POELs with the HLB values of 6.3, 9.6 and 11.3 are called as POEL(1), POEL(2), POEL(3), respectively. Chitosan (Nacalai Tesque Ind. Co., Ltd., Kyoto, Japan) was used to coat the first microcapsules with the layer-by-layer method. Acetic acid (Wako Pure Chemical Ind. Co., Ltd., Tokyo, Japan) was used to dissolve chitosan.

2.2. Preparation of Microcapsules

a) Spray drying method

Figure 1 shows the flow chart for preparing the first microcapsules with the spray drying method, where the spray drying machine equipped with the nozzle of 700 μm inner diameter (DL-41: Yamato Science Ind. Co., Tokyo, Japan) was used. The oil solution was prepared by the following two ways.

First, palmitic acid (PA) and grape polyphenol (GP) of a given weight were directly dissolved in ethanol to prepare the oil solution. Second, POEL was dissolved in the oil solution prepared just above in order to stabilize GP and to increase the microencapsulation efficiency. Each oil solution was spray dried by changing the spraying pressure and the inlet temperature to prepare the first microcapsules. **Table 1** shows the experimental conditions.

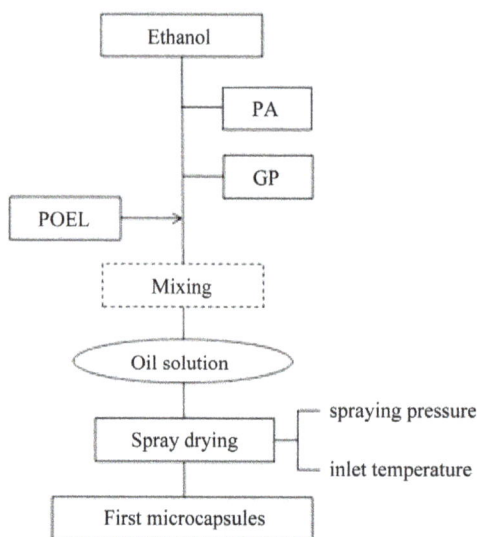

Figure 1. Flow chart for preparing first microcapsules with spray drying.

Table 1. Experimental conditions for preparing first microcapsules.

Oil solution	
Ethanol	200 ml
Palmitic acid (PA)	10 g
Grape polyphenol (GP)	2.5 g
Surfactant (POEL)	1.0 g
HLB of POEL	6.3: POEL(1), 9.6: POEL(2), 11.3: POEL(3)
Spray drying	
Feed velocity	0.6 m^3/min
Spraying pressure	P = 0.5, 1.0, 1.5, 2.0 kgf/cm^2
Inlet temperature	T_{in} = 80, 100, 120, 140°C

b) Layer-by layer method

Figure 2 shows the schematic diagram for preparing the second microcapsules with the layer-by-layer method. Chitosan of a given weight was added into the acetic acid aqueous solution (1 w/vol%) and dissolved. Then, the first microcapsules of a given weight were added into this acetic acid aqueous solution under stirring due to the magnetic stirrer for 20 min. As chitosan is polycation and the first microcapsules charge negatively, chitosan may adsorb and coat the surface of first microcapsule due to hetero-coagulation. After this operation, the second microcapsules were separated out with filtration paper, dried at room temperature and characterized. The second microcapsules were prepared by changing the chitosan concentration (C_S).

Table 2 shows the experimental conditions for preparing the second microcapsules with the layer-by-layer method.

2.3. Characterization

Mean diameter and Zeta potential

The mean diameters and Zeta potential of microcapsules were measured by Particle Size Analyzer (SALD-3000; Shimazu Seisakusho Ind. Co., Kyoto, Japan). Here, the mean diameters were the Sauter mean diameters.

Yield of microcapsules

The yield (Y) of first microcapsules was obtained by the following Equation (1).

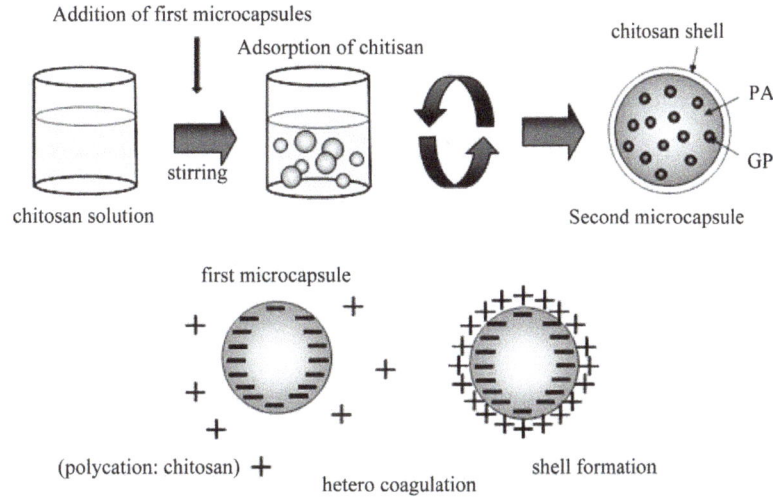

Figure 2. Flow chart for preparing first microcapsules with spray drying.

Table 2. Experimental conditions for preparing second microcapsules.

Distilled water	
Acetic acid	200 ml
First microcapsules	10 g
Chitosan	C_S = 1.0 g (1.0 w/v%), 2.0 g (2.0 w/v%), 3.0 g (3.0 w/v%)
Stirring velocity	1.0 g
Microencapsulation time	6.3: POEL(1), 9.6: POEL(2), 11.3: POEL(3)

$$Y = \frac{\text{weight of microcpsules collected}}{\text{weight of}\left(GP + PA + POEL\right)} \times 100 \tag{1}$$

Microencapsulation efficiency

The microencapsulation efficiency (λ) was measured as follows. The first microcapsules of a given weight were added into distilled water and stirred by the magnetic stirrer for 10 min in order to dissolve the unmicroencapsulated GP. Then, the microcapsules washed with distilled water were added into distilled water of 100 cm^3 and broken by the rotor stator homogenizer under the conditions of stirring velocity of 2000 rpm for 10 min. Furthermore, the microcapsule slurry prepared just above was stirred by the ultrasonic homogenizer for 10min in order to perfectly dissolve GP in water. The concentration of GP in water was measured by the absorption spectrophotometer (UV-160A, Shimazu Seisakusho, Ind. Co., Kyoto, Japan). For this measurement, the calibration curve between the concentration of GP and the absorption degree was obtained beforehand. Then, the microencapsulation efficiency (λ) was calculated by the following Equation (2).

$$\lambda = \frac{\text{weight of GP measured}}{\text{weight of GP in feed}} \times 100 \tag{2}$$

Alcohol resistance

The second microcapsules of a given weight were added in ethylalcohol under stirring due to the magnetic stirrer. Then, the photographs of second microcapsules were taken by the optical microscope at the constant time intervals.

The transient mean diameters of microcapsules were measured from these photographs. Then, the alcohol solution was sampled out and the concentration of GP was measured by the same method as stated above.

Observation

The microcapsules were observed by scanning electron microscope (SEM: JSM-5800) and optical microscope (DP10, OLYMPUS Ind. Co., Ltd., Tokyo, Japan).

3. Results and Discussion

3.1. Effects of Spraying Pressure and Inlet Temperature

Figure 3 shows the SEM photographs of first microcapsules prepared by changing the spraying pressure (a) and the inlet temperature (b). The spherical and irregular microcapsules with the wider diameter distributions are observed. The diameters of microcapsules decreased with the spraying pressure (P) and increased with the inlet temperature (T_{in}).

In order to know the dependence of mean diameters on the spraying conditions in detail, the dependences of mean diameters and standard deviations of microcapsules on the spraying pressure (P) and the inlet temperature (T_{in}) are shown in **Figure 4**. With increasing the spraying pressure, the mean diameters drastically decreased

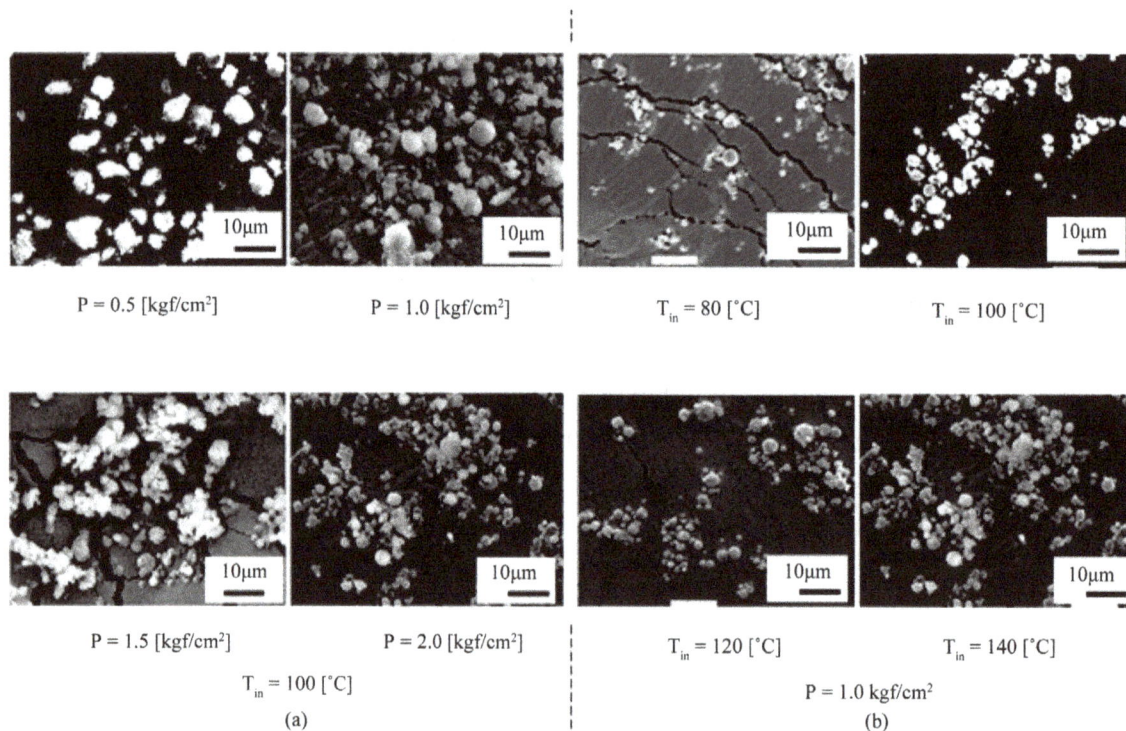

P = 0.5 [kgf/cm²]   P = 1.0 [kgf/cm²] T_{in} = 80 [°C] T_{in} = 100 [°C]

P = 1.5 [kgf/cm²]   P = 2.0 [kgf/cm²] T_{in} = 120 [°C] T_{in} = 140 [°C]

T_{in} = 100 [°C]

P = 1.0 kgf/cm²

(a)   (b)

Figure 3. SEM photographs of microcapsules (effects of spraying pressure (a) and inlet temperature (b)).

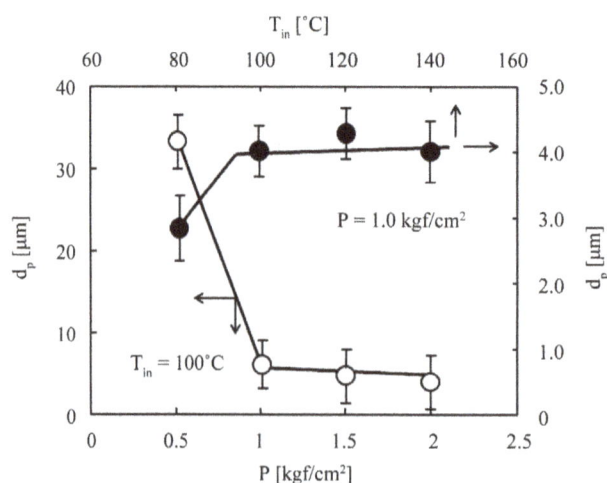

Figure 4. Dependences of mean diameters and standard deviation on spraying pressure and inlet temperature.

from 35 μm at P = 0.5 kgf/cm^2 to 5 μm at P = 1.0 kgf/cm^2 and then gradually decreased. While, with increasing the inlet temperature, the mean diameters slightly increased from 3.2 μm at T_{in} = 80°C to 4.5 μm at T_{in} = 100°C and then kept almost constant. Also, as the dispersion degree (standard deviation/mean diameter) changed from 0.3 to 0.65, the diameter distributions were found to be wider. The higher the inlet temperature, the faster the evaporation speed of ethanol and the faster the preparation of microcapsules. However, the volcanic phenomenon on the surface of oil droplets may occur due to fast evaporation, leading to the unstability of oil droplets [10]. As a result, the first microcapsules may become easy to adhere or coalesce and the diameters of microcapsules may become larger.

Figure 5 and **Figure 6** show the effects of spraying pressure and inlet temperature on the yield (Y) and the microencapsulation efficiency (λ), respectively. With increasing the spraying pressure, the yield and the microencapsulation efficiency increased from Y = 15% at P = 0.5 kgf/cm^2 to Y = 55% at P = 2.0 kgf/cm^2 and from λ = 7% at P = 0.5 kgf/cm^2 to λ = 75% at P = 2.0 kgf/cm^2, respectively.

On the other hand, with increasing the inlet temperature, the yield (Y) and the microencapsulation efficiency (λ) increased from Y = 8% at T_{in} = 80°C to Y = 56% at T_{in} = 140°C and λ = 60% at T_{in} = 80°C to λ = 75% at T_{in} = 140°C, respectively. When the inlet temperature and the spray drying pressure are lower, the sound oil droplets may not be prepared through the nozzle because of higher viscosity of oil solution.

Also, as the diameters of first microcapsules become larger at the low spraying pressure of P = 0.5 kgf/cm^2, the yield and the microencapsulation efficiency may become lower because of the insufficient drying at the lower inlet temperature.

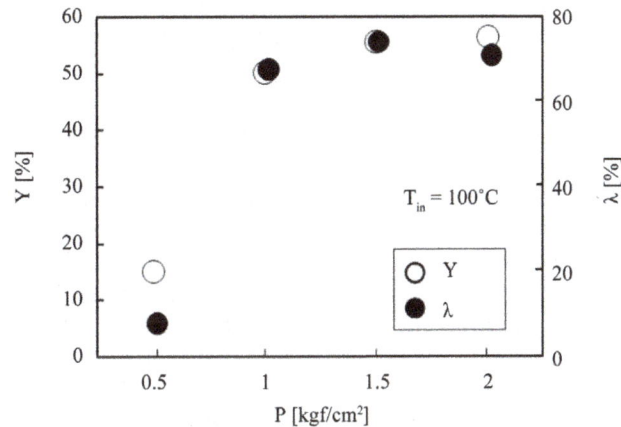

Figure 5. Effect of spraying pressure on yield and microencapsulation efficiency.

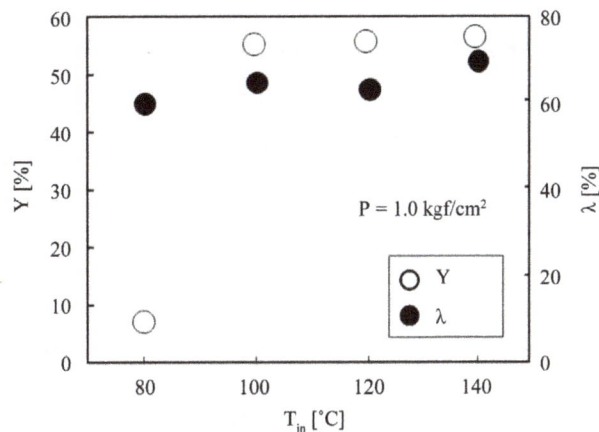

Figure 6. Effect of inlet temperature on yield and microencapsulation efficiency.

3.2. Effect of Addition of Oil Soluble Surfactant

As the low microencapsulation efficiencies were obtained, the oil soluble surfactants with the different HLB values were added to stabilize GP in the oil solution. The effect of oil soluble surfactants on the mean diameters, the yield and the microencapsulation efficiency of microcapsules were investigated, where the first microcapsules were prepared at P = 1.5 kgf/cm^2 and T_{in} = 100°C.

Figure 7 shows the dependencies of the yield, the microencapsulation efficiency and the mean diameters on the oil surfactant species. From **Figure 7**, the following fundamental informations could be obtained. The mean diameters slightly decreased by addition of oil soluble surfactant, but the difference in the mean diameters due to the surfactant species was not clear. And, the diameter distributions become narrower than without the surfactant. The yield increased from Y = 55% without the surfactant to Y = 72% with POEL(3). The microcapsulation efficiency increased λ = 75% without the surfactant to λ = 92% with POEL(3). Increase in the microencapsulation efficiency may be due to increase in the stability of GP in the oil solution. Namely, GP might be stabilized with the wrapping effect due to the hydrophilic group of oil soluble surfactant [11] [12]. As the hydrophilic group of POEL(3) is larger than those of POEL(1) and POEL(2), the stabilization of GP due to the wrapping effect may become stronger.

3.3. Alcohol Resistance

As, generally, the microcapsules prepared by the spray drying were multi core type, it can be expected that the core materials are on the surface of microcapsules [5]-[7]. If the core materials were on the surface of microcapsules, the core materials could not be prevented the microcapsules from contacting with circumstance. In order to solve these troubles, the emulsions were stabilized by adding some surfactants and proteins [4] [7] [8] [13]. Similarly, in this study, the first microcapsules prepared by the spray drying method were coated with the layer-by-layer method.

Namely, in order to give the microcapsules alcohol resistance, the first microcapsules were coated with chitosan by the layer-by-layer method.

Figure 8 shows the optical microscopic photographs of the transient features of first microcapsules (a) and the second microcapsules (b). It was found that the first microcapsules disappeared at 60 min, but the second microcapsules could be observed even at 48 h.

Also, **Figure 9** shows the transient features of the ratios (d_{pt}/d_{po}) of mean diameters, where d_{po} and d_{pt} are the mean diameters at t = 0 and t = t from adding the second microcapsules in ethyl alcohol, respectively. In **Figure 9**, d_{pt}/d_{po} = 1 means that the microcapsules in ethyl alcohol are kept without dissolution. Also, the smaller the values of ratios, the lower the alcohol resistance because of dissolution of microcapsules. The first microcapsules rapidly dissolved in ethanol and disappeared at ca. 1h. Meanwhile, the second microcapsules coated with the chitosan concentration (C_S) of 1.0 w/v% gradually dissolved with elapsing time. However, the second microcapsules coated with the chitosan concentration (C_S) of 2.0 w/v% and 3.0 w/v% did not dissolve and remained even at 48 h.

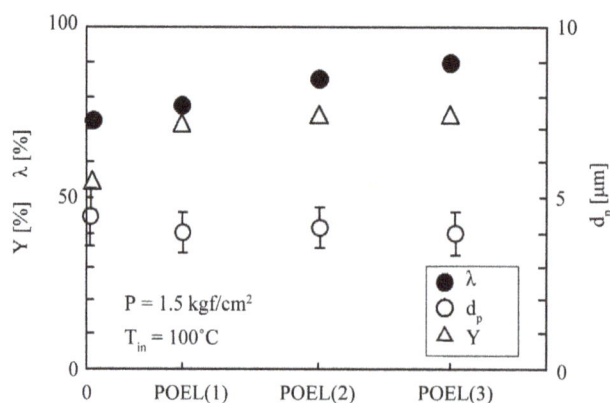

Figure 7. Dependences of microencapsulation efficiency, yield and mean diameter on oil soluble surfactant species.

| 0min | 10min | 30min | 60min |

(a)

| 0min | 10min | 30min | 60min |

| 6h | 12h | 24h | 48h |

(b)

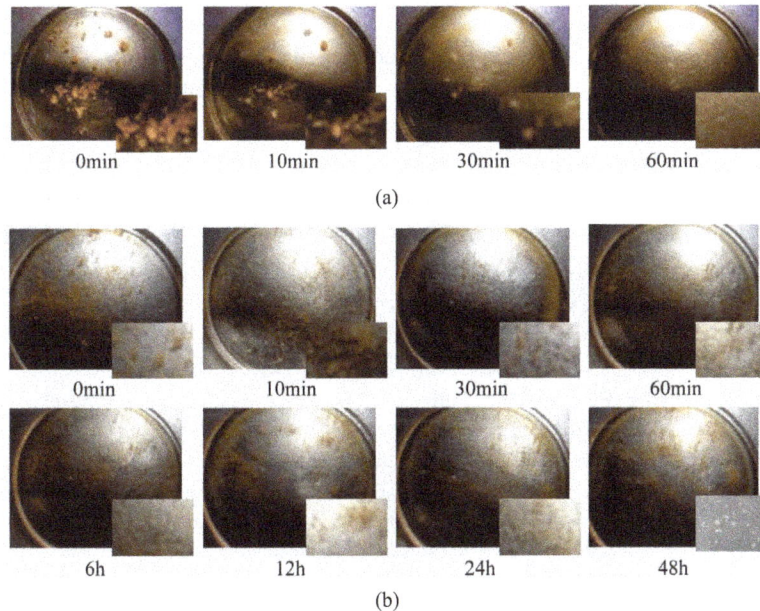

Figure 8. Observation of microcapsules in ethanol. (a) First microcapsules; (b) Second microcapsules (2.0 w/v% of chitosan concentration).

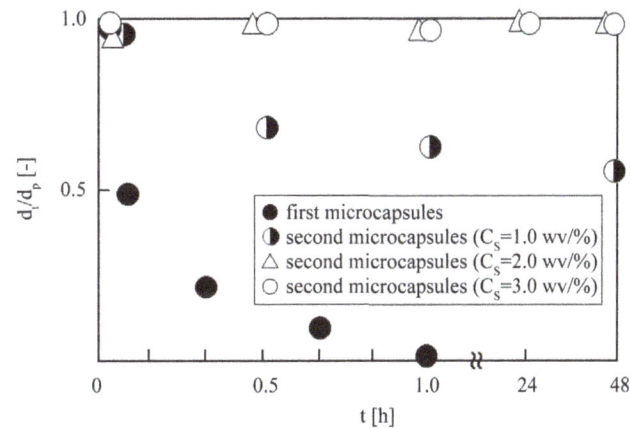

Figure 9. Transient features of ratios of mean diameters of microcapsules.

From these results it was confirmed that the second microcapsules were given alcohol resistance by the chitosan coating. The first microcapsules have the negative surface charge (−5.3 mV) due to the carboxylic group and chitosan is polycation. As a result, chitosan may adsorb on the surface of first microcapsules to form the chitosan shell with alcohol resistance.

4. Conclusions

The palmitic acid microcapsules containing grape polyphenol were prepared with the spray drying method followed by the layer-by-layer method using chitosan. The following fundamental results could be obtained.

1) The microcapsules with the mean diameters from 5 μm to 35 μm could be prepared by changing the spraying pressure and the inlet temperature.

2) The yield and the microencapsulation efficiency could be increased by increasing the spraying pressure and the inlet temperature.

3) The yield and the microencapsulation efficiency could be considerably increased by the addition of oil so-

luble surfactant.

4) The larger the HLA values, the higher the microencapsulation efficiency due to the wrapping effect.

5) The second microcapsules could be given alcohol resistance by chitosan coating.

References

[1]   Tanaka, M. (2008) Key Point of Preparation of Nano/Microcapsules. Techno System Publishing Co. Ltd., Tokyo.

[2]   Kondo, T. (1967) Saishin Maikurokapseruka Gijutsu (Microencapsulation Technique). TES, Tokyo.

[3]   Koishi, M., Eto, K. and Higure, H. (2005) (Preparation + Utilization) Microcapsules. Kogyo Chosakai, Tokyo.

[4]   Shirokawa, K., Taguchi, Y., Yokoyama, H., Ono, F. and Tanaka, M. (2013) Preparation of Temperature and Water Responsive Microcapsules Containing Hydroquinone with Spray Drying Method. *Journal of Cosmetics, Dermatological Sciences and Applications*, **3**, 49-54. http://dx.doi.org/10.4236/jcdsa.2013.33A2012

[5]   Soottitantawat, A., Bigeard, F., Uoshii, H., Furuta, T., Ohkawara, A. and Linko, P. (2005) Influence of Emulsion and Powder Size on the Stability of Encapsulated D-Limonene by Spray Drying. *Innovative Food Science and Emerging Technologies*, **6**, 107-114. http://dx.doi.org/10.1016/j.ifset.2004.09.003

[6]   Polavarapu, S., Oliver, C.M., Ajlouni, S. and Augustin, M.A. (2012) Impact of Extra Virgin Olive Oil and Ethylenediaminetetraacetic Acid (EDTA) on the Oxidative Stability of Fish Oil Emulsions and Spray-Dried Microcapsules Stabilized by Sugar Beet Pectin. *Journal of Agricultural and Food Chemistry*, **60**, 444-450. http://dx.doi.org/10.1021/jf2034785

[7]   Laohasongkram, K., Mahamaktudsanee, T. and Chaiwanichsiri, S. (2011) Microencapsulation of Macadamia Oil by Spray Drying. *Procedia Food Science*, **1**, 1660-1665. http://dx.doi.org/10.1016/j.profoo.2011.09.245

[8]   Gharsallaoui, A., Roudaut, G., Beney, L., Chambin, O., Voilley A. and Saurel, R. (2012) Properties of Spray-Dried Food Flavours Microencapsulated with Two-Layered Membranes: Roles of Interfacial Interactions and Water. *Food Chemistry*, **132**, 1713-1720. http://dx.doi.org/10.1016/j.foodchem.2011.03.028

[9]   Xia, E.Q., Deng, G.F., Guo, Y.J. and Li, H.B. (2010) Biological Activities of Polyphenols from Grapes. *International Journal of Molecular Sciences*, **11**, 622-646. http://dx.doi.org/10.3390/ijms11020622

[10] Yokoyama, H., Mo, L., Taguchi, Y. and Tanaka, M. (2008) Effect of Viscosity of Shell Solution on the Content of Solid Powder as Core Material in Microencapsulation by the Drying-in-Liquid Method. *Journal of Applied Polymer Science*, **109**, 1585-1593. http://dx.doi.org/10.1002/app.24765

[11] Kobayashi, S., Taguchi, Y. and Tanaka, M. (2005) Preparation of Nanospheres Containing Dye by Mini Emulsion Polymerization. *Journal of the Japan Society of Colour Material*, **78**, 260-264. http://dx.doi.org/10.4011/shikizai1937.78.260

[12] Erdem, B., Sudol, E.D., Dimonie, V.L. and El-Aasser, M.S. (2000) Encapsulation of Inorganic Particles via Miniemulsion Polymerization. *Macromolecular Symposia*, **155**, 181-198. http://dx.doi.org/10.1002/1521-3900(200004)155:1<181::AID-MASY181>3.0.CO;2-2

[13] Gharsallaoui, A., Saurel, R., Chambin, O., Cases, E., Voilley, A. and Cayot, P. (2010) Utilisation of Pectin Coating to Enhance Spray-Dry Stability of Pea Protein-Stabilised Oil-in-Water Emulsions. *Food Chemistry*, **122**, 447-454. http://dx.doi.org/10.1016/j.foodchem.2009.04.017

14

Anti-M$_3$ Muscarinic Acetylcholine Receptor Antibodies in Systemic Lupus Erythematosus

Silvia Reina[1,2], Cecilia Pisoni[3], Alicia Eimon[3], Carolina Carrizo[3], Roberto Arana[3], Enri Borda[1,2]*

[1]Pharmacology Unit, School of Dentistry, University of Buenos Aires, Buenos Aires, Argentina
[2]National Research Council of Argentina (CONICET), Buenos Aires, Argentina
[3]Section of Rheumatology and Immunology, Department of Internal Medicine, CEMIC, Buenos Aires, Argentina
Email: *enri@farmaco.odon.uba.ar

Abstract

Background: Evidences have shown that anti-M$_3$ muscarinic acetylcholine receptor IgG (anti-M$_3$ mAChR IgG) are clinically useful autoantibody that exert a cholinergic pharmacologic effect binding and interacting with M$_3$ mAChR at the level of exocrine gland (salivary and ocular). *Aims*: The aim of this study was to determine the associations between serum level of anti-M$_3$ mAChR IgG in patients with systemic lupus erythematosus (SLE) and other autoantibodies, serum prostaglandin E$_2$ (PGE$_2$), and clinical manifestations. *Methods*: Serum autoantibodies against M$_3$ mAChR synthetic peptide were measured by enzyme-linked immuno absorbent assay (ELISA) using, as an antigen, a 25-mer peptide K-R-T-V-P-D-N-Q-C-F-I-Q-F-L-S-N-P-A-V-T-F-G-T-A-I corresponding to the amino acid sequence of the second extracellular loop of the human M$_3$ mAChR. Serum levels of antinuclear antibodies (ANA), anti-Smith (Sm) antibodies, anti-phospholipid (APL) antibodies, and PGE$_2$ were determined by ELISA in patients with SLE. *Results*: We found significantly enhanced titers of anti-M$_3$ mAChR IgG in sera from SLE patients compared with healthy individuals (control). In addition, serum levels of PGE$_2$ were significantly higher in SLE patients than in control patients and were significantly higher in active than in non-active SLE. No correlation was found with other autoantibodies present in SLE. By contrast, a positive correlation was found between anti-M$_3$ mAChR IgG and PGE$_2$ serum levels in SLE. *Conclusions*: As anti-M$_3$ mAChR antibodies present in the sera of SLE patients may be another factor in the pathogenesis of this disease, and the increment of PGE$_2$ in the sera of SLE has a modulatory action on the inflammatory process, suggesting that the presence of these autoantibodies against M$_3$ mAChR may contribute to sustained immune deregulation and the strong inflammatory component observed in SLE.

---

*Corresponding author.

Keywords

Anti-M$_3$ mAChR Antibodies, Systemic Lupus Erythematosus, Prostaglandin E$_2$

1. Introduction

The onset and development of autoimmune disease (AID) are the consequence of interactions between genetic and environmental factors, which result in dysregulation of the immune system, and are characterized by the presence of autoantibodies and autoreactive T cells. Under these circumstances, immune system antimicrobial defenses react against normal components of the body and result in organ-specific or systemic immunopathology. Autoantibodies may also appear in the blood of healthy individuals or in some special situations, such as infection and the pre-clinical phase of infectious diseases [1]-[3].

Systemic lupus erythematosus (SLE) is an autoimmune disease characterized by the production of multiple autoantibodies [4]-[8], with an inflammatory/necrotic phenomenon in different tissues [9] [10]. This condition is associated with hyperactivity of B cells, and different immuno-regulatory abnormalities [11] [12]. In addition, T cells from SLE patients exhibit defects in early activation events as well as an impaired proliferative response to mitogenic lectins [12] [13]. Furthermore, anti-nuclear (ANA), anti-Smith (anti-Sm), anti-phospholipid (APL), and other autoantibodies are detected in patients with SLE [4] [14] [15]. One early study, in which 23 asymptomatic pregnant women with positive anti-Ro or anti-La titers were followed for many years, reported that four subjects developed SLE, which suggested that anti-Ro or anti-La antibodies preceded the development of SLE [16]. In another study, Aho *et al.* reported that SLE patients were positive for ANA before the onset of SLE and the percentage was much higher than that of controls which was a much higher rate than controls [17]. Moreover, the results from the United States Department of Defense Serum Repository showed that the presence of ANA, anti-Ro, anti-La, anti-double strain deoxyribonucleic acid (anti-ds DNA), anti-Sm, APL, anti-ribonucleo protein (anti-nRNP) antibodies and rheumatoid factor (RF) preceded the onset of SLE [18]-[20]. Among SLE patients, 88% were positive for at least one of these autoantibodies, which was a much higher percentage than healthy controls, and the prevalence of these autoantibodies increased after diagnosis [21] [22]. Anti-Ro, anti-La, and APL antibodies were the earliest detectable autoantibodies during the pre-clinical phase of rheumatoid arthritis (RA) [18]-[22]. In addition, the presence of these autoantibodies was associated with incipient severe SLE. For example, patients who were positive for anti-ds DNA antibodies often developed renal disease [22] [23], patients who were positive for IgG RF were more likely to develop arthritis [18], and positive APL was associated with malar rash and photosensitivity [19]. In addition, regular patterns exist among these autoantibodies. The majority of La-positive pre-clinical SLE patients were also Ro-positive, and a significant overlap was observed between patients positive for anti-ds DNA antibody and those positive for anti-chromatin antibody [20].

A recently published nested case-control study showed that 66% of Sjögren Syndrome (SS) patients were positive for ANA, RF, and anti-La or anti-Ro antibodies approximately 5 years before the onset of SS. A maximum of 18 years elapsed between positivity for these antibodies and the onset of SS in these subjects [23]. The seropositive rate for these antibodies and the anti-M$_3$ muscarinic acetylcholine receptor (mAChR) autoantibodies increased as the onset of SS neared [24]-[26]. In conclusion, the evidence suggests that these autoantibodies are predictors of SS. Moreover, the presence of these autoantibodies in the serum of patients with SLE is another topic of discussion in SLE pathogenesis.

The autoimmune nature of lupus and its predominant inflammatory component was accompanied by the expression of cyclo-oxygenase-2 (COX-2) in the inflammatory areas, with the subsequent release of arachidonic acid via membrane-bound phospholipase A$_2$. The biosynthesis of arachidonic acid by COX-2 led to an enhancement of prostanoid production of PGE2 serie, which conduct to the dysregulation in the production of proinflammatory cytokines (IL-6, IL-10, and nitric oxide) [27] [28]. Therefore, we focused on the family of prostaglandins (PG), which are the result of the oxidative modification of arachidonic acid and its cascade products through COX-2 expression and activation in patients with SLE.

2. Aim

The aim of our preliminary study was to investigate the inflammatory status in SLE patients compared to active and non-active groups by assessing the generation of PGE$_2$ and its association with the presence or absence of anti M_3 mAChR autoantibodies and SLE disease activity index (SLEDAI).

3. Methodology

3.1. Patients

Blood samples from 30 patients with SLE, according to the classification criteria of the American College of Rheumatology (ACR) [29] were obtained. A total of 26 women subjects and four men subjects with a mean age of 41.4 ± 11.9 years were included in the study. Also, blood samples of 30 healthy women subjects with a mean age of 39.6 ± 10.2 years were used as controls. Fifteen patients had non-active disease (<3) and 15 were considered to have active disease (≥3), according to the SLEDAI measured [30] [31]. Most patients were receiving low to moderate doses of glucocorticoids as well as immunosuppressive drugs-mainly cyclophosphamide, methotrexate, azathioprine, and chloroquine. No patients with renal failure or conditions different from SLE were included in the study. The demographic and clinical characteristics of the study population (SLE patients) and normal individuals (controls) are shown in **Table 1**. All of the patients signed an informed consent form to participate in the study, and the investigation was conducted according to the tenets of the Declaration of Helsinki of 1975, as revised in 2000.

3.2. Autoantibody Detection

ELISAs were performed to measure ANA, anti-Sm, and APL using commercially available ELISA kits (INOVA Diagnostic, Inc., San Diego, CA, USA). ELISAs were performed according to the manufacturers' instructions. Values of optical density (OD) at 450 nm were obtained, and the IgG antibody concentrations were calculated by extrapolating OD_{450} values to a standard curve.

3.3. M_3 mAChR Autoantibodies

The IgG fraction from 30 patients with SLE and 30 normal subjects was independently subjected to affinity chromatography on the synthesized peptide covalently linked to AffiGel 15 gel (Bio-Rad, Richmond, CA, USA) as described previously [25]. Briefly, the IgG fraction was loaded onto the affinity column equilibrated with phosphate-buffered saline (PBS). The non-peptide fraction was first eluted with the same buffer. Specific anti-

Table 1. Demographic and clinical characteristics of SLE patients and healthy individuals.

Clinical characteristics		
	SLE patients	Normal individuals
Number	30	30
Current age, mean years ± SD	41.4 ± 11.9	39.6 ± 10.2
Disease duration, mean years ± SD	7.88 ± 10.6	N/A
Female gender, n (%)	26 (86.7)	30 (100)
Organ/system involved		
Malar rash, n (%)	18 (60.0)	N/A
Photosensitivity, n (%)	17 (56.7)	N/A
Hematological, n (%)	23 (76.6)	N/A
Renal, n (%)	13 (43.4)	N/A
Current antibodies		
ANA positive, n (%)	30 (100)	N/A
Anti-Sm positive, n (%)	5 (16.6)	N/A
Anti-phospholipid (APL) positive, n (%)	6 (20.0)	N/A
Anti-M3 synthetic peptide IgG, n (%)	13 (43.3)	3 (10.0)

peptide antibodies were then eluted with 3 M potassium thiocyanate (KSCN) and 1 M sodium chloride (NaCl), followed by immediate extensive dialysis against PBS. The IgG concentrations of non-anti-peptide antibodies and specific anti-muscarinic receptor peptide IgG were determined by a radial immunodiffusion assay, and their immunological reactivity against muscarinic receptor peptides was evaluated by ELISA. The concentration of the affinity-purified anti-M_3 peptide IgG (1×10^{-7} M) that maximally increased optical density (OD: 2.4 ± 0.2) corresponded to a total IgG concentration of 1×10^{-6} M (OD: 2.2 ± 0.2). The normal IgG fraction purified by affinity column chromatography gave a negative result (OD: 0.24 ± 0.03).

3.4. ELISA Assay

Fifty microlitres of M_3 mAChR peptide solution in 0.1 M sodium carbonate (Na_2CO_3) buffer (pH = 9.6) was used to coat microtiter plates (Corning Costar, Tewksbury, MA, USA) at 4°C overnight as decribed [25]. After blocking the wells, varying concentrations of purified IgG from patients with SLE and healthy individuals were allowed to react with the antigens for 2 h at 37°C. The wells were then thoroughly washed with Tween® 20 in PBS. Goat anti-human IgG avidin-alkaline phosphatase (50 μl) was added and incubated for 1 h at 37°C. After several washing steps, p-nitrophenyl phosphate (1 mg·mL^{-1}) was added as the substrate; the reaction was terminated at 30 min. OD values were measured using an ELISA reader (Uniskan Laboratory System, Helsinki, Finland). As negative controls, non-antigen paired wells and wells with no primary antiserum were also tested.

3.5. PGE$_2$ Procedure

Serum PGE$_2$ was measured by ELISA according to the manufacturer's protocol (PGE$_2$ Biotrack Enzyme Immune Assay System; Amersham Bioscience, Piscataway, NJ, USA). The OD cutoff value for PGE$_2$ was 4.4 ± 0.33 ng/ml. All serum samples were frozen promptly after collection and kept at −80°C until used for PGE$_2$ determination. The PGE$_2$ results are expressed as ng/mL.

3.6. Statistical Analysis

Statistical analysis was performed using GraphPad Prism (GraphPad, San Diego, CA, USA). Statistical significance was determined by the two-tailed t test for independent populations. Analysis of variance (ANOVA) and Dunn's and Kruskal-Wallis tests were employed for multiple comparisons. Pearson's analysis was applied to establish correlation. Differences between means were considered significant at $P \leq 0.05$.

3.7. Ethical Approval of the Study Protocol

The study was approved by the Ethics Committee of the School of Dentistry at Buenos Aires University (Buenos Aires, Argentina). The studies were conducted according to the tenets of the Declaration of Helsinki. All participants provided written informed consent to participate in the study.

4. Results

ELISA assays were performed to determine whether a correlation exists between serum IgG against M_3 mAChR synthetic peptide (**Figure 1(a)**) as well as serum PGE$_2$ levels (**Figure 1(b)**) in SLE patients compared with normal individuals. **Figure 1(a)** shows the optical density (OD) values for each studied serum from SLE patients and normal subjects. Also, **Figure 1(b)** shows serum PGE$_2$ levels in SLE patients and normal subjects. The cut-off values obtained with SLE patient sera were always greater than two standard deviations (SD) from those from normal individuals. In **Figure 1(c)**, a positive correlation is shown between serum PGE$_2$ levels and anti-M_3 synthetic peptide titers (see table insert) of the individual sera from SLE patients.

Additionally, **Table 2** shows the comparison and a statistical analysis of different autoantibodies from sera of SLE patients, showing that anti-M_3 synthetic peptide IgG was significantly different from anti-Sm antibodies and APL antibodies. No significant values were obtained when we compared anti-M_3 synthetic peptide IgG with ANA.

The possible association between SLE disease activity, according to the SLEDAI and levels of anti-M_3 synthetic peptide IgG and serum PGE$_2$ levels (expressed as optical density values or ng/ml, respectively) was tested. Accordingly, when SLE patients were grouped on the basis of the disease status (active or non-active), no sig-

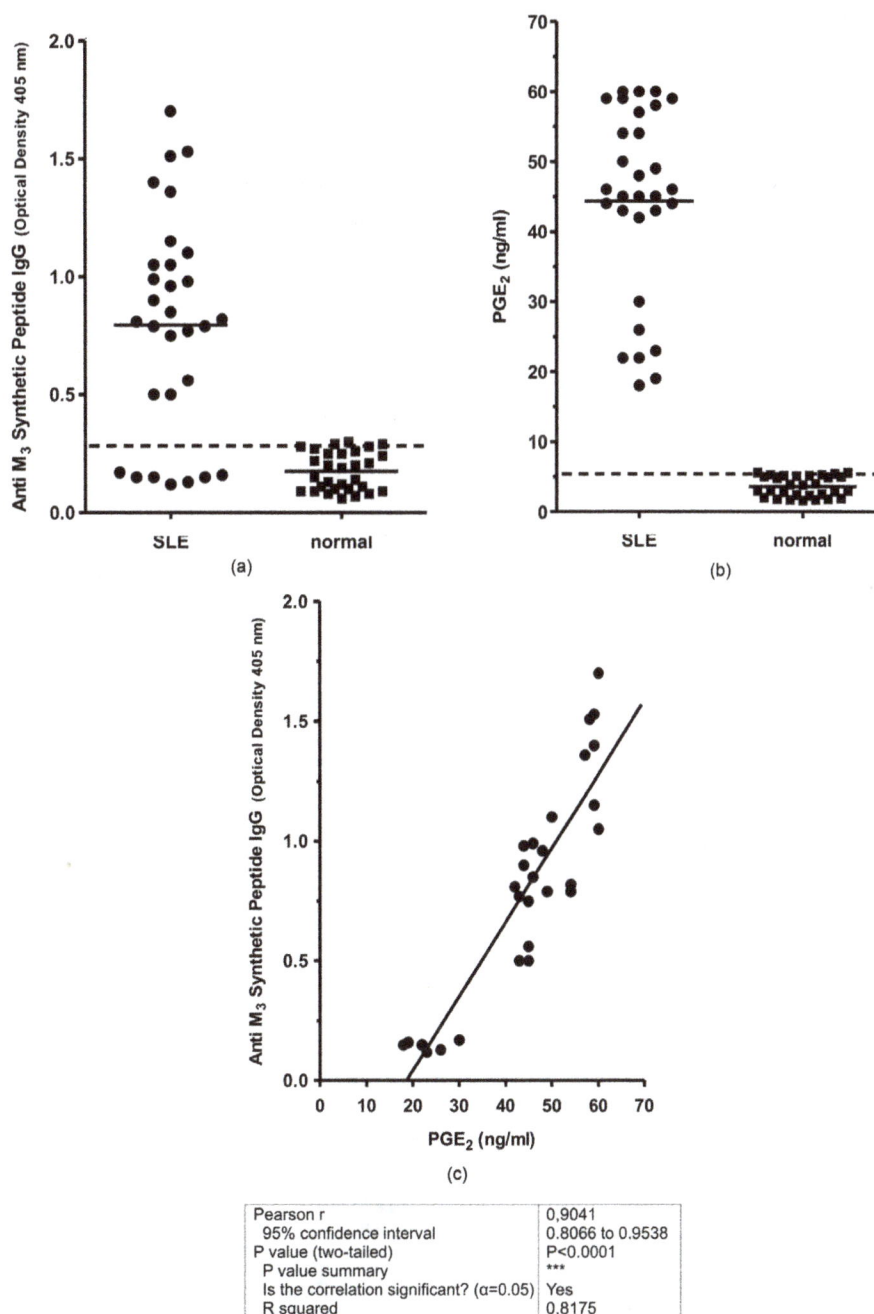

Figure 1. Scattergram showing immunoreactivity of circulating IgG antibodies against M_3 mAChR synthetic peptide (a) and serum PGE_2 (b). The individual optical density (OD) values for each serum sample (1:30 dilution) from 30 SLE patients and 30 normal individuals. Dotted/dashed line: cutoff values of OD 0.24 and 4.40 for anti-M_3 mAChR synthetic peptide IgG and serum PGE_2, respectively. Solid lines, median OD values. $P < 0.0001$ between groups, and (c) correlation between the anti-M_3 synthetic peptide IgG and serum PGE_2 levels.

nificant differences were found for the anti-M_3 synthetic peptide IgG (**Figure 2(a)**). On the contrary, a significant association between active or non-active status of SLE patients was observed when we analyzed serum PGE_2 levels (**Figure 2(b)**).

Finally, when we examined the possible association among the three parameters tested (SLEDAI, anti-M_3 synthetic peptide IgG levels, and serum PGE_2 levels) in this study, a highly significant association was found

Table 2. Comparison between anti-M₃ synthetic peptide IgG and different antibodies in SLE patients.

Variable	Dunn's multiple comparison test	Number of patients
Anti-M3 synthetic peptide IgG versus ANA	ns	30
Anti-M3 synthetic peptide IgG versus anti-Sm	Yes ($P < 0.05$)	30
Anti-M3 synthetic peptide IgG versus APL	Yes ($P < 0.05$)	30

Results were analyzed by one-way ANOVA followed by Kruskal-Wallis tests ($P < 0.0001$).

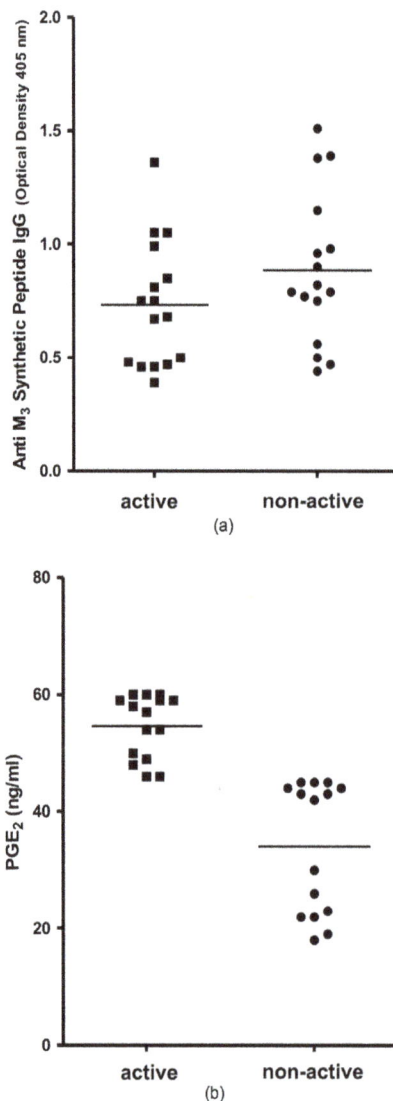

Figure 2. Scattergram showing immunoreactivity of circulating IgG antibodies against M₃ mAChR synthetic peptide (a) and serum PGE₂ (b) in active and non-active forms of SLE disease. Values are the individual OD values for each serum sample from 30 SLE patients and 30 healthy volunteers. Dotted/dashed line: cutoff values of OD 0.24 and 4.40 for anti-M₃ mAChR synthetic peptide IgG and serum PGE₂, respectively. Solid lines, median OD values. $P < 0.0001$ between groups.

only between the levels of PGE₂ and the active and non-active SLE disease status (SLEDAI) (**Table 3**).

5. Discussion

Systemic lupus erythematosus (SLE) is a challenging disease to assess and manage. Much progress in our un-

Table 3. Association between disease activity (SLEDAI) and levels of autoantibodies and serum PGE$_2$.

Conditions	Active SLE	Non-active SLE	P values
SLEDAI	6.51 ± 0.90	0.53 ± 0.23	<0.0001
Anti-M3 synthetic peptide IgG (optical density 405 nm)	0.73 ± 0.10	0.88 ± 0.22	0.0876
PGE2 (ng/mL)	54.60 ± 1.39	34.07 ± 2.89	<0.0001
Number of patients	15	15	N/A

Values represent the mean ± SEM of 30 patients grouped according to disease activity.

derstanding of its etiopathogenesis has been made. Moreover, differences in the clinical interpretation of the signs and symptoms are attributable to the complexity of the disorder and the likely diverse mechanisms that contribute to its clinical expression. This extra challenge complicates the work of scientists who seek to understand the disease more fully and clinicians treating patients with SLE.

SLE is an autoimmune disease that not only can have very different manifestations, but may also share some pathogenic mechanisms that may help to identify therapeutic targets.

In this study, we have shown the differential expression of some autoantibodies, such as ANA, anti-Sm, and APL [18] [19], is present at a much higher percentage in sera from SLE patients than in sera from healthy individuals. In addition, we detected for the first time the presence of anti-M$_3$ synthetic peptide IgG in the serum of SLE patients. This autoantibody was significantly associated with anti-Sm and APL antibodies but was unassociated with ANA. In previous studies was reported that ANA has the highest sensitivity in patients with SLE [32]. Moreover, the anti-M$_3$ synthetic peptide IgG was unassociated with malar rash, photosensitivity, or hematologic and renal alterations.

All of these autoantibodies are also associated with the clinical characteristics in the development of different clinical forms of SLE detected both in initial and chronic disease.

SLE is characterized not only by a dysregulatory immune response including overactive B-cells but is also always accompanied by an inflammatory process with T cell hyperactivity, where PGE$_2$ is increased in the serum of SLE patients. That, in turn, not only modulates the immune processes at the sites of inflammation but also has the ability to generate other inflammatory cytokines [28]. However, the increased serum levels of PGE$_2$ in SLE patients reveal that this prostanoid mediates the inflammatory process observed in this disease; under identical experimental conditions, a significant correlation between PGE$_2$ levels and anti-M$_3$ synthetic peptide IgG was found.

These results appear to be a pivotal factor mediated at the level of inflammatory site, maintaining and increasing the production of other proinflammatory cytokines, such as IL-6, IL-10, and nitric oxide [33]. Therefore, PGE$_2$ and the anti-M$_3$ synthetic peptide antibody could be jointly responsible for the dysregulated production of proinflammatory cytokines that maintains the immune-inflammatory process characteristic of this disease.

In previous works patients with active discoid SLE were shown to have a strong expression of COX-2 in the inflammatory areas [27].

When SLE patients were grouped on the basis of disease activity (active and non-active disease), no significant differences were found for anti-M$_3$ synthetic peptide IgG titers, though a significant difference in serum PGE$_2$ levels was observed. Perhaps the increase in PGE$_2$ is necessary to maintain the active inflammatory process in the course of SLE disease.

Although a possible association exists between the presence of elevated levels of anti-M$_3$ synthetic peptide IgG and many different clinical and laboratory parameters, we failed to find a significant correlation with most of these parameters. However, a significant correlation between the titer of this cholinergic autoantibody and the production of PGE$_2$ was detected. These data suggest that, first, the anti-M$_3$ synthetic peptide IgG may participate in the onset of the disease, and second, these autoantibodies may contribute to the generation of other proinflammatory cytokines.

6. Conclusion

On the basis of our results, we have demonstrated significantly enhanced titers of anti-M$_3$ synthetic peptide IgG in patients with SLE, as well as significantly higher levels of serum PGE_2. We consider that PGE_2 and these cholinergic autoantibodies may contribute, in part, to the pathogenesis of the autoreactive and inflammatory phenomenon described here and observed in SLE patients.

Acknowledgements

This study was supported by grants from the University of Buenos Aires (UBACyT 2011-2014) and CONICET (PIP 2014).

Conflict of Interest

The authors declare that they have no vested interest that could be constructed to have inappropriately influenced this study.

References

[1]   Deane, K.D. (2014) Preclinical Rheumatoid Arthritis (Autoantibodies): An Updated Review. *Current Rheumatology Report*, **16**, 419-422. http://dx.doi.org/10.1007/s11926-014-0419-6

[2]   Bizzaro, N. (2007) Autoantibodies as Predictors of Disease: The Clinical and Experimental Evidence. *Autoimmunity Review*, **6**, 325-333. http://dx.doi.org/10.1016/j.autrev.2007.01.006

[3]   Bizzaro, N. (2008) The Predictive Significance of Autoantibodies in Organ-Specific Autoimmune Diseases. *Clinical Reviews in Allergy & Immunology*, **34**, 326-331. http://dx.doi.org/10.1007/s12016-007-8059-5

[4]   Sherer, Y., Gorstein, A., Fritzler, M.J. and Shoenfeld, Y. (2004) Autoantibody Explosion in Systemic Lupus Erythematosus: More than 100 Different Antibodies Found in SLE Patients. *Seminars in Arthritis and Rheumatism*, **34**, 501-537. http://dx.doi.org/10.1016/j.semarthrit.2004.07.002

[5]   Li, Q.Z., Zhou, J., Wandstrat, A.E., Carr-Johnson, F., Branch, V. and Karp, D.R. (2007) Protein Array Autoantibody Profiles for Insights into Systemic Lupus Erythematosus and Incomplete Lupus Syndromes. *Clinical Experimental Immunology*, **147**, 60-70.

[6]   Mansour, R.B., Lassoued, S., Gargouri, B., El Gaid, A., Attia, H. and Fakhfakh, F. (2008) Increased Levels of Autoantibodies against Catalase and Superoxide Dismutase Associated with Oxidative Stress in Patients with Rheumatoid Arthritis and Systemic Lupus Erythematosus. *Scandinavian Journal of Rheumatology*, **37**, 103-108. http://dx.doi.org/10.1080/03009740701772465

[7]   Magalhaes, M.B., da Silva, L.M., Voltarelli, J.C., Donadi, E.A. and Louzada-Junior, P. (2007) Lymphocytotoxic Antibodies in Systemic Lupus Erythematosus Are Associated with Disease Activity Irrespective of the Presence of Neuropsychiatric Manifestations. *Scandinavian Journal of Rheumatology*, **6**, 442-447. http://dx.doi.org/10.1080/03009740701482768

[8]   Braun, A., Sis, J., Max, R., Mueller, K., Fiehn, C., Zeier, M. and Andrassy, K. (2007) Anti-Chromatin and Anti-C1q Antibodies in Systemic Lupus Erythematosus Compared to Other Systemic Autoimmune Diseases. *Scandinavian Journal of Rheumatology*, **36**, 291-298. http://dx.doi.org/10.1080/03009740701218717

[9]   D'Cruz, D.P., Khamashta, M.A. and Hughes, G.R. (2007) Systemic Lupus Erythematosus. *Lancet*, **369**, 587-596. http://dx.doi.org/10.1016/S0140-6736(07)60279-7

[10] Rahman, A. and Isenberg, D.A. (2008) Systemic Lupus Erythematosus. *New England Journal of Medicine*, **358**, 929-939. http://dx.doi.org/10.1056/NEJMra071297

[11] Pugh-Bernard, A.E. and Cambier, J.C. (2006) B Cell Receptor Signaling in Human Systemic Lupus Erythematosus. *Current Opinion in Rheumatology*, **18**, 451-455. http://dx.doi.org/10.1097/01.bor.0000240353.99808.5f

[12] Nagy, G., Koncz, A. and Perl, A. (2005) T- and B-Cell Abnormalities in Systemic Lupus Erythematosus. *Critical Reviews in Immunology*, **25**, 123-140. http://dx.doi.org/10.1615/CritRevImmunol.v25.i2.30

[13] Ishikawa, S., Akakura, S., Abe, M., Terashima, K., Chijiiwa, K., Nishimura, H., Hirose, S. and Shirai, T. (1998) A Subset of CD4$^+$ T Cells Expressing Early Activation Antigen CD69 in Murine Lupus: Possible Abnormal Regulatory Role for Cytokine Imbalance. *Journal of Immunology*, **161**, 1267-1273.

[14] Bohm, I. (2004) Apoptosis: The Link between Autoantibodies and Leuko-/Lymphocytopenia in Patients with Lupus Erythematosus. *Scandinavian Journal of Rheumatology*, **33**, 409-416. http://dx.doi.org/10.1080/03009740410006907

[15] Reichlin, M. (1993) Antibodies to Defined Antigens in the Systemic Rheumatic Diseases. *Bulletin on the Rheumatic Diseases*, **42**, 4-6.

[16] Waltuck, J. and Buyon, J.P. (1994) Autoantibody-Associated Congenital Heart Block: Outcome in Mothers and Child-

ren. *Annals of Internal Medicine*, **120**, 544-551. http://dx.doi.org/10.7326/0003-4819-120-7-199404010-00003

[17] Aho, K., Koskela, P., Makitalo, R., Heliovaara, M. and Palosuo, T. (1992) Antinuclear Antibodies Heralding the Onset of Systemic Lupus Erythematosus. *Journal of Rheumatology*, **19**, 1377-1379.

[18] Heinlen, L.D., McClain, M.T., Merrill, J., Akbarali, Y.W., Edgerton, C.C., Harley, J.B. and James, J.A. (2007) Clinical Criteria for Systemic Lupus Erythematosus Precede Diagnosis, and Associated Autoantibodies Are Present before Clinical Symptoms. *Arthritis & Rheumatism*, **56**, 2344-2351. http://dx.doi.org/10.1002/art.22665

[19] McClain, M.T., Arbuckle, M.R., Heinlen, L.D., Dennis, G.J., Roebuck, J., Rubertone, M.V., Harley, J.B. and James, J.A. (2004) The Prevalence, Onset, and Clinical Significance of Antiphospholipid Antibodies Prior to Diagnosis of Systemic Lupus Erythematosus. *Arthritis & Rheumatism*, **50**, 1226-1232. http://dx.doi.org/10.1002/art.20120

[20] Heinlen, L.D., McClain, M.T., Ritterhouse, L.L., Bruner, B.F., Edgerton, C.C., Keith, M.P., James, J.A. and Harley, J.B. (2010) 60 kD Ro and nRNP A Frequently Initiate Human Lupus Autoimmunity. *PLoS ONE*, **5**, e9599. http://dx.doi.org/10.1371/journal.pone.0009599

[21] Arbuckle, M.R., McClain, M.T., Rubertone, M.V., Scofield, R.H., Dennis, G.J., James, J.A. and Harley, J.B. (2003) Development of Autoantibodies before the Clinical Onset of Systemic Lupus Erythematosus. *New England Journal of Medicine*, **349**, 1526-1533. http://dx.doi.org/10.1056/NEJMoa021933

[22] Arbuckle, M.R., James, J.A., Kohlhase, K.F., Rubertone, M.V., Dennis, G.J. and Harley, J.B. (2001) Development of Anti-dsDNA Autoantibodies Prior to Clinical Diagnosis of Systemic Lupus Erythematosus. *Scandinavian Journal of Immunology*, **54**, 211-219. http://dx.doi.org/10.1046/j.1365-3083.2001.00959.x

[23] Jonsson, R., Theander, E., Sjöström, B., Brokstad, K. and Henriksson, G. (2013) Autoantibodies Present before Symptom Onset in Primary Sjögren Syndrome. *JAMA*, **310**, 1854-1855. http://dx.doi.org/10.1001/jama.2013.278448

[24] Tzioufas, A.G., Kapsogeorgou, E.K. and Moutsopoulos, H.M. (2012) Pathogenesis of Sjögren's Syndrome: What We Know and What We Should Learn. *Journal of Autoimmunity*, **39**, 4-8. http://dx.doi.org/10.1016/j.jaut.2012.01.002

[25] Reina, S., Sterin-Borda, L., Orman, B. and Borda, E. (2004) Autoantibodies against Cerebral Muscarinic Cholinoceptors in Sjögren Syndrome: Functional and Pathological Implications. *Journal of Neuroimmunology*, **150**, 107-115. http://dx.doi.org/10.1016/j.jneuroim.2004.01.019

[26] Reina, S., Sterin-Borda, L. and Borda, E. (2012) Anti-M$_3$ Peptide IgG from Sjögren's Syndrome Triggers Apoptosis in A253 Cells. *Cellular Immunology*, **275**, 33-41. http://dx.doi.org/10.1016/j.cellimm.2012.03.006

[27] Chae, B.S., Shin, T.Y., Kim, D.K., Eun, J.S., Leem, J.Y. and Yang, J.H. (2008) Prostaglandin E$_2$-Mediated Dysregulation of Proinflammatory Cytokine Production in Pristane-Induced Lupus Mice. *Archives of Pharmacal Research*, **31**, 503-510. http://dx.doi.org/10.1007/s12272-001-1185-6

[28] Abreu-Velez, A.M., Smith Jr., G. and Howard, M.S. (2011) Activation of the Signaling Cascade in Response to T Lymphocyte Receptor Stimulation and Prostanoids in a Case of Cutaneous Lupus. *North American Journal of Medical Sciences*, **3**, 251-254. http://dx.doi.org/10.4297/najms.2011.3251

[29] Tan, E.M., Cohen, A.S., Fries, J.F., Masi, A.T., McShane, D.J., Rothfield, N.F., Schaller, J.G., Talal, N. and Winchester, R.J. (1982) The 1982 Revised Criteria for the Classification of Systemic Lupus Erythematosus. *Arthritis & Rheumatism*, **25**, 1271-1277. http://dx.doi.org/10.1002/art.1780251101

[30] Bombardier, C., Gladman, D.D., Urowitz, M.B., Caron, D., Chang, C.H., *et al.*, The Committee on Prognosis Studies in SLE (1992) Derivation of the Sledai. A Disease Activity Index for Lupus Patients. *Arthritis & Rheumatism*, **35**, 630-640. http://dx.doi.org/10.1002/art.1780350606

[31] Guzman, J., Cardiel, M.H., Arce-Salinas, A., Sánchez-Guerrero, J. and Alarcón-Segovia, D. (1992) Measurement of Disease Activity in Systemic Lupus Erythematosus. Prospective Validation of 3 Clinical Indices. *Journal of Rheumatology*, **19**, 1551-1558.

[32] Eriksson, C., Kokkonen, H., Johansson, M., Hallmans, G., Wadell, G. and Rantapaa-Dahlqvist, S. (2011) Autoantibodies Predate the Onset of Systemic Lupus Erythematosus in Northern Sweden. *Arthritis Research & Therapy*, **13**, R30-R34. http://dx.doi.org/10.1186/ar3258

[33] Tsai, C.Y., Wu, T.H., Tsai, S.T., Chen, K.H., Thajeb, P., Lin, W.M., Yu, H.S. and Yu, C.L. (1994) Cerebrospinal Fluid Interleukin-6, Prostaglandin E$_2$, and Autoantibodies in Patients with Neuropsychiatric Systemic Lupus Erythematosus and Central Nervous System Infections. *Scandinavian Journal of Rheumatology*, **23**, 57-63. http://dx.doi.org/10.3109/03009749409103028

15

Study of *in Vitro* Interaction of Sildenafil Citrate with Bovine Serum Albumin by Fluorescence Spectroscopy

Md. Abdus Salam[1], Md. Rokonujjaman[1], Asma Rahman[2], Ummay Nasrin Sultana[2], Md. Zakir Sultan[2]*

[1]Department of Chemistry, University of Dhaka, Dhaka, Bangladesh
[2]Centre for Advanced Research in Sciences (CARS), University of Dhaka, Dhaka, Bangladesh
Email: *zakir.sultan@du.ac.bd

Abstract

In vitro interaction of sildenafil citrate (SC) with bovine serum albumin (BSA) was investigated at two excitation wavelengths of BSA (280 nm and 293 nm) at two different temperatures (298 K and 308 K) by fluorescence emission spectroscopy. The study showed that quenching of BSA fluorescence by sildenafil citrate was the result of formation BSA-SC complex with probable involvement of both tryptophan and tyrosine residues of BSA. Fluorescence quenching constant was determined from Stern-Volmer equation, and both static quenching and dynamic quenching were showed for BSA by SC at the conditions. Van't Hoff equation was used to measure the thermodynamic parameters ΔG, ΔH, and ΔS at the temperatures which indicated that the hydrogen bond and the hydrophobic forces played major roles for BSA-SC complexation. The binding number (n) was found to be ≈1 indicating that one mole BSA bound with one mole SC. The binding affinity of SC to BSA was calculated at different temperatures. The binding constant was decreased with increasing temperatures indicating that stability of BSA-SC complex decreased with increasing temperatures.

Keywords

Sildenafil Citrate, Bovine Serum Albumin, Quenching, Fluorescence Spectroscopy

1. Introduction

Sildenafil citrate (**Figure 1**) is a drug used to treat erectile dysfunction and pulmonary arterial hypertension (PAH)

---
*Corresponding author.

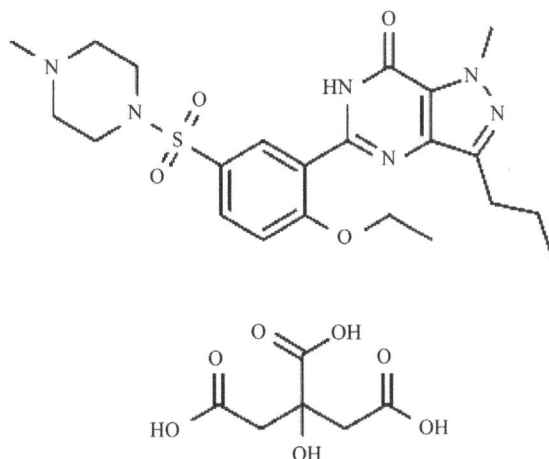

Figure 1. Chemical structure of sildenafil citrate (SC).

[1]. It acts by inhibiting cGMP-specific phosphodiesterase type 5 (PDE5), an enzyme that promotes degradation of cGMP, which regulates blood flow in the smooth muscle. Sildenafil has no direct relaxant effect on isolated human corpus cavernosum, but enhances the effect of nitric oxide (NO) by inhibiting phosphodiesterase type 5 (PDE5), which is responsible for degradation of cGMP in the corpus cavernosum.

Serum albumin is the most abundant soluble protein in human blood plasma and they are serving as deport protein and binding of numerous ligands, such as fatty acids, drugs, and metal ions, in the bloodstream to their target organs [2] [3]. Therefore, serum albumin is considered as a model to study the drug-protein interaction *in vitro* [4]. Bovine serum albumin (BSA) is an extensively studied ideal protein model of albumin group since it displays 80% homology with human serum albumin (HSA) [5]. BSA is an ideal protein of a single polypeptide chain of 583 amino acid residues and three structurally homologous domains (I-III) which are divided into nine loops (L1-L9) by 17 disulfide bonds, and each domain is further divided into two sub-domains (A and B) [6]. It is a convenient protein for intrinsic fluorescence measurement due to the presence of two intrinsic tryptophan (Trp) residues which is highly sensitive to its local environment, and can be used to observe changes in the fluorescence emission spectra due to protein conformational changes, binding to substrates, and denaturation [7]. There are also numerous tyrosine residues of BSA depending on the excitation wavelength selected which have minor contribution for intrinsic fluorescence. Trp-212, located within the hydrophobic binding pocket of sub-domain IIA (site-I), and Trp-134, located on the surface of sub-domain IB (site-II) [8]-[10]. The binding sites of BSA for endogenous and exogenous ligands may be in these domains, and some ligands specifically bind to the different domains of serum albumin [11]. However, BSA plays an important role in binding of numerous drugs in the bloodstream to their target organs for understanding the pharmacokinetics and pharmacodynamics properties of drug candidates.

Drugs bound at molecular level to proteins are acted as carriers which lead to the interpretation of the metabolism, distribution, free concentration, efficacy and transporting process of drugs [12]. Moreover, investigation of drug-protein interaction provides the information of structural features determining the therapeutic effect of drugs helping to understand the drug toxicity and playing a key role in the researching pharmacology, pharmacodynamics and biochemistry. Therefore drug-protein binding has become an important research field in life sciences, chemistry and clinical medicine [13] [14].

There are some popular techniques which have been used to investigate the interaction between drugs and BSA. Fluorescence spectroscopy is one of the powerful techniques to study molecular interactions which change local environment of fluorophore and help to predict the binding phenomenon of drugs to BSA [15]. However, the *in vitro* mechanism of interactions of SC with BSA in presence has not been explored. So it is significant to study the interaction between SC and BSA by fluorescence spectroscopy.

In the present study, *in vitro* interaction of SC with BSA has been studied by fluorescence emission spectroscopy at two excitation wavelengths of BSA (280 nm and 293 nm) at two different temperatures. For this study, participating residues, quenching constant, thermodynamic parameters and forces, binding constant and binding number at mentioned conditions were measured.

2. Materials and Method

2.1. Reagent and Materials

All chemicals and reagents were of analytical grade and doubly distilled water was used throughout the study. BSA (fatty acid free, fraction V, 96% - 98%), sodium dihydrogen phosphate (NaH_2PO_4), potassium dihydrogen phosphate (KH_2PO_4) were purchased from Sigma Chemical Co., USA., and sildenafil citrate (99.4%) was kind gift from the ACI Ltd., Bangladesh.

2.2. Apparatus

All fluorescence spectra were recorded on fluorescence spectrophotometer (Model: F-7000, Hitachi, Japan) equipped with 1.0 cm quartz cell. For different temperatures a thermostat bath (Unitronic Orbital, P-Spectra, Spain) was used.

2.3. Sample Preparation

Five mL of previously prepared 20×10^{-6} mol·L^{-1} BSA in phosphate buffer of pH 7.4 was taken in each of the eight test tubes. Sildenafil citrate was added in different volumes to seven out of eight test tubes to have the following concentrations: (20, 40, 80, 120, 160, 240 and 320) $\times 10^{-6}$ mol·L^{-1}, respectively. The ratio of SC and BSA ([SC]/[BSA]) in BSA-SC system of seven test tubes were 1:1, 2:1, 4:1, 6:1, 8:1, 12:1 and 16:1, respectively. The mixture solutions of BSA and SC must be hatched at least 5 min before the spectroscopic measurements.

2.4. Spectroscopic Measurement

The fluorescence emission spectra for BSA-SC system were recorded at the two excitation wavelengths of BSA (280 nm and 293 nm) at two different temperatures (298 K and 308 K). The widths of both entrance and exit slit were set to 5 nm. These emission spectra were recorded for three times for each treatment in the range of 320 - 460 nm for BSA at same experimental conditions since there were no emission spectra of SC in this range.

3. Results and Discussion

3.1. The Interaction of SC with BSA

When BSA is excited by appropriate wavelength of light, all of its fluorophores (tryptophan, tyrosine and phenylalanine) can emit fluorescence. When 280 nm excitation wavelength is used, fluorescence of albumin comes from both tryptophan and tyrosine residues, whereas 293 nm wavelength only excites tryptophan residues [16]. It was compared the fluorescence of BSA excited at 280 nm and 293 nm in the presence of SC that would be determined the interactions residues of BSA with SC. The plots F/F_o against [SC]/[BSA] at excitation wavelengths 280 nm and 293 nm were compared at 298 K, respectively. Here, F_o is the fluorescence intensity of BSA, F is the fluorescence intensity of BSA in presence of SC.

Figure 2 indicates that the fluorescence of BSA excited at 280 nm obviously differed from that excited at 293 nm in the presence of SC. This difference between quenching of serum albumin fluorescence showed that the both tyrosine and tryptophan residues participated in the molecular interactions between BSA and SC.

3.2. Effect of SC on the Fluorescence Emission Spectra of BSA

In order to determine the effect of SC with BSA, the fluorescence emission spectra were measured at two excitation wavelengths of BSA (280 nm and 293 nm) at two different temperatures (298 K and 308 K).

Figure 3 shows the fluorescence of BSA gradually decreased with the increasing concentration of SC, indicating that there was a strong interaction and energy transfer between SC and BSA at the both excitation wavelengths of BSA (λEx_{max} of BSA = 280 nm and 293 nm) at two different temperatures (298 K and 308 K). As a result, there were quenching of intrinsic fluorescence of BSA but no significant shift of the emission maximum wavelength was observed.

3.3. Fluorescence Quenching Analysis

Quenching refers to any process which decreases the fluorescence intensity of a given substance (fluorophore)

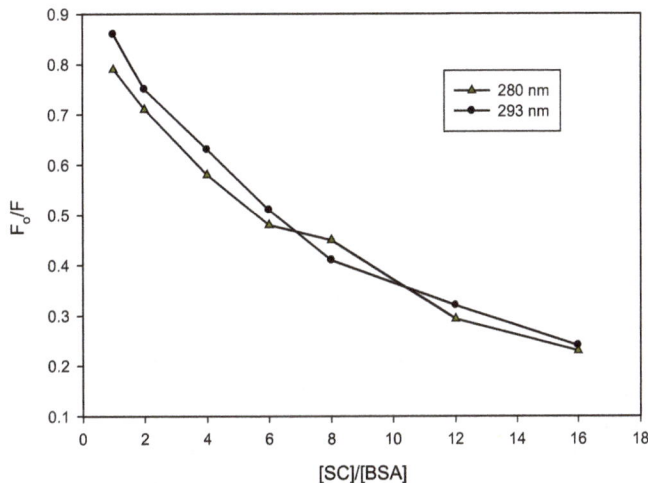

Figure 2. Fluorescence titration curve of BSA in presence of SC at the excitation wavelength of 280 nm and 293 nm at 298 K.

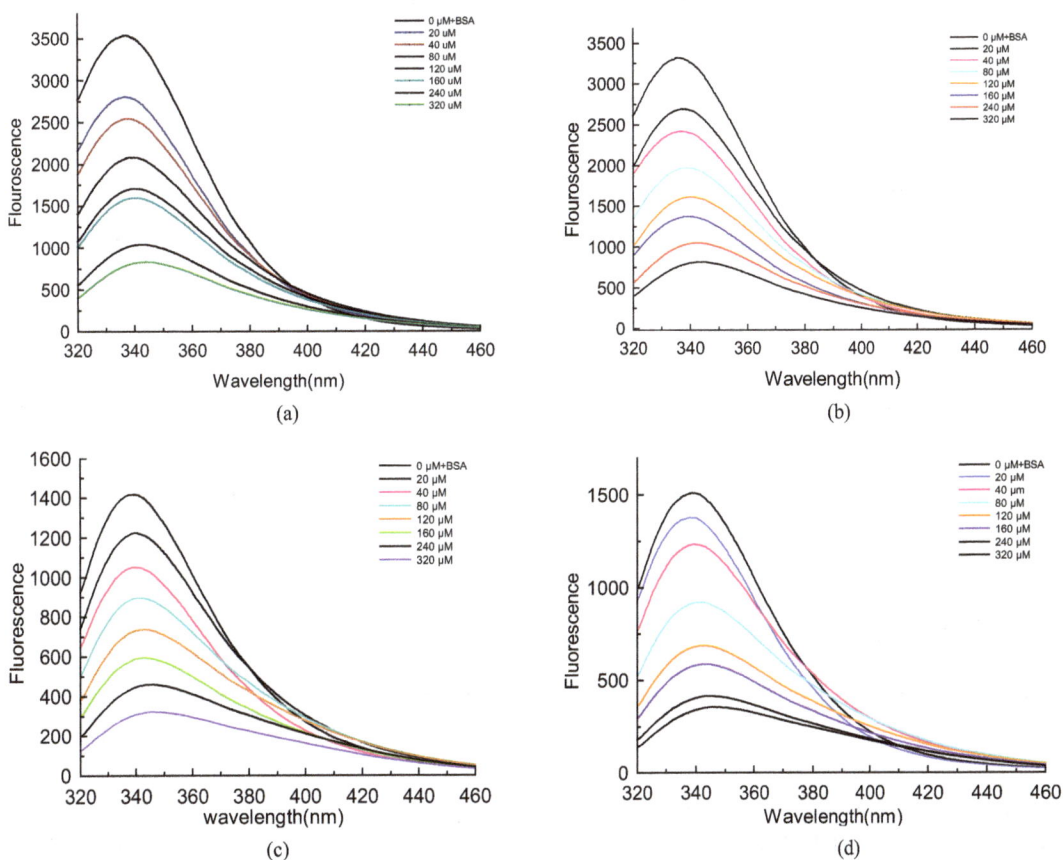

Figure 3. Fluorescence emission spectra of BSA-SC system at the excitation of (a) 280 nm at 298 K; (b) 280 nm at 308 K; (c) 293 nm at 298 K; (d) 293 nm at 308 K.

induced by a variety of molecular interactions with quencher molecule [17]. A variety of processes can result in quenching, such as excited state reactions, energy transfer, complex-formation and collisional quenching. Formation of complex between quencher and the fluorophore refers to static quenching. On the other hand, collision of the quencher and fluorophore during the excitation refers to dynamic quenching [18]. The fluorescence quenching data are usually analyzed by Stern-Volmer equation [7].

$$F_o/F = 1 + Ksv[Q]$$

where, F_o and F are the fluorescence intensities in the absence and presence of quencher, [Q] is the quencher concentration and Ksv is the Stern-Volmer quenching constant which indicates the strength of interaction between albumin protein and quencher molecule. Hence, this equation was applied to determine Ksv by linear regression of a plot of F_o/F against [Q]. The static quenching distinguished from dynamic quenching by their differing dependence of temperature [7]. Dynamic quenching depends upon diffusion and higher temperatures result in larger diffusion coefficients. As a result, the Stern-Volmer quenching constants (Ksv) were expected to increase with increasing temperature. In contrast, increased temperature is likely to result in decreasing stability of complexes, and thus lower value of static quenching constants [19].

The pattern of quenching of BSA fluorescence by SC was determined by measuring the value of Stern-Volmer quenching constant (Ksv) at the excitation wavelength of BSA (280 nm and 293 nm) at two different temperatures (298 K and 308 K). Ksv was calculated from the slope of the plot of F/F_o versus concentration of SC based on the fluorescence data (**Figure 4**) at the conditions.

Figure 4 displays the Stern-Volmer plots of the quenching of BSA fluorescence by SC at two excitation wavelength of BSA (280 nm and 293 nm) at two different temperatures (298 K and 308 K). The plots showed that within the experimental concentrations, the results were good agreement with the Stern-Volmer equation. The plots were linear and Stern-Volmer quenching constants were obtained from the slopes at two different temperatures; these are mentioned in **Table 1**. The Stern-Volmer quenching constant decreased with increasing temperature for static quenching while for dynamic quenching the reverse effect was observed [20]. It was seen from the **Table 1** that the Ksv decreased by increasing temperature at 280 nm but increased by increasing temperature at 293 nm. So it was observed that both dynamic and static quenching were present of BSA by SC at two different temperatures.

3.4. Thermodynamic Parameters and Nature of Binding Forces

There are many interaction forces (e.g. hydrophobic force, electrostatic interactions, Vander Waals interactions,

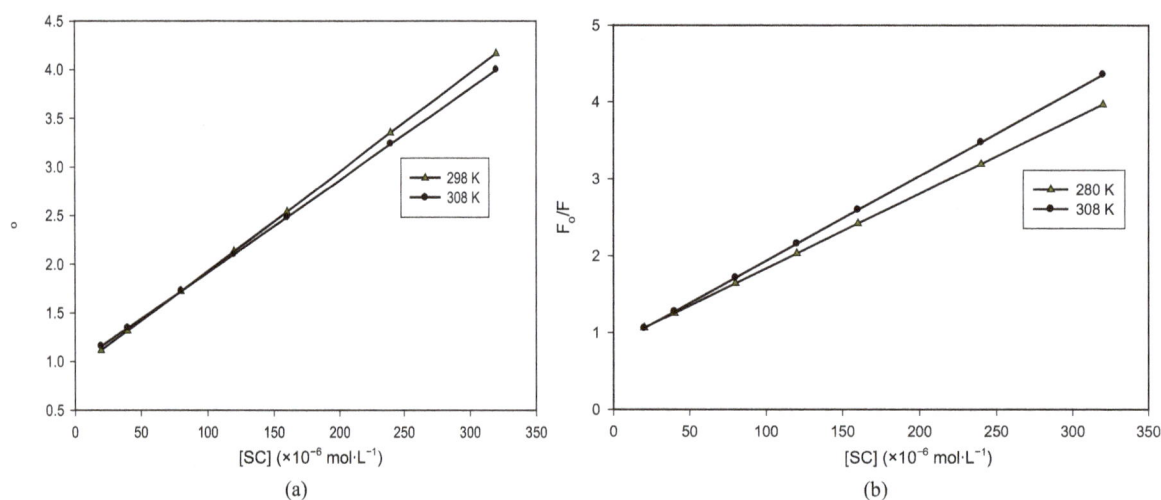

Figure 4. The Stern-Volmer plots for BSA-SC system at the excitation wavelength of BSA (a) 280 nm and (b) 293 nm at two different temperatures (298 K and 308 K).

Table 1. The Stern-Volmer quenching constant (Ksv) for BSA-SC system at 280 nm and 293 nm at two different temperatures (298 K and 308 K).

T (K)	Ksv ($\times 10^3$ L·mol^{-1}) at 280 nm	Ksv ($\times 10^3$ L·mol^{-1}) at 293 nm
298	10.2	9.7
308	9.5	11.0

hydrogen bonds, etc.) between quencher and fluorescence active molecule [10]. The thermodynamic parameters were calculated in order to elucidate the interaction between the drug and BSA, which can be determined from the Van't Hoff equation:

$$\ln Ka = -(\Delta H/RT) + (\Delta S/R)$$

where, ΔS = entropy change, ΔH = enthalpy change, R = universal gas constant and Ka = analogous to the Stern-Volmer quenching constants Ksv at the corresponding temperature [21].

The enthalpy change (ΔH) and the entropy change (ΔS) can be determined from the slope and intercept of the fitted curve of lnKsv against 1/T, respectively (**Figure 5**). The free energy, ΔG can be estimated from the following relationship:

$$\Delta G = \Delta H - T\Delta S$$

Table 2 shows that ΔS was a positive value, and ΔH was a small negative value. The negative value of ΔH reveals that the formation of BSA-SC complex was an exothermic reaction. Moreover, the negative sign for ΔG indicates the spontaneity of the binding process of SC with BSA. According to the views of Ross and Subramanian [22], the model of interaction between drug and biomolecule can be summarized as follows: 1) the positive ΔS value is frequently regarded as the evidence for a hydrophobic interaction [23] because the water molecules arranged in an orderly fashion around the drug and protein establish a more random configuration; 2) the negative value of ΔH can be obtained whenever there is a possibility of hydrogen bonding [22]. Thus both hydrogen bonding and hydrophobic interactions were present in the SC-BSA binding at 280 nm at both temperatures.

3.5. Binding Constant and Binding Points

When sildenafil citrate binds independently to a set of equivalent sites on BSA, the equilibrium between free and bound sildenafil citrate is given by the following equation [24]

$$\log[(F_o - F)/F] = \log K + n\log[Q]$$

where, K = binding constant to site of albumin, n = number of binding sites for drug per albumin.

The values of K and n are calculated from the values of intercept and slope of the plot of $\log[(F_o - F)/F]$ versus log[Q].

Table 3 contains the values of binding constant (K) and binding number (n), at two excitation wavelength of BSA (280 nm and 293 nm) which were obtained from the intercept and slope of **Figure 6**. It was observed that

Table 2. Thermodynamic parameters for BSA-SC system at 280 nm at two different temperatures (298 K and 308 K).

T (K)	ΔH (KJ/mol)	ΔS (J/mol)	ΔG (KJ/mol)
298	−5.89	57.01	−22.87
308			−23.44

Table 3. Binding constant and binding points for BSA-SC system at two excitation wavelength of BSA at two different temperatures.

T (K)	K (×10³ mol·L⁻¹) at 280 nm	n	K (×10³ mol·L⁻¹) at 293 nm	n
298	14.32		6.22	
308	12.37	0.9411	5.62	1.064

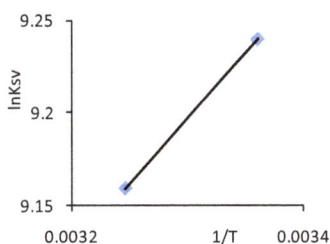

Figure 5. The Van't Hoff plot for BSA-SC system at 280 nm at two different temperatures (298 K and 308 K).

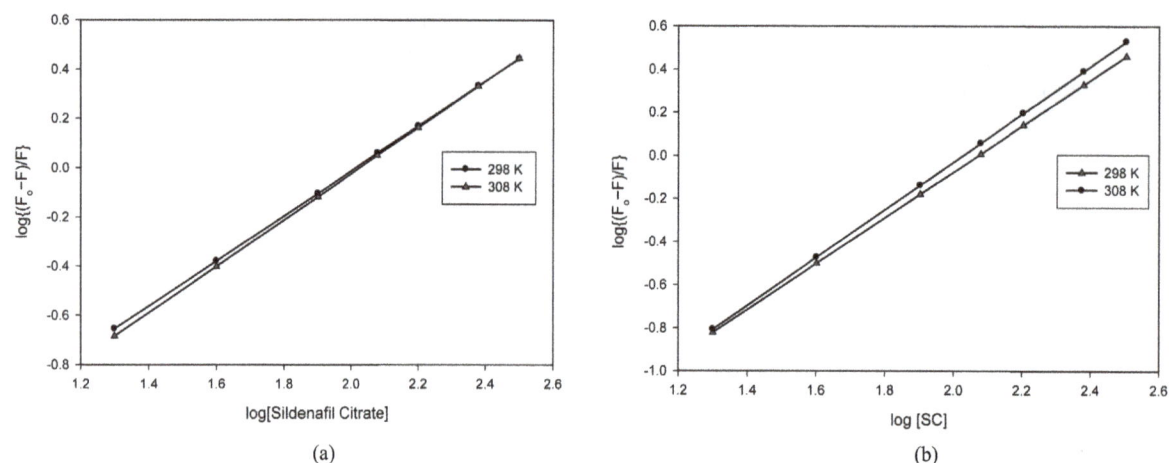

(a)   (b)

Figure 6. Plot for binding constant and binding points for BSA-SC system (a) at 280 nm (b) 293 nm at two different temperatures.

the binding constant decreases with the increase in temperature of the BSA-SC complex resulting in the reduction of stability of the complex. The values of n were found to be ≈1 at both excitation wavelength of BSA at two different temperatures. The molar ratio of the BSA-SC system at 280 nm and 293 nm was 1:1 indicated that one mole SC bound with 1 mole of BSA.

4. Conclusion

Drug-drug or drug-protein interactions produce an increase or a decrease in the therapeutic action, or produce various adverse effects that are not normally associated with the drugs [25]-[27]. Interaction of BSA with SC was successfully investigated by fluorescence spectroscopy. Experimental result showed both tryptophan and tyrosine residues of BSA participated in the interactions with SC [27]. The quenching mechanism of fluorescence of BSA by SC was both static and dynamic quenching process results of BSA-SC complex formation. The study of thermodynamic parameters showed that interactions between drugs and BSA were hydrophobic and hydrogen bonding. The stability of BSA-SC complex was decreased with increasing temperatures and it was found that sildenafil citrate bound with BSA with a mole ratio of 1:1.

References

[1]   Boolell, M., Allen, M.J., Ballard, S.A., Gepi-Attee, S., Muirhead, G.J., Naylor, A.M., Osterloh, I.H. and Gingell, C. (1996) Sildenafil: An Orally Active Type 5 Cyclic GMP-Specific Phosphodiesterase Inhibitor for the Treatment of Penile Erectile Dysfunction. *International Journal of Impotence Research*, **8**, 47-52.

[2]   Tian, J.N., Liu, J.Q., He, W.Y., Hu, Z.O., Yao, X.J. and Chen, X.G. (2004) Probing the Binding of Scutellarin to Human Serum Albumin by Circular Dichroism, Fluorescence Spectroscopy, FTIR and Molecular Modeling Method. *Biomacromolecules*, **5**, 1956-1961. http://dx.doi.org/10.1021/bm049668m

[3]   Malonga, H., Neault, J.F. and Tajmir-Riahi, H.A. (2006) Transfer RNA Binding to Human Serum Albumin: A Model for Protein-RNA Interaction. *DNA Cell Biology*, **25**, 393-398. http://dx.doi.org/10.1089/dna.2006.25.393

[4]   Ahmad, B., Parveen, S. and Khan, R.H. (2006) Effect of Albumin Conformation on the Binding of Ciprofloxacinto Human Serum Albumin: A Novel Approach Directly Assigning Binding Site. *Biomacromolecules*, **7**, 1350-1356. http://dx.doi.org/10.1021/bm050996b

[5]   Mallick, A., Haldar, B. and Chattopadhyay, N. (2005) Spectroscopic Investigation on the Interaction of ICT Probe 3-Acetyl-4-oxo-6,7-dihydro-12H Indolo-[2,3-a] Quinolizine with Serum Albumins. *Journal of Physical Chemistry B*, **109**, 14683-14690. http://dx.doi.org/10.1021/jp051367z

[6]   Carter, D. and Ho, J.X. (1994) Structure of Serum Albumin. *Advances in Protein Chemistry*, **45**, 153-203. http://dx.doi.org/10.1016/S0065-3233(08)60640-3

[7]   Lakowicz, J.R. (1999) Principles of Fluorescence Spectroscopy. 2nd Edition, Plenum Press, New York. http://dx.doi.org/10.1007/978-1-4757-3061-6

[8]   Peters Jr., T. (1985) Serum Albumin. *Advances in Protein Chemistry*, **37**, 161-245.

http://dx.doi.org/10.1016/S0065-3233(08)60065-0

[9] Moriyama, Y., Ohta, D., Hachiya, K., Mitsui, Y. and Takeda, K. (1996) Fluorescence Behavior of Tryptophan Residues of Bovine and Human Serum Albumins in Ionic Surfactant Solutions: A Comparative Study of the Two and One Tryptophan(s) of Bovine and Human Albumins. *Journal of Protein Chemistry*, **15**, 265-272. http://dx.doi.org/10.1007/BF01887115

[10] Papadopoulou, A., Green, R.J. and Franzier, R.A. (2005) Interaction of Flavonoids with Bovine Serum Albumin: A Fluorescence Quenching Study. *Journal of Agricultural and Food Chemistry*, **53**, 158-163. http://dx.doi.org/10.1021/jf048693g

[11] Zhang, J., Yin, Z., Wu, W., Wang, Z., He, R. and Wu, Z. (2012) Characterization of Interaction between Raltitrexed and Bovine Serum Albumin by Optical Spectroscopic Techniques. *Chemical Research in Chinese Universities*, **28**, 963-970.

[12] Mostafa, S., EL-Sadek, M. and Alla, E.A. (2002) Spectrophotometric Determination of Ciprofloxacin, Enrofloxacin and Pefloxacin through Charge Transfer Complex Formation. *Journal of Pharmaceutical and Biomedical Analysis*, **27**, 133-142. http://dx.doi.org/10.1016/S0731-7085(01)00524-6

[13] Ni, Y., Liu, G.L. and Kokot, S. (2011) Competitive Binding of Small Molecules with Biopolymers: A Fluorescence Spectroscopy and Chemometrics Study of the Interaction of Aspirin and Ibuprofen with BSA. *Analyst*, **136**, 4794-4801. http://dx.doi.org/10.1039/c1an15550d

[14] Gentili, P.L., Ortica, F. and Favaro, G. (2008) Static and Dynamic Interaction of a Naturally Occurring Photochromic Molecule with Bovine Serum Albumin Studied by UV-Visible Absorption and Fluorescence Spectroscopy. *Journal of Physical Chemistry B*, **112**, 16793-16801. http://dx.doi.org/10.1021/jp805922g

[15] Kwon, S. and Carson, J.H. (1998) Fluorescence Quenching and Dequenching Analysis of RNA Interactions *in Vitro* and *in Vivo*. *Analytical Biochemistry*, **264**, 133-140. http://dx.doi.org/10.1006/abio.1998.2846

[16] Steinhardt, J., Krijn, J. and Leidy, J.G. (1971) Differences between Bovine and Human Serum Albumins: Binding Isotherms, Optical Rotatory Dispersion, Viscosity, Hydrogen Ion Titration, and Fluorescence Effects. *Biochemistry*, **10**, 4005-4015. http://dx.doi.org/10.1021/bi00798a001

[17] Bhattacharyya, M., Chaudhuri, U. and Poddar, R.K. (1990) Evidence for Cooperative Binding of Chlorpromazine with Hemoglobin: Equilibrium Dialysis, Fluorescence Quenching and Oxygen Release Study. *Biochemical and Biophysical Research Communications*, **167**, 1146-1153. http://dx.doi.org/10.1016/0006-291X(90)90643-2

[18] Rasoulzadeh, F., Asgari, D., Naseri, A. and Rashidi, M.R. (2010) Spectroscopic Studies on the Interaction between Erlotinib Hydrochloride and Bovine Serum Albumin. *DARU Journal of Pharmaceutical Sciences*, **18**, 179-184.

[19] Kaushelendra, M., Himesh, S., Govind, N., Sita, S.P. and Singhai, A.K. (2011) Method Development and Validation of Metformin Hydrochloride in Tablet Dosage Form. *E-Journal of Chemistry*, **8**, 1309-1313.

[20] Kandagal, P.B., Seetharamappa, J., Shaikh, S.M.T. and Manjunatha, D.H. (2007) Binding of Trazodone Hydrochloride with Human Serum Albumin: A Spectroscopic Study. *Journal of Photochemistry and Photobiology A*: Chemistry, **185**, 239-244. http://dx.doi.org/10.1016/j.jphotochem.2006.06.015

[21] Sun, S-F., Zhou, B., Hou, H-N., Liu, Y. and Xiang, G-Y. (2006) Studies on the Interaction between Oxaprozin-E and Bovine Serum Albumin by Spectroscopic Methods. *International Journal of Biological Macromolecules*, **39**, 197-200. http://dx.doi.org/10.1016/j.ijbiomac.2006.03.020

[22] Ross, P.D. and Subramanian, S. (1981) Thermodynamics of Protein Association Reactions: Forces Contributing to Stability. *Biochemistry*, **20**, 3096-3102. http://dx.doi.org/10.1021/bi00514a017

[23] Li, D., Zhu, J., Jin, J. and Yao, X. (2007) Studies on the Binding of Nevadensin to Human Serum Albumin by Molecular Spectroscopy and Modeling. *Journal of Molecular Structure*, **846**, 34-41. http://dx.doi.org/10.1016/j.molstruc.2007.01.020

[24] Sultana, S., Bin Sayeed, M.S., Ahamed, M.U., Islam, M.S., Bahar, A., Sultan, M.Z. and Hasnat, A. (2013) Interaction of Nalbuphine Hydrochloride with Deoxyribonucleic Acid Measured by Fluorescence Quenching. *Drug Research*, **63**, 224-227. http://dx.doi.org/10.1055/s-0033-1334874

[25] Rahman, M.A., Salam, M.A., Sultan, M.Z., Hossain, K., Rahman, A. and Rashid, M.A. (2014) DSC and HPLC Studies of Some Common Antidiabetic and Antihypertensive Drugs. *Bangladesh Pharmaceutical Journal*, **17**, 123-127.

[26] Ahsan, M.R., Sultan, M.Z., Amjad, F.M., Sultana, S., Baki, M.A., Hossain, M.A., Hossain, M.A. and Amran, M.S. (2012) The Study of *in Vitro* Interaction of Ciprofloxacin with Paracetamol and Zinc in Aqueous Medium. *Journal of Scientific Research*, **4**, 701-708. http://dx.doi.org/10.3329/jsr.v4i3.8709

[27] Rokonujjaman, M., Salam, M.A. and Sultan, M.Z. (2015) *In Vitro* Study of Interactions of Sildenafil Citrate with Bovine Serum Albumin in Presence of Bisoprolol Fumarate and Metformin Hydrochloride by Fluorescence Spectrophotometry. *British Journal of Medicine & Medical Research*, **5**, 362-375. http://dx.doi.org/10.9734/BJMMR/2015/11655

16

In Vivo and *in Vitro* Evaluation of Permethrin, Cypermethrin or Zeta-Cypermethrin Mixed with Plant Extracts against Susceptible and Resistant (San Alfonso) *Rhipicephalus* (*Boophilus*) *microplus* (Acari: Ixodidae) Strains

Froylán Ibarra-Velarde*, Yazmin Alcala-Canto, Yolanda Vera-Montenegro

Department of Parasitology, Faculty of Veterinary Medicine and Zoothecnics, National University Autonomous of Mexico, Mexico City, Mexico
Email: *ibarraf@unam.mx

Abstract

Acaricide resistance is a major problem that hinders the control of the cattle tick *Rhipicephalus* (*Boophilus*) *microplus* in Mexico. Permethrin (P), cypermethrin (C) and zeta-cypermethrin (Z) have been used to control *R.* (*B.*) *microplus*, and tick populations have developed resistance to these acaricides. The aim of the present study was to evaluate the effectiveness of a mixture containing P, C, or Z mixed with plant extracts through *in vitro* laboratory bioassays, using susceptible and triple resistant (San Alfonso) *R. microplus* strains. Untreated controls received only water. Results of laboratory bioassays using larval packet tests revealed an efficacy of 100% (P), 100% (Z), and 98.03% (C) using susceptible larvae, and an efficacy of 88.67% (P), 91.51% (C), and 99.27% (Z) on triple-resistant larvae. Egg laying, larvae hatching and efficacy was assessed using ticks collected from treated and untreated animals. Product Z produced a 92.04% efficacy on engorged ticks collected from experimentally-infested cattle, whereas C and P exerted 80.66% and 20.04% efficacy, respectively. Engorged females collected exclusively from control animals were challenged *in vitro* with the experimental products, and efficacy was as follows: 91.37% (Z), 85.95% (C), and 13.58% (P). Adding plant extracts to a pyrethroid formulation led to dramatic increases of percent reduction of both susceptible and resistant immature ticks in contrast to untreated larvae and susceptible adults. Results from this study may lead to suggesting the adoption of an acaricide-botanical mixture strategy for tick control worldwide.

*Corresponding author.

Keywords

Rhipicephalus (*Boophilus*) *microplus*, Efficacy, Pyrethroids + Plant Extracts, *In Vitro, In Vivo*

1. Introduction

Ticks are ectoparasites which frequently attacks cattle located in tropical or subtropical areas worldwide. In Mexico, *Boophilus microplus* causes strong economical losses to cattle because they play an important role on the transmision of babesiosis and anaplasmosis. In our country, from over 30 million cattle heads, 75% of them are located in tropical or subtropical areas and therefore susceptible to suffer the mentioned diseases.

Recent data indicates that 17% of Mexican cattle exported to the USA are rejected because it is infested with ticks [1]. During decades, the most used ixodicides for tick control have been organophosphates, pyrethroids and amidins [2]. Nevertheless, treatment costs are high, the use of chemical acaricides increases the risk of leaving drug residues in meat, milk as well as the environment, and some *R.* (*Boophilus*) *microplus* strains have developed acaricide resistance [3]. Studies reporting the acaricidal activity of plant extracts against *R.* (*Boophilus*) *microplus* have encouraged the use of natural active compounds that could be used as an alternative because of their lower environmental impact and cost; e.g., the extracts of *Hypericum polyanthemum* [4], limonene [5], plants from the Meliaceae family [6] [7], *Copaifera reticulata* [8], *Eucalyptus* spp. [9], *Anona squamosa*, *Azadirachta indica* [10], among others have been evaluated for their potential efficacy against *R.* (*Boophilus*) *microplus*. Natural extracts, whether alcoholic or water-based, have a longstanding historic tradition in Mexico and are regarded as a danger-free approach to treat and/or control infectious diseases. Although this might be an overstatement, it may be true for some chemical groups. In the search for these control alternatives, it is believed that some plant extracts mixed with some known ixodicides could enhance the ixodicidal effect. The aim of the present study was to evaluate the effectiveness of a mixture containing Permethrin (P), cypermethrin (C) and zeta-cypermethrin (Z) mixed with plant extracts through *in vitro* laboratory bioassays, using susceptible and triple resistant (San Alfonso) *R. microplus* strains.

2. Materials and Methods

2.1. *In Vivo* Test against *R.* (*Boophilus*) *microplus* Susceptible Larvae in Cattle

Compounds-Permetrin (P), cypermethrin (C) or Z-Cypermethrin (Z) extracts were mixed with plant extracts (Monocotyledons) at 25%. (Registration under patent regulation IK33/Power X21 initially authorized by the Federal Commission for the Protection of Sanitary Risks (Cofepris-Mexico in spanish), No. 113300CO220103/ 2012.

Animals

Animals used in this study were managed according to bioethical regulations according to the animal welfare Committee of our institution. Twenty-four european mixed race, steers with an average weight of 275 Kg, were used. They were kept on non-infested pads during the experiment. They were fed on commercial food and water was supplied *ad libitum*.

2.2. *R.* (*Boophilus*) *microplus* Strain

R. (*B.*) *microplus* susceptible and San Alfonso (resistant to amitraz, pyrethroids and organophosphates) strain larvae were kindly donated by the National Center of Parasitology (CENAPA) located in Morelos, Mexico and kept under biosecurity measures at the parasitology laboratory of our institution.

2.3. Infestation

On day 0, 1 g of 15-day-old susceptible larvae (equivalent to aproximately 20,000 larvae), were placed on the back of each animal. They remained on the experimental cattle until day 21 after infestation when ticks were engorged and fell to the floor for hatching.

2.4. Treatment

All animals were divided in 4 groups (G) of 6 animals each according to the average counts of ticks. G1 served as untreated control (T), G2 received permetrin (P), G3 was treated with cypermethrin (C) and G4 received Z-Cypermethrin (Z). Treatment was applied by aspersion using 5 litters of compound/animal. The untreated control was aspersed only with tap water using also 5 l/animal.

Twenty-four hours after treatment, engorged female ticks were collected from each group. They were placed in a sieve (100 microns mesh) and washed out with tap water. Afterwards, they were dried and placed in a Petri dish. Ticks isolated per group were transported to the parasitology laboratory and incubated at 27°C and 80% humidity to allow continuation of the development cycle. Weight of ova and percentage of eclosion from these specimens was estimated.

The obtained data on the pre and postreatment of all experimental groups were compared with regard to the untreated control group.

2.5. Larval Immersion *in Vitro* Assay

The larval immersion technique proposed by [11] was used to test acaricidal efficacy *in vitro*. Fifteen-day old larvae from susceptible and resistant San Alfonso (Triple Resistant: Amidins, Organophosphates and Piretroids) were used. Then larvae were divided for testing in four groups: Untreated Control (T); Permethrin (P); Cypermethrin (C) and Z-cypermethrin (Z). To assess the mortality percentage, live and dead larvae were counted. Each concentration was tested in three replicates.

2.6. Obtention of Ova

Engorged R. (*Boophilus*) *microplus* were collected from the four experimental groups. They were washed and dried on absorbent paper, weighed individually in an analytical weighing scale. Four groups (T, P, C, Z) of 20 ticks each were placed in Petri dishes and incubated at 27°C and 85% relative humidity to assess egg laying and larval hatching.

2.7. Percentage of Egg Hatching

Eggs were incubated by standard procedures at 27°C and 85% humidity during 21 days. The eclosion percentage was estimated by counting the eggs and larvae contained in each tube with the aid of an stereoscopic microscope. The index of egg laying (IE) was calculated as follows:

Index of Egg Laying $(IE) = $ Weight of eggs laid $(g)/$Weight of females (g)

The percentage (%) inhibition of egg-laying was therefore determined with the following formulae: [12].

% inhibition of egg laying $= ($IE control group $-$ IE treated group/E control group$) \times 100$

The efficacy of treatment was calculated according to formulae proposed by Drummond and Whetstone (1973) where:

Estimated reproduction (ER) = [(Weight of eggs (g)/Weight of females (g)] × % eclosion × 20,000 (estimate of the number of larvae in 1 g of eggs)

Once the ER was calculated in both treated and control groups, the control % was estimated:

Effectiveness of treatment $= \left[($ER control $-$ ER treated$)/$ER control$\right] \times 100$

2.8. Challenge of Engorged Females *in Vitro*

Engorged adult ticks were evaluated using the immersion test according to [13]. Eighty ticks were collected from the untreated controls, washed, dried on absorbent paper and weighed individually in an analytical weighing scale. Four groups of 20 ticks with similar weights each were immersed during 5 minutes in 1 ml of water, P, C or Z diluted in 0.5 l water. Ticks from each group were recovered from the solutions, dried and placed in a 9 cm Petri dish padded with Whatmann filter paper. Petri dishes were incubated at 27°C - 28°C and 75% - 85% relative humidity. The effect of the experimental products on tick mortality was recorded 24 h after treatment. After 14 days, the number of females laying eggs was recorded and eggs were collected, weighed and incubated at 27°C - 28°C and 75% - 85% relative humidity up to the hatching of the larvae. ER was estimated as mentioned previously.

2.9. Probit Analysis

After susceptible and triple-resistant larvae were exposed to filter paper circles impregnated with different water-based concentrations of permethrin, cypermethrin, or Z-cypermethrin prepared from stock solutions of 10,000 ppm, results were subjected to Probit analysis using the POLO-PC software, provided by the Department of Pharmacology and Physiology of the FMVZ-UNAM. The LC_{50} of permethrin, cypermethrin and Z-cypermethrin were determined by an analysis of regression to the Probit-transformed data of death larvae with 95% confidence limits.

3. Results

3.1. *In Vitro* Efficacy against *R.* (*Boophilus*) *microplus* Susceptible Larvae

The obtained results showed that permethrin killed all larvae on the assay generating a 100% efficacy. Cipermethrin reached a 98.0% efficacy and Z-Cypermethrin generated a 100% mortality. The larvae from the untreated control remained healthy and active and no mortality was observed (**Table 1**).

3.2. *In Vitro* Efficacy against San Alfonso Triple Resistant Strain of *R.* (*Boophilus*) *microplus* Larvae

The average efficacy exerted by permethrin was 88.6%, cypermethrin produced a 91.5% mortality and Z-Cypermethrin caused a 99.2% efficacy. The untreated control group remained healthy with no mortality (**Table 2**).

3.3. Effectiveness of Treatment

As shown in **Table 3**, product Z produced a 92.04% efficacy against engorged ticks collected from experimentally-infested cattle, whereas C and P exerted 80.66% and 20.04% efficacy, respectively. Regarding adult ticks challenged *in vitro* with the experimental products, efficacy was as follows: 91.37% (Z), 85.95% (C), and 13.58% (P) (**Table 4**).

Table 1. Efficacy of three compounds against larvae of a susceptible strain of *Rhipicephalus* (*Boophilus*) *microplus* according to the Shaw assay.

GROUP (n = 3)	Alive (mean)	Dead (mean)	Mortality %
Untreated controls	100	0	0
Permethrin	0	100	100
Cypermethrin	1	50	98.03
Z-Cypermethrin	0	100	100

Table 2. Efficacy of three compounds against larvae of a triple-resistant (San Alfonso) strain of *Rhipicephalus* (*Boophilus*) *microplus* using the Shaw assay.

GROUP (n = 6)	Alive (mean)	Dead (mean)	Mortality %
Untreated controls	100	0	0
Permethrin	10	78	88.67
Cypermethrin	4.6	50	91.51
Z-Cypermethrin	1	182	99.27

Table 3. Effectiveness of *in vitro* treatment against engorged *Riphicephalus* (*Boophilus*) *microplus* adult females.

Group	Estimated reproduction	Efficacy (%)
Untreated	19.41	0
Permethrin	15.52	20.04
Cypermethrin	3.75	80.66
Z-Cypermethrin	1.54	92.04

Table 4. Effectiveness of *in vitro* treatment (Drummond assay) against engorged *Riphicephalus* (*Boophilus*) *microplus* adult females.

Group	Estimated reproduction	Efficacy (%)
Untreated	18.96	0
Permethrin	16.39	13.58
Cypermethrin	2.66	85.95
Z-Cypermethrin	1.63	91.37

After subjecting data of the susceptible strain of *Rhipicephalus* (*Boophilus*) *microplus* larvae mortality to Probit analysis, the LC50 of permethrin, cypermethrin, and Z-cypermethrin were determined. The LC_{50} were 1015.78 ppm with 95% confidence intervals (415.82 - 1618.25) for permethrin, 436.2 (404.10 - 468.57) for cypermethrin, and 258.54 (243.76 - 273.84) por Z-cypermethrin (**Table 5**).

Regarding the San Alfonso strain larvae, the LC_{50} were 8353.7 (7956.8 - 8750.42) for permethrin, 3235.19 (3069.09 - 3419.28) for cypermethrin, and 345.08 (329.3 - 363.48) for Z-cypermethrin (**Table 6**).

4. Discussion

Most cattle located in the tropics, are at risk from being infested by various tick species as well as tick-borne diseases [14], *R. Boophilus microplus* (Canestrini) is an ectoparasite of cattle that causes significant economic losses in several tropical and subtropical countries of Africa, Latin America, Northern and Eastern Australia. It represents one of the main constraints to cost-effective production due to its direct parasitic action and to the fact that it is the vector of important pathogens.

In the present study, results of *in vitro* bioassays using larval packet tests revealed an efficacy of 100% (P), 98.03% (C) and 100% (Z), using susceptible larvae, and an efficacy of 88.67% (P), 91.51% (C), and 99.27% (Z) on triple-resistant larvae. Data obtained strongly suggests that adding plant extracts to a pyrethroid formulation led to dramatic increases of percent reduction of both susceptible and resistant immature ticks in contrast to untreated larvae. Regarding adult females, a desirable efficacy of over 90% was assessed only with product Z. It is therefore tempting to speculate that the lower level of efficacy observed in adult ticks treated with pyrethroid-derived products in contrast to results observed in larvae, might be caused by a lower penetration of the experimental plant-derived products to the harder cuticle present in adults, or to the contribution of more developed metabolic pathways involved in pyrethroid resistance.

A variation of LC_{50} values for pyrethroids has been documented [15]. This variation might be due to the difference in strains and performed methodology. In this study, a significant difference in LC_{50} values was observed between permethrin, cypermethrin and Z-cypermethrin in biossays carried out on susceptible strains. It is therefore reasonable to suggest that the latter products have a higher efficacy than permethrin. Moreover, the resistant strain required a higher concentration to achieve the LC_{50} value for the three acaricides. This value was significantly higher for the experimental permethrin and cypermethrin; which prompt the need of further studies to determine the resistance to these products.

In addition efficacy on larvae of the experimental pyrethroids used in the present study was similar to pyrethroid-based commercial products, which has been determined as 100% [16]. In contrast, the same authors reported a higher efficacy (92% - 99%) on engorged females than the one determined in the present study. Thus, studies are required to improve the pharmacological design of these compounds in order to enhance their efficacy on adult ticks.

Willadsen and Kemp [17] have regrettably discussed the impact that decades of scientific advances have had on tick control for farming and animal husbandry practices. In Australia, for example, adoption of acaricide-based tick control programs among cattle producers ranged from 19% to as low as 6% of farms surveyed. Contributing factors include the complexity of the livestock-tick interactions, the cost of implementation, and the limited success rates of the various tick control strategies available. Nari and Hansen [18] mentioned that the cost of development of a new ixodicide can be in excess of 100 to 230 million US dollars and that this process might take more than 10 years from the discovery of a candidate to the launching on the market. Furthermore, selection of resistance genes in ticks against current ixodicides is an increasing problem [19]. Therefore, new

Table 5. Lethal concentration of permethrin, cypermethrin and Z-cypermethrin on a suceptible strain of *Riphicephalus* (*Boophilus*) *microplus* larvae.

Group	Slope ± S.E.	R2	LC50 (ppm) (95% confidence limit)
Permethrin	2.86 ± 0.310	0.91	1015.78 (415.82 - 1618.25)
Cypermethrin	3.04 ± 0.149	0.89	436.2 (404.10 - 468.57)
Z-cypermethrin	3.32 ± 0.673	0.97	258.54 (243.76 - 273.84

Table 6. Lethal concentration of permethrin, cypermethrin and Z-cypermethrin on San Alfonso strain of *Riphicephalus* (*Boophilus*) *microplus* larvae.

Group	Slope ± S.E.	R2	LC50 (ppm) (95% confidence limit)
Permethrin	0.35 ± 0.20	0.92	8353.7 (7956.8 - 8750.42)
Cypermethrin	1.22 ± 0.68	0.95	3235.19 (3069.09 - 3419.28)
Z-cypermethrin	2.86 ± 0.02	0.99	345.08 (329.3 - 363.48)

strategies for tick control should be undertaken to optimize the use of available drugs. The success of some experimental acaricides obtained from natural extracts has prompted research on active phytochemicals that might have efficacy against ticks. There are many studies on the activity of plants against engorged females and larvae most of which show the reduction in the egg-laying capacity of ticks exposed to different natural extracts [8]-[20].

The present findings highly suggest to undertake broader bioassays in order to elucidate the role of natural compounds combined with current ixodicides in the larvicidal and anti-fertility outcomes described in the present paper and to improve acaricidal effectiveness, particularly in resistant strains. Results from this study may lead to suggest the adoption of an acaricide-botanical mixture strategy for the control of triple-resistant *R. microplus* in Mexico and elsewhere.

5. Conclusion

The mixture of three pyrethroids with plant extracts exerted higher acaricidal efficacy under *in vitro* and *in vivo* conditions.

Acknowledgements

The authors are indebted to Ing. Alejandro Canales-Farías from Laboratorios Shark, S.A. de C.V for kind donation of the compounds.

References

[1]   Bram, R.A., George, J.E., Reichar, R.E. and Tabaciinic, W.J. (2002) Threat of Foreign Arthropod-Borne Pathogens to Livestock in the United States. *Journal of Medical Entomology*, **39**, 405-416. http://dx.doi.org/10.1603/0022-2585-39.3.405

[2]   Rodriguez-Vivas, I., Rivas, A.L., Chowell, G., Fragoso, S.H., Rosario, C.R., Garcia, Z., Smith, S.D., Williams, J.J. and Schwager, S.J. (2007) Spatial Distribution of Acaricide Profiles (*Boophilus microplus* Strains Susceptible or Resistant to Acaricides) in Southeastern Mexico. *Veterinary Parasitology*, **146**, 158-169. http://dx.doi.org/10.1016/j.vetpar.2007.01.016

[3]   Miller, R.J., Davey, R.B. and George, J.E. (2002) Modification of the Food and Agriculture Organization Larval Packet Test to Measure Amitraz Susceptibility against Ixodidae. *Journal of Medical Entomology*, **39**, 645-651. http://dx.doi.org/10.1603/0022-2585-39.4.645

[4]   Ribeiro, V.L.S., Toigo, E., Bordignon, S.A.L., Gonçalves, K. and von Poser, G. (2007) Acaricidal Properties of Extracts from the Aerial Parts of *Hypericum polyanthemum* on the Cattle Tick *Boophilus microplus*. *Veterinary Parasitology*, **147**:199-203. http://dx.doi.org/10.1016/j.vetpar.2007.03.027

[5]   Ferrarini, S.R., Oliveira, D.M., da Rosa, R.G., Rolim, V., Eifler-Lima, V.L., von Poser, G. and Ribeiro, V.L.S. (2008) Acaricidal Activity of Limonene, Limonene Oxide And β-Amino Alcohol Derivatives on *Rhipicephalus* (*Boophilus*)

microplus. Veterinary Parasitology, **157**, 149-153. http://dx.doi.org/10.1016/j.vetpar.2008.07.006

[6] Mulla, M.S. and Su, T. (1999) Activity of Biological Effects of Neem Products against Arthropods of Medical and Veterinary Importance. *American Mosquito Control Association*, **15**, 133-152.

[7] Borges, M.F., Ferri, P.H., Silva, W.J., Silva, W.C. and Silva, J.G. (2003) *In Vitro* Efficacy of Extracts of *Melia azedarach* against the Tick *Boophilus microplus. Medical and Veterinary Entomology*, **17**, 228-231. http://dx.doi.org/10.1046/j.1365-2915.2003.00426.x

[8] Fernandes, F.F. and Freitas, E.P.S. (2007) Acaricidal Activity of an Oleoresinous Extract from *Copaifera reticulata* (Leguminosae: Caesalpinioideae) against Larvae of the Southern Cattle Tick, *Rhipicephalus (Boophilus) microplus* (Acari: Ixodidae). *Veterinary Parasitology*, **147**, 150-154. http://dx.doi.org/10.1016/jj.vetpar.2007.02.035

[9] Chagas, A.C.S., Passos, M.W.M., Prates, H.T., Leite, R.C., Furlong, J. and Fortes, I.C.P. (2002) Acaricidal Effect of Essential Oils and Emulsion Concentrates of *Eucalyptus* spp on *Boophilus microplus. Brazilian Journal of Veterinary Research and Animal Science*, **39**, 247-253. http://dx.doi.org/10.1590/S1413-95962002000500006

[10] Magadum, S., Mondal, D.B. and Ghosh, S. (2009) Comparative Efficacy of *Annona squamosa* and *Azadirachta indica* Extracts against *Boophilus microplus* Izatnagar Isolate. *Parasitology Research*, **105**, 1085-1091. http://dx.doi.org/10.1007/s00436-009-1529-3

[11] Shaw, R.D. (1966) Culture of an Organophosphorus-Resistant Strain of *Boophilus microplus* (Can.) and an Assessment of Its Resistance Spectrum. *Bulletin of Entomological Research*, **56**, 389-405.

[12] Sardá Ribeiro, V., Avancini, C., Goncalves, K., Toigo, E. and Von Poser, G. (2008) Acaricidal Activity of *Calea serrata* (Asteraceae) on *Boophilus microplus* and *Rhipicephalus sanguineus. Veterinary Parasitology*, **151**, 351-354.

[13] Drummond, R.O. and Whetstone, T.M. (1973) Lone Star Tick: Laboratory Tests of Acaricides. *Journal of Economic Entomology*, **66**, 1274-1276. http://dx.doi.org/10.1093/jee/66.6.1274

[14] Bock, R., Jackson, L., De Vos, A. and Jorgensen, W. (2004) Babesiosis of Cattle. *Parasitology*, **129**, S247-S269.

[15] Sharma, A.K., Kumar, R., Kumar, S., Nagar, G., Kumar, S.N., Sing Rawat, S., Dhakad, M.L., Rawat, A.K.S., Ray, D.D. and Ghosh, S. (2012) Deltamethrin and Cypermethrin Resistance Status of *Rhipicephalus (Boophilus) microplus* Collected from Six Agro-Climatic Regions of India. *Veterinary Parasitology*, **188**, 337-345. http://dx.doi.org/10.1016/j.vetpar.2012.03.050

[16] Fragoso, H., Martinez, I., Ortiz, N. and Osorio, M. (2006) Comparison of the Efficacy of Organofosfates, Piretroids and Amidines Ixodicides against a *Boophilus microplus* Ticks Reinfestation in Naturally Infested Cattle. XXX National Congress of Buiatrícs, Mexico.

[17] Willadsen, P. and Kemp, D.H. (1988) Vaccination with Concealed Antigens for Tick Control. *Parasitology Today*, **4**, 196-198. http://dx.doi.org/10.1016/0169-4758(88)90084-1

[18] Nari, A. and Hansen, H.J. (1999) Resistance of the Ecto and Endoparasites: Actual and Future Solutions. 67th General Session, International Organization of Epizootias, París.

[19] Fernandes, F.F. (2001) Toxicological Effects and Resistance to Pyretroids in *Boophilus microplus* from Goiás, Brasil. *Arquivo Brasileiro de Medicina Veterinária e Zootecnia*, **53**, 548-552. http://dx.doi.org/10.1590/S0102-09352001000500004

[20] Fernandes, F.F., Freitas, E.P.S., Costa, A.C. and Silva, I.G. (2005) Larvicidal Potential of *Sapindus saponaria* to Control the Cattle Tick *Boophilus microplus. Pesquisa Agropecuária Brasileira*, **40**, 1243-1245. http://dx.doi.org/10.1590/S0100-204X2005001200013

17

Protective Effect of Ketamine against Acetic Acid-Induced Ulcerative Colitis in Rats

Esraa Elsayed Ashry, Rasha Bakheet Abdellatief, Abeer Elrefaiy Mohamed, Hassan Ibrahim Kotb

Faculty of Medicine, Assiut University, Assiut, Egypt
Email: esraaashry@yahoo.co.uk, r_bakheet@yahoo.com, Abeer_refaiy@yahoo.com, kotbhi@yahoo.com

Abstract

Objective: Inflammatory bowel diseases (IBD), including Crohn's disease and ulcerative colitis (UC), are chronic and recurrent disorders of the gastrointestinal tract with unknown etiology. Considering the adverse effects and incomplete efficacy of currently administered drugs, it is crucial to explore new drugs with more desirable therapeutic profiles. As non-competitive N-methyl-D-aspartate (NMDA) receptor antagonists have shown analgesic and anti-inflammatory properties *in vitro* and *in vivo*, this study aims to investigate the role of ketamine, a noncompetitive NMDA receptor antagonist, in acetic acid-induced rat colitis. Methods: Ketamine (10, 50 mg/kg), and dexamethasone (1 mg/kg) were given intraperitoneally 30 min before induction of colitis which was done by instillation of 2 mL of 4% acetic acid (vol/vol). At the 4th day of colitis induction, animals were sacrificed and distal colons were assessed macroscopically and microscopically. Furthermore, the mucosal contents of lipid peroxidation (LPO), reduced glutathione (GSH), nitric oxide (NO) and tumor necrosis factor-α (TNF-α) were assessed. Results: Ketamine (50 mg/kg) and dexamethasone significantly ($p < 0.05$) improved macroscopic and histologic scores, diminished colonic levels of MDA, NO and TNF-α and elevated GSH levels. Conclusion: Our data suggest that ketamine has valuable protective effects in acetic acid colitis and it may be a new therapy target in ulcerative colitis patients, possibly by regulating antioxidants and inflammatory mediators.

Keywords

Ketamine, Ulcerative Colitis, Rats

1. Introduction

Ulcerative colitis is a chronically recurrent inflammatory bowel disease. Although its etiology remains essentially unknown, yet studies suggest that genetic susceptibility, altered immune response and environmental factors are involved in both initiation and progression of colitis. Despite the great deal of attention for this disease during the past years, its pharmacological treatment is still unsatisfactory [1] [2].

The acetic acid-induced ulcerative colitis is a widely used animal model of ulcerative colitis [3]-[5]. This experimental model resembles ulcerative colitis in histology, eicosanoid production and response to sulfasalazine [6].

Management of inflammatory bowel diseases (IBD) is based on aminosalicylates, glucocorticoids, immunomodulators and more recently monoclonal antibodies. Nevertheless, the high incidences of adverse effects together with the failure to be generally efficacious make it indispensable to explore new candidates with more desirable therapeutic profiles [7].

Ketamine, a noncompetitive N-methyl-D-aspartate (NMDA) receptor antagonist, is commonly used as an intravenous or intramuscular anesthetic. Several investigators show that administration of ketamine has protective effects against polymicrobial sepsis in rats. Ketamine probably inhibits NF-κB activation and attenuates the proinflammatory cytokine response. It was reported that ketamine has inhibitory effects on lipopolysaccharide (LPS)-induced TNF-α production in endotoxin-induced shock in rats [8] [9]. Others have documented that ketamine could suppress proinflammatory cytokines production in human whole blood *in vitro* [10] [11].

In the present study, we have evaluated the protective effects of ketamine, a noncompetitive N-methyl-D-aspartate (NMDA) receptor antagonist, against acetic acid-induced colitis in rats.

2. Materials and Methods

2.1. Materials

Animals: Adult male Wistar rats (200 - 250 g) (n = 30) were purchased from Animal house of faculty of Medicine, Assiut University. The animal room was maintained at 22°C - 24°C and a lighting regimen of 12 hour light/ 12 hour dark. Rats were fed with standard house chow and water *ad libitum*. All animal experiments were performed after getting prior approval from the Institutional Animal Ethics Committee Assiut University.

Drugs: Ketamine (1867-66-9) and Dexamethasone (50-02-2) were purchased from Sigma-Tec Pharmaceutical Industries Egypt-S.A.E.

2.2. Experimental Design

Rats were divided into five groups (n = 6 per group). Group I kept as control and received no treatment. Group II, III, IV, V were subjected to the induction of ulcerative colitis by intracolonic injection of 2 ml acetic acid (4% v/v). Thirty min before induction of colitis, group II was given normal saline (i.p.); group III was treated with dexamethasone (1 mg/kg, i.p.); Group IV, V were treated with ketamine (10 and 50 mg/kg, i.p.) respectively.

2.2.1. Induction of Colonic Inflammation

All animals (except group I) were fasted for 6h prior to study, with access to water *ad libitum* and anesthetized by an intraperitoneal injection of 1% sodium pentobarbital in a dose of 50 mg/kg before induction of colitis, 2 ml acetic acid (4% v/v) in 0.9% saline were infused for 30s using a soft pediatric catheter size of 6F 2 mm in diameter, inserted through rectum into the colon up to a distance of 8cm and maintained in a supine Trendelenburg position for 30 s to prevent leakage of the intracolonic instill. On the 4th day after operation, colon were collected after sacrificing the animals, portions of colon specimens were dissected out, washed with physiological saline and kept in 10% formalin for macroscopic and histological studies [3] [12].

2.2.2. Assessments of Colitis

Macroscopic scoring: For each animal, the distal 10 cm portions of the colon were removed cut longitudinally and cleaned with physiological saline to remove fecal residues. Macroscopic inflammation scores are assigned based on the clinical features of the colon using a scale ranging from 0 - 4 as follows: 1, intact epithelium with no damage; 2, patch type superficial hyperemia; 3, generalized patch type hyperemic regions; 4, generalized hyperemia and hemorrhage [13].

Histological analysis: The colon specimens (2 cm) collected from the animals were fixed in 10% formalin, embedded in paraffin and cut into 4 μm sections. The paraffin sections were deparafinized with xylene, hydrated and stained with hematoxylin and eosin for studying mucosal damage assessment. The assessment was done as previously described by Noronha *et al.*, [14] according to following scale: 0, intact epithelium, no leukocyte or hemorrhage; 1, <25% disrupted epithelium, focal leukocyte infiltrates and focal hemorrhage; 2, 25% disrupted epithelium, focal leukocyte infiltrates and focal hemorrhage; 3, 50% disrupted epithelium, widespread leuko-cytes, and hemorrhage; 4, >50% disrupted epithelium, extensive leukocyte infiltration and hemorrhage.

Biochemical measurements: The colon tissue were homogenized in 10 mmol Tris-HCl buffer (pH 7.4) and the homogenate were used for the measurement of Nitric oxide (NO), lipid peroxidation (LPO), reduced glutathione (GSH) and TNF-α.

Malondialdehyde measurement: Lipid peroxidation, a major indicator of oxidative stress, was determined by measuring MDA level in tissue homogenate. MDA is a byproduct of the arachidonate cycle, its level was deter-mined spectrophotometrically by using the thiobarbituric acid reactive substances method previously described by Ohkawa et al., (1979) [15]. A standard curve was run simultaneously with each set of samples by using 1, 1, 3, 3-tetramethoxypropane as an external standard. The results are expressed as nmol/gm wet tissue weight.

NO measurement: Nitric oxide formation was measured in tissue samples by assaying nitrite, one of the stable end products of NO oxidation, serum nitrite concentration was assayed spectrophotometrically by using Griess reaction according to the standard method described by Green et al. (1982) [16].

GSH measurements: The colon GSH content was determined using Ellman's reagent (5, 5-dithio-bis-2-nitro-benzoic acid) according to the method of Griffith (1980) [17]. A standard curve was prepared for each assay. The results are expressed as μmol/gm wet tissue weight.

Determination of TNF-α: The colon tissue was used for measurement of TNF-α level according to the manu-facturer's instructions using an immuno assay kit (Assaypro, LTA, Italy).

2.3. Statistical Analysis

Results are expressed as mean ± SD. The data was analyzed by one way ANOVA followed by Dennett's test with post-hoc was employed. A p value < 0.05 was considered significant.

3. Results

3.1. Effect of Ketamine on Macroscopic Features

Colonic instillation of acetic acid triggered an intense inflammatory response on the 4th day of colitis induction, the distal colon showed severe macroscopic edematous inflammation. The mucosa was inflamed, ulcerated, hyperemic and hemorrhagic compared to normal control group. However, intracolonic treatment with dexame-thasone and ketamine (50 mg/k) 30 min before induction of ulcerative colitis attenuated the macroscopic dam-age and improved macroscopic scores. Ketamine (50 mg/kg) was found to be satisfactory in the protection of the rat colon against acetic-acid induced injury. No significant differences were seen between ketamine (50 mg/kg) and dexamethasone. However, low dose of ketamine (10 mg/kg) failed to improve macroscopic scores (**Table 1**).

3.2. Effect of Ketamine on Histopathological Features

Colonic mucosa of rats in the control group had a normal architecture with intact epithelium, signs of inflamma-tion or necrosis were not observed (**Figure 1(A)**). Four days subsequent to the induction of colitis, the micro-scopic inspection of the colon revealed multifocal areas of necrosis, hemorrhage, submucosal edema, extensive polymorphonuclear granulocyte infiltration in the mucosa, the inflammation extended through the muscularis mucosae and submucosa, distorted crypts as well as massive necrotic destruction of the epithelium was observed

Table 1. Protective effects of ketamine (10, 50 mg/kg, ip) on macroscopic and histologic features of the colon 4 days after induction of colitis.

No.	Group	Macroscopic damage score	Histologic score
I	Control	1 ± 0.00^c	0 ± 0.00^c
II	Acetic acid control	4 ± 0.1^b	3.9 ± 0.3^b
III	Dexamethasone (1 mg/kg, ip)	1.3 ± 0.9^c	1.4 ± 0.3^c
IV	Ketamine (10 mg/kg, ip)	2.95 ± 0.4	2.8 ± 0.2
V	Ketamine (50 mg/kg, ip)	1.78 ± 0.6^c	1.6 ± 0.4^c

Values are expressed as mean ± SD; n = 6; ^{b}p < 0.05 in comparison to control group; ^{c}p < 0.05 in comparison to acetic acid control group.

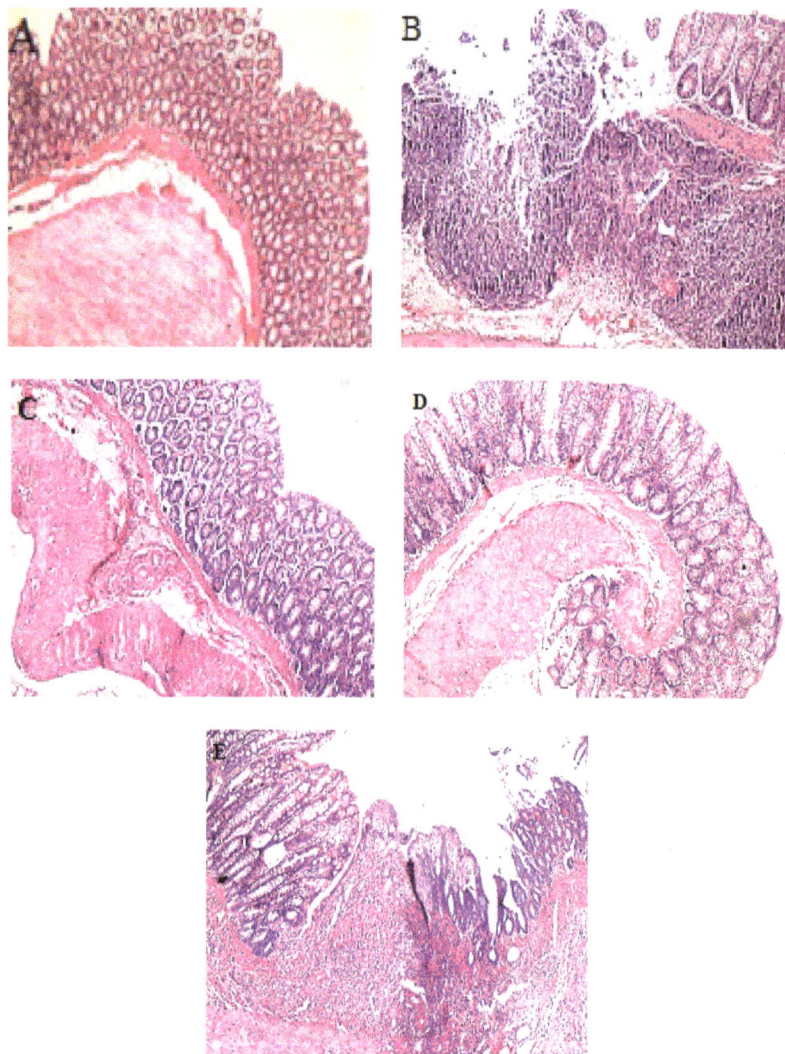

Figure 1. Effect of ketamine on colon histology. (A) Specimen from a normal rat showing colon with normal mucosa; (B) Control specimen from acetic acid induced rats showing colitis with large necrotic destruction of epithelial cells, areas of hemorrhage, submucosal edema and inflammatory cellular infiltration; (C) Colitis + Dexamethasone (1 mg/kg B. wt); (D) Colitis + Ketamine (50 mg/kg B. wt) + (E) Colitis + Ketamine (10 mg/kg B. wt) (100× magnification).

(**Figure 1(B)**). In ketamine (50 mg/kg) and dexamethasone treated groups, the histopathological changes were significantly attenuated, as judged by epithelization of the mucosa, reduction of edema and inflammatory cells recruitment (**Figure 1(C)**, **Figure (D)**). No significant difference was observed between ketamine (50 mg/kg) and dexamethasone treated groups, both of them showed a significant decrease in the pathological scores in acetic acid-induced colitis rats as compared with the colitis control group. However, low dose of ketamine (10 mg/kg) showed focal disruption of epithelium and focal inflammatory cells in the lamina propria of all rats in this group (**Figure 1(E)**, **Table 1**).

3.3. Effect of Ketamine on Malondialdehyde Level

Effect of ketamine on malondialdehyde level is shown in **Figure 2**. Administration of ketamine (50 mg/kg) or dexamethasone to acetic acid treated rats significantly reduced lipid peroxidation ($p < 0.05$) compared to colitis group. However, ketamine (10 mg/kg) didn't show any significant differences in comparison to the colitis group.

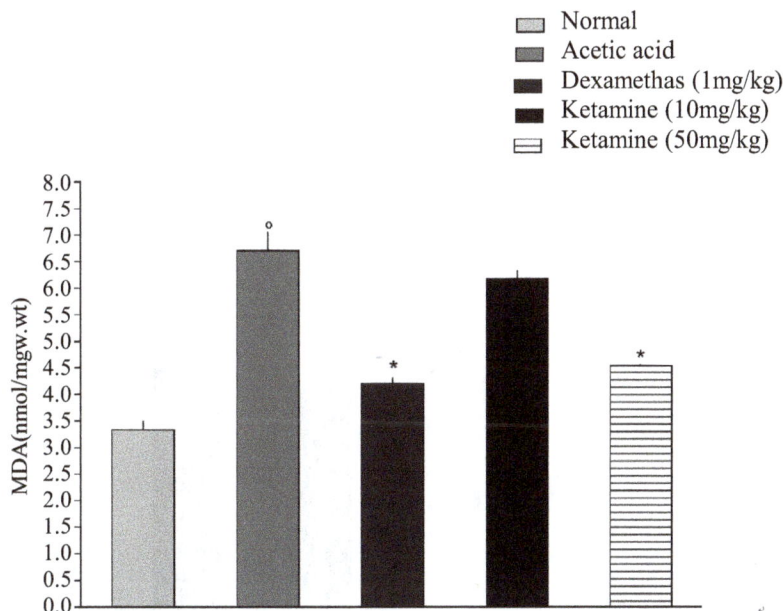

Figure 2. Effect of ketamine on MDA level in the colonic tissue. Ketamine (50 mg/kg) or dexamethasone treatment significantly reduced MDA levels. Values are expressed as mean ± SD, *p < 0.05 vs. acetic acid group, colitis significantly increased MDA levels, °p < 0.05 vs. control group.

3.4. Effect of Ketamine on Nitrite Level

Nitrite was markedly enhanced in the inflamed colon after intrarectal acetic acid instillation. Treatment with either ketamine (50 mg/kg) or dexamethasone significantly (p < 0.05) inhibited acetic acid induced NO production in tissue (**Figure 3**).

3.5. Effect of Ketamine on GSH Level

Effect of ketamine on colon GSH level is shown in **Figure 4**. The decreased colonic GSH in the colitis group was found to be significantly (p < 0.05) increased after ketamine (50 mg/kg) and dexamethasone treatment.

3.6. Effect of Ketamine on TNF-α

Colonic levels of TNF-α show drastic rise after acetic acid introduction compared with those of control group. In contrast these values were significantly lower in rats treated with ketamine (50 mg/kg) or dexamethasone. There were no significant differences in TNF-α levels between ketamine (50 mg/kg) and dexamethasone treated animals (**Figure 5**).

4. Discussion

Our study was focused on studying the effects of ketamine on acetic acid-induced colitis and our results clearly show that ketamine could inhibit experimental colitis. Ketamine administered 30 min before intracolonic instillation of 4% acetic acid caused a dramatic reduction in the severity of colitis which was comparable to dexamethasone. This effect is possibly attributed to its anti-inflammatory and antioxidant properties as indicated by improved macroscopic and histological features, correction of the increased biochemical markers MDA, nitrite, GSH and a decrease in colonic content of TNF-α.

Ketamine is a noncompetitive N-methyl-D-aspartate (NMDA) receptor antagonist, extensively used as a safe and adequate intravenous or intramuscular anesthetic in various clinical situations. Ketamine is recommended for use in cases with a high risk of septicemia. It was reported that in addition to its anesthetic activity, it has novel anti-inflammatory properties [18]. However, no clear definitive mechanism for the anti-inflammatory action of ketamine has been suggested.

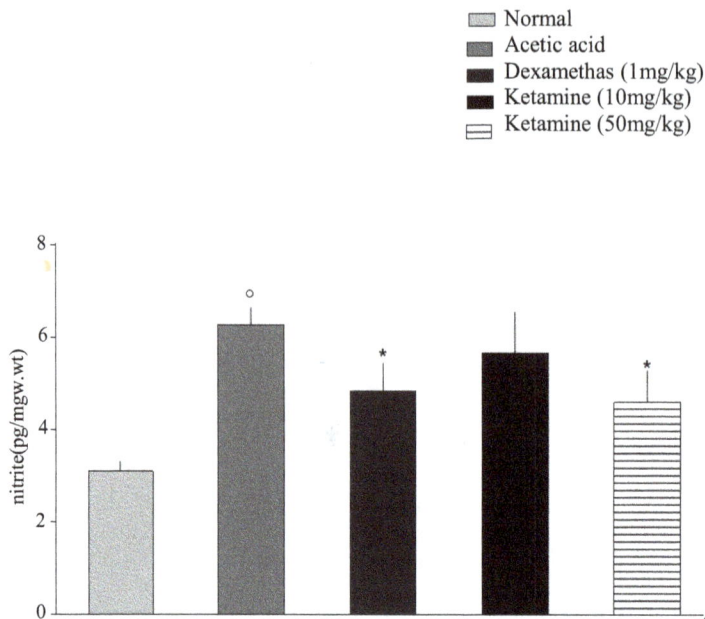

Figure 3. Effect of ketamine on NO level in the colonic tissue. Ketamine (50 mg/kg) or dexamethasone treatment significantly reduced NO levels. Values are expressed as mean ± SD, $^*p < 0.05$ vs. colitis group. Colitis significantly increased NO levels, $^{\circ}p < 0.05$ vs. control group.

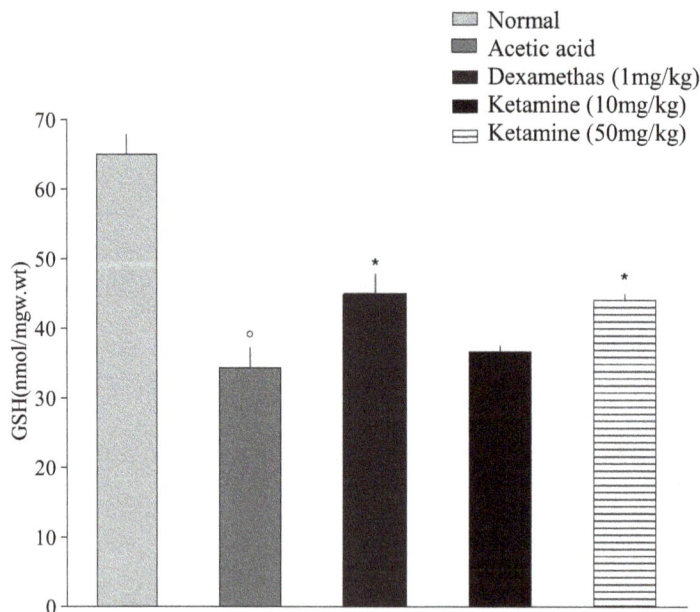

Figure 4. Effect of ketamine on GSH level in the colonic tissue ketamine (50 mg/kg) or dexamethasone treatment significantly elevated GSH levels. Values are expressed as mean ± SD, $^*p < 0.05$ vs. colitis group. Colitis significantly reduced GSH levels, $^{\circ}p < 0.05$ vs. control group.

It was reported that ROS (reactive oxygen species) generated in the inflamed mucosa can modulate many inflammatory events.ROS produce several inflammatory cytokines in various tissues which aggravate tissue damage. The free radicals produced during oxidative damage attack polyunsaturated fatty acids in plasma membrane leading to membrane lipid peroxidation and severe cell damage. This process plays a significant role in the pathogenesis of the disease [19]. In this study colitis control animals exhibited increased levels of MDA in colon

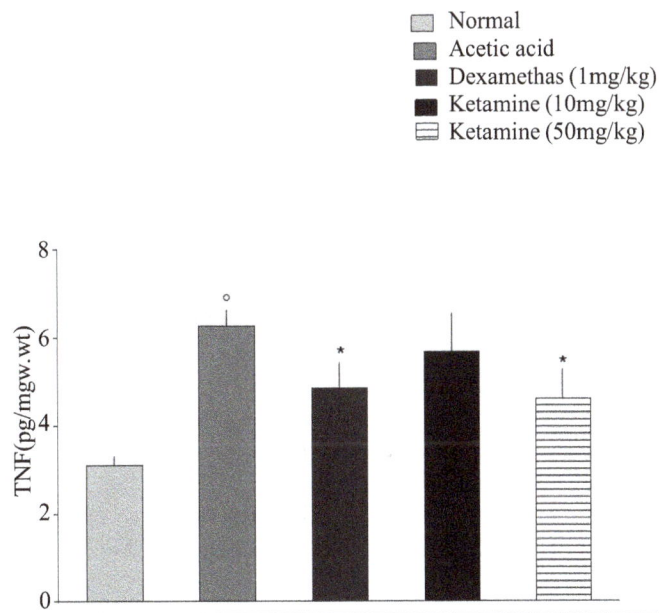

Figure 5. Effect of ketamine on TNF-α level in the colonic tissue. Ketamine (50 mg/kg) or dexamethasone treatment significantly reduced TNF-α levels. Values are expressed as mean± SD, $^{*}p < 0.05$ vs. colitis group. Colitis significantly increased TNF-α levels, $^{\circ}p < 0.05$ vs. control group.

tissue. Ketamine treatment dramatically reduced the increased MDA levels. A significant reduction in MDA by treatment with ketamine exhibits the anti-inflammatory effect in the experimental colitis model and this may be related to the antioxidant and free radical scavenging ability of ketamine.

GSH is an important intracellular antioxidant agent in mammalian gut. It is involved in the repair mechanism as it inhibits mucosal damage by free radicals. During inflammation, GSH level decreases resulting in severe degradation of colon mucosa. Therefore GSH plays an important role in protecting the intestinal cells and as a defense mechanism against inflammation [20]. Treatment with ketamine significantly increased the colonic GSH level, reasonably, the mitigation of macroscopic and histopathologic indices.

NO is an important proinflammatory mediator. The nitric oxide and iNOS has been reported as potential mediators for colitis. During colitis, the observed inflammatory reactions as enhanced interstitial edema, increased arteriolar blood flow, fluid exudation across intestinal capillaries, thickening of the intestinal wall, are all associated with inflammatory mediators such as NO [21]. The present study showed that administration of ketamine significantly inhibited NO production which prevented peroxynitrite formation from inflammatory cells and countered inflammation.

The relationship between NMDA receptors and peripheral inflammatory responses has not been completely understood. Érces *et al.* 2012 [22], have proposed that Ca^{2+} over influx via the receptor associated ion channel activates excessive NO generation by NOS isoforms which mediate the downstream signal transduction of the NMDA receptors with subsequent excitotoxic neuronal cell death and intestinal malfunction. They postulated that reduction of the excessive NO generation by direct or indirect inhibition of NOS may be an appropriate approach for the treatment of intestinal inflammatory changes.

Ulcerative colitis has been associated with an intense local immune response which is associated with recruitment of lymphocytes and macrophages followed by release of soluble cytokines. Cytokines are crucial elements in gastrointestinal inflammation, however, their overproduction result injurious events.TNF is an important proinflammatory cytokine released from the macrophages and lymphocytes in the early inflammatory response. It has been reported to play an integral role in the pathogenesis of inflammatory bowel disease [23]. Blocking of TNF has been shown to inhibit colitis in animal models. It was increased following acetic acid instillation in our experiment. Ketamine treatment inhibits TNF production which may be due to inhibition of its synthesis or release. Our results parallel recent investigations showing anti-inflammatory properties of ketamine [24].

The anti-inflammatory effect of ketamine subanesthetic doses has been demonstrated in various animal models. It was found that ketamine produced a dose-dependent decrease in mortality with a significant reduction in the production of tumour necrosis factor-α (TNF-α) and IL-6 after stimulation of lipopolysaccharide in carrageenan-sensitized mice injected with endotoxin [25]. Recent studies have demonstrated that ketamine inhibited the leucocyte production and release of various cytokines as TNF-α, IL-6, IL-8 and nitric oxide and inhibited oxygen radical generation of isolated human neutrophils [18] [26] [27].

Guzman *et al.*, 2010 [28], found that ketamine protection against intestinal I/R injury was related to a reduction of leukocytes, and particularly the infiltration of neutrophils. They reported that Ketamine pretreatment lowered inflammatory cell infiltration, sP-selectin serum levels, and reduced ATIII depletion. Moreover, Zahler *et al.*, 1999 [29] have reported that ketamine alters neutrophil function and endothelial-neutrophil interactions, and some of its anti-inflammatory properties are related to its inhibitory effect on leukocyte reactivity [29] [30].

In 2005, Mazar *et al.*, [18] have proposed the protective anti-inflammatory effects of ketamine are mediated by adenosine. They reported that ketamine administration causes release of adenosine in the periphery, and adenosine through A2A receptors, reduces the systemic inflammatory response by inhibition of secretion of proinflammatory cytokines as well as leukocyte activation and recruitment.

In clinical settings, the anti-inflammatory effect of ketamine has also been found. A low dose of ketamine (0.25 mg/kg) in patients undergoing coronary artery bypass surgery (CABG) has significantly suppressed intraoperative and postoperative increases in serum IL-6, IL-9 and C-reactive protein [31] [32]. This dose also significantly decreased superoxide production after on-pump coronary artery bypass graft surgery (CABG) [33].

The involvement of NMDA receptors in IBD has received little attention. Erces *et al.*, 2012 [22] have reported that, NMDA antagonist treatment resulted in significantly reduced TNF-α and IL-6 levels 6 day after trinitrobenzesulfonic acid (TNBS) administration. Moreover, it was found that treatment with the endogenous NMDA receptor antagonist Kynurenic acid in the early phase of acute experimental colitis in rats reduced significantly plasma levels of (TNF-α), inflammatory enzyme activities xanthine oxidoreductase (XOR), myeloperoxidase (MPO) and nitric oxide synthase (NOS), and colonic motility. They proposed that inhibition of the enteric NMDA receptors may provide a novel therapeutic option via which to influence intestinal hypermotility and inflammatory processes [34] [35].

5. Conclusion

We can conclude that, ketamine may be a new and effective therapy target in IBD patients. Further human studies would be beneficial elucidating the effect of ketamine more clearly and the possible therapeutic efficacy of ketamine in the treatment of UC, as well as the precise molecular basis of the protection it exerts over the intestinal mucosa.

References

[1] Nagib, M.M., Tadros, M.G., Elsayed, M.I. and Khalifa, A.E. (2013) Anti-Inflammatory and Antioxidant Activities of Olmesartan Midoxomil Ameliorates Experimental Colitis in Rats. *Toxicology and Applied Pharmacology*, **271**, 106-113. http://dx.doi.org/10.1016/j.taap.2013.04.026

[2] Sotnikova, R., Nosalova, V. and Navarova, J. (2013) Efficacy of Quercetin Derivatives in Prevention of Ulcerative Colitis in Rats. *Interdisciplinary Toxicology*, **6**, 9-12. http://dx.doi.org/10.2478/intox-2013-0002

[3] MacPherson, B.R. and Pfeiffer, C.J. (1978) Experimental Production of Diffuse Colitis in Rats. *Digestion*, **17**, 135-150. http://dx.doi.org/10.1159/000198104

[4] Noa, M., Mas, R., Carbaja, D. and Valdes, S. (2000) Effect of D-002 on Acetic Acid-Induced Colitis in Rats at Single and Repeated Doses. *Pharmacological Research*, **41**, 391-395. http://dx.doi.org/10.1006/phrs.1999.0596

[5] Nosal'ova, V., Zeman, M., Černa, S., Navarova, J. and Zakalova, M. (2007) Protective Effect of Melatonin in Acetic Acid Induced Colitis in Rats. *Journal of Pineal Research*, **42**, 364-370. http://dx.doi.org/10.1111/j.1600-079X.2007.00428.x

[6] Keshavarzian, A., Haydek, J., Zabihi, R., Doria, M., D'Astice, M. and Sorensen, J.R.J. (1992) Agents Capable of Eliminating Reactive Oxygen Species: Catalase, WR-2721, Cu(II)$_2$(3,5-DIPS)$_4$ Decrease Experimental Colitis. *Digestive Diseases and Sciences*, **37**, 1866-1873.

[7] Baumaqart, D.C. and Sandbom, W.J. (2007) Inflammatory Bowel Disease: Clinical Aspects and Established and Evolving Therapies. *Lancet*, **369**, 1641-1657. http://dx.doi.org/10.1016/S0140-6736(07)60751-X

[8]   Takenaka, I., Ogata, M., Koga, K., Matsumoto, T. and Shigematsu, A. (1994) Ketamine Suppresses Endotoxin-Induced Tumor Necrosis Factor Alpha Production in Mice. *Anesthesiology*, **80**, 402-408. http://dx.doi.org/10.1097/00000542-199402000-00020

[9]   Taniguchi, T., Shbata, K. and Yamamoto, K. (2001) Ketamine Inhibits Endotoxin-Induced Shock in Rats. *Anesthesiology*, **95**, 928-932. http://dx.doi.org/10.1097/00000542-200110000-00022

[10]   Kawasaki, T., Ogata, M., Kawasaki, C., Ogata, J., Inoue, Y. and Shgemastu, A. (1999) Ketamine Suppresses Proinflammatory Cytokine Production in Human Whole Blood *in Vitro*. *Anesthesia & Analgesia*, **89**, 665-669.

[11]   Kawasaki, C., Kawasaki, T., Ogata, M., Nandate, K. and Shgemastu, A. (2001) Ketamine Isomers Suppress Superantigen-Induced Proinflammatory Cytokine Production in Human Whole Blood. *Canadian Journal of Anesthesia*, **48**, 819-823. http://dx.doi.org/10.1007/BF03016701

[12]   Fabia, R., Willén, R., Ar'Rajab, A., Andersson, R., Ahrén, B. and Bengmark, S. (1992) Acetic Acid-Induced Colitis in the Rat: A Reproducible Experimental Model for Acute Ulcerative Colitis. *European Surgical Research*, **24**, 211-225. http://dx.doi.org/10.1159/000129209

[13]   Kuralay, F., Yildiz, C., Ozutemiz, O., Islekel, H., Caliskan, S., Bingol, B. and Ozkal, S. (2003) Effects of Trimetazidine on Acetic Acid-Induced Colitis in Female Swiss Rats. *Journal of Toxicology and Environmental Health*, **66**, 169-179. http://dx.doi.org/10.1080/15287390306402

[14]   Noronha-Blob, L., Lowe, V.C., Muhlahauser, R.O. and Bruch, R.M. (1993) NPC 15669, an Inhibitor of Neutrophil Recruitment Is Efficacious in Acetic Acid-Induced Colitis in Rats. *Gastroenterology*, **104**, 1021-1029.

[15]   Ohkawa, H., Ohishi, N. and Yagi, K. (1979) Assay for Lipid Peroxides in Animal Tissues by Thiobarbituric Acid Reaction. *Analytical Biochemistry*, **95**, 351-358. http://dx.doi.org/10.1016/0003-2697(79)90738-3

[16]   Green, L.C., Wagner, D.A., Glogowski, J., Skipper, P.L., Wishnok, J.S. and Tannenbaum, S.R. (1982) Analysis of Nitrate, Nitrite, and [^{15}N] Nitrate in Biological Fluids. *Analytical Biochemistry*, **126**, 131-138.

[17]   Grififith, O.W. (1980) Determination of Glutathione and Glutathione Disulfide Using Glutathione Reductase and 2-Vinylpyridine. *Analytical Biochemistry*, **106**, 207-212. http://dx.doi.org/10.1016/0003-2697(80)90139-6

[18]   Mazar, J., Rogachev, B., Shaked, G., Ziv, N.Y., Czeiger, D., Chaimovitz, C., Zlotnik, M., Mukmenev, I., Byk, G. and Douvdevani, A. (2005) Involvement of Adenosine in the Anti-Inflammatory Action of Ketamine. *Anesthesiology*, **102**, 1174-1181. http://dx.doi.org/10.1097/00000542-200506000-00017

[19]   Jena, G., Trivedi, P.P. and Sandala, B. (2012) Oxidative Stress in Ulcerative Colitis: An Old Concept but a New Concern. *Free Radical Research*, **46**, 1339-1345. http://dx.doi.org/10.3109/10715762.2012.717692

[20]   Chavan, S., Sava, L., Saxena, V., Pillai, S., Sontakke, A. and Ingole, D. (2005) Reduced Glutathione: Importance of Specimen Collection. *Indian Journal of Clinical Biochemistry*, **20**, 150-152. http://dx.doi.org/10.1007/BF02893062

[21]   Gillberg, L., Varsanyi, M., Sjostrom, M., Lordal, M., Lindholm, J. and Hellstrom, P.M. (2012) Nitric Oxide Pathway-Related Gene Alterations in Inflammatory Bowel Disease. *Scandinavian Journal of Gastroenterology*, **47**, 1283-1297. http://dx.doi.org/10.3109/00365521.2012.706830

[22]   Érces, D., Varga, G., Fazekas, B., Kovacs, T., Tőkés, T., Tiszlavicz, L., Fülöp, F., Vécsei, L., Boros, M. and Kaszaki, J. (2012) N-Methyl-D-Asparate Receptor Antagonist Therapy Suppresses Colon Motility and Inflammatory Activation Six Days after the Onset of Experimental Colitis in Rats. *European Journal of Pharmacology*, **692**, 225-234. http://dx.doi.org/10.1016/j.ejphar.2012.06.044

[23]   Popivanova, B.K., Kitamura, K., Wu, Y., Kondo, T., Kagaya, T., Kaneko, S., *et al.* (2008) Blocking TNF-Alpha in Mice Reduces Colorectal Carcinogenesis Associated with Chronic Colitis. *Journal of Clinical Investigation*, **118**, 560-570.

[24]   Gokcinar, D., Ergin, V., Cumaoglu, A., Menevse, A. and Aricioglu, A. (2013) Effects of Ketamine, Propofol, and Ketofol on Proinflammatory Cytokines and Markers of Oxidative Stress in a Rat Model of Endotoxemia-Induced Acute Lung Injury. *Acta Biochimica Polonica*, **60**, 451-456.

[25]   Koga, K., Ogata, M., Takenaka, I., Matsumoto, T. and Shigematsu, A. (1994) Ketamine Suppresses Tumor Necrosis Factor-Alpha Activity and Mortality in Carrageenan Sensitized Endotoxin Shock Model. *Cardiogenic Shock*, **44**, 160-168.

[26]   Shimaoka, M., Iida, T., Ohara, A., Taenaka, N., Mashimo, T., Honda, T. and Yoshiya, I. (1996) Ketamine Inhibits Nitric Oxide Production in Mouse-Activated Macrophage-Like Cells. *British Journal of Anaesthesia*, **77**, 238-242. http://dx.doi.org/10.1093/bja/77.2.238

[27]   Yu, Y., Zhou, Z., Xu, J., Liu, Z. and Wang, Y. (2002) Ketamine Reduces NF-κB Activation and TNF-α Production in Rat Mononuclear Cells Induced by Lipopolysaccharide *in Vitro*. *Annals of Clinical & Laboratory Science*, **32**, 292-298.

[28]   Guzman-DeLaGarza, F.J., Camara-Lemarroy, C.R., Ballesteros-Elizondo, R.G., Alarcon-Galvan, G., Cordero-Perez, P.

and Fernandez-Garza, N.E. (2010) Ketamine Reduces Intestinal Injury and Inflammatory Cell Infiltration after Ischemia/Reperfusion in Rats. *Surgery Today*, **40**, 1055-1062.

[29] Zahler, S., Heindl, B. and Becker, B.F. (1999) Ketamine Does Not Inhibit Inflammatory Responses of Cultured Human Endothelial Cells but Reduces Chemotactic Activation of Neutrophils. *Acta Anaesthesiologica Scandinavica*, **3**, 1011-1016.

[30] Buras, J.A. and Reenstra, W.R. (2007) Endothelial-Neutrophil Interactions during Ischemia and Reperfusion Injury: Basic Mechanisms of Hyperbaric Oxygen. *Neurological Research*, **29**, 127-131.
http://dx.doi.org/10.1179/016164107X174147

[31] Roytblat, L., Talmor, D., Rachinsky, M., *et al.* (1998) Ketamine Attenuates the Interleukin-6 Response after Cardiopulmonary Bypass. *Survey of Anesthesiology*, **87**, 266-271.

[32] Bartoc, C., Frumento, R.J., Jalbout, M., Bennett-Guerrero, E., Du, E. and Nishanian, E. (2006) A Randomized, Double-Blind, Placebo-Controlled Study Assessing the Anti-Inflammatory Effects of Ketamine in Cardiac Surgical Patients. *Journal of Cardiothoracic and Vascular Anesthesia*, **20**, 217-222. http://dx.doi.org/10.1053/j.jvca.2005.12.005

[33] Zilberstein, G., Levy, R., Rachinsky, M., *et al.* (2002) Ketamine Attenuates Neutrophil Activation after Cardiopulmonary Bypass. *Anesthesia & Analgesia*, **95**, 531-536.

[34] Varga, G., Érces, D., Fazekas, B., Fülöp, M., Kovacs, T., Kaszaki, J., Fülöp, F., Vécsei, L. and Boros, M. (2010) N-Methyl-D-Asparate Receptor Antagonism Decreases Motility and Inflammatory Activation in the Early Phase of Acute Experimental Colitis in the Rats. *Neurogastroenterology & Motility*, **22**, 217-225.
http://dx.doi.org/10.1111/j.1365-2982.2009.01390.x

[35] Hirota, K. and Lambert, D.J. (2011) Ketamine: New Uses for an Old Drug. *BJA*, **107**, 123-126.
http://dx.doi.org/10.1093/bja/aer221

18

Deterioration in Hemodynamics Reaction, Baroreflex Sensitivity, Sympathetic Nerve Activity and Redox State of Thoracic Aorta in the Experimental Model of Nitrate Tolerance and Its Pharmacological Correction

Nikoloz V. Gongadze[1], Tamara D. Kezeli[2], Galina V. Sukoyan[1,3]*, Zaza Chapichadze[4], Nino M. Dolidze[2], Makrine Mirziashvili[1], Mariam Chipashvili[2]

[1]Department of Medical Pharmacology and Pharmacotherapy, Tbilisi State Medical University, Tbilisi, Georgia
[2]Department of Pharmacology, Faculty of Medicine, I. Javakhishvili Tbilisi State University, Tbilisi, Georgia
[3]International Scientific Centre of Introduction of New Biomedical Technology, Tbilisi, Georgia
[4]Department of Pharmacology, State Regulation Agency for Medical Activities Ministry of Health and Social Affairs of Georgia, Tbilisi, Georgia
Email: *galinasukoian@mail.ru

Abstract

Continuous treatment with organic nitrates causes nitrate tolerance and provides evidence for a relationship between mitochondrial complex 1 activity and mitochondrial aldehyde dehydrogenase-2 (ALDH-2) with disturbances of the hemodynamics reaction during nitroglycerin (NTG) tolerance (NTGT). The purpose of this study was the evaluation of efficacy of original oxidized form NAD-containing drug, NADCIN®, on hemodynamic reactions, baroreflex sensitivity (BRS) and reflex control of splanchnic sympathetic nerve activity (SSNA), level of redox-potential, activity of ALDH-2 and superoxide anion generation in aortic tissue in rat model of NTGT. Five groups (7 - 9 each) of male Wistar rats, including control, acute i.v. NTG (150 mcg/kg) administration, NTG tolerance NTGT treatment with NADCIN® 8 mg/kg and methylene blue (MB, 2.5 mg/kg) were used. NTGT in rats was accompanied with the greatly attenuation of hemodynamics reaction, BRS, the decreasing of the ability to reflex control of SSNA without pronounce overexpression of endothelin-1 in vessels (aorta). In NTGT rats i.v. NTG along induced less hypotensive reactions and alterations in

heart period vs single NTG treated group, more expressively decreased BRS (−34%) and reflex control of SSNA (−18%). NADCIN® significantly inhibits tolerance-inducing properties of the prolonged nitroglycerin infusion (max decrease of blood pressure response to nitroglycerin injection, % of normal controls: NTGT 51.2%, NADCIN® 91.6%, MB 55.8%). NADCIN® in NTGT rats after NTG i.v. administration increased reduced BRS (+37.8%, p < 0,05), reflex control of SSNA (+29.4%, p < 0.05) and reversed the decreasing of NAD/NADH ratio, ALDH-2 activity and decreasing in superoxide generation in thoracic aortic tissue. Thus, course treatment with NADCIN® of NTGT rats restores hemodynamics changes, BRS and SSNA throughout the increasing of redox-potential NAD/NADH and cessates the NTGT developing.

Keywords

Experimental Model of Nitroglycerin Tolerance, Baroreflex Sensitivity, Aldehyde Dehydrogenase, Redox-Potential, Splanchnic Sympathetic Nerve Activity

---

1. Introduction

Organic nitrates and nitroglycerin (glyceryl trinitrate, GTN) in particularly, has long been one of the key medicines for cardiovascular diseases including coronary artery disease, acute myocardial infarction and congestive heart failure for more than 100 years. The anti-ischemic effect of NTG is believed to be based on the drug-induced decrease in preload and afterload, improvement of coronary collateral flow, dilatation of stenotic coronary arteries, and the inhibition of platelet aggregation. GTN, along with other lower potency nitrates induces coronary vasodilatation throughout to its bioconversion into relaxant agent nitric oxide (NO) [1]. Propose mechanisms include neurohormonal counterregulatory mechanisms to maintain blood pressure [2], increased production of superoxide anions [3]-[5] and oxidative stress as a result, reduced biotransformation of NTG to NO, and alterations in cyclic GMP metabolism [6], endothelial dysfunction, inhibition of nitroglycerin metabolizing enzyme, changes in GNT-signaling or endogenous active substances, and so on [7]. However, long-term administration of nitroglycerin results in progressive loss of vascular sensitivity to nitrate in rodents and humans, but diminished bioactivation of GTN by deterioration in ALDH2 activity appears to be the most plausible cause [8]-[10], and that this reaction is accelerated by an allosteric action of NAD^+ [11]. The dysfunction of Complex I (presumably through the generation of NAD^+ deficit and/or altered $NADH/NAD^+$ ratio) exerts an inhibitory effect on ALDH independently of any reactive oxygen species (ROS) participation. It is thus likely that prolonged exposure to GTN tolerance manifested as increased ROS generation accompanied by alterations in NAD^+ availability and/or altered $NADH/NAD^+$ ratio, might provoke conformational (and other) changes in ALDH-2 undermining its activity [11] [12]. In according with this, the aim of the study was to investigated the ability of original reduced form NAD-containing drug, NADCIN®[1] [13], on the hemodynamic reactions, baroreflex sensitivity, reflex control of sympathetic nerve activity and level of redox-potential, NAD/NADH and NADP/NADPH and ALDH activity in thoracic aorta tissue in nitroglycerin-induced tolerant rats.

2. Materials and Methods

2.1. Experimental Design

Experiments were carried out in 76 male Wistar rats weighing 250 - 300 g. Animals received humane care in compliance with "Guide for the Care and Use of Laboratory animals" (National Institutes of Health publication 86-23, Revised 1996) and was performed with approval of the local Interinsitutional (International Scientific Centre of Introduction of New Biomedical Technology, Department of Pharmacology, Faculty of Medicine, I.Javakhishvili Tbilisi State University and Department of Medical Pharmacology and Pharmacotherapy, Tbilisi State Medical University, Tbilisi) Animal Care and Use Committee. Nitroglycerin-induced tolerance was re-

---

[1]NADCIN®, lyophylizate for preparation salin for i/v and i/m injection, containing 0.5 mg oxidized form of NAD, inosine 80.0 mg and 10.0 mg os sodium chloride, in 5 ml ampoule (patent WO 200789166 A1 Sukoyan G.V. Medicinal preparation for regulating a systemic inflammatory response syndrome. 2007-08-09), manufactured by "Biotechpharm GE", Ltd, Georgia.

produced by treatment with NTG (10 mg/kg, s.c.) three times a day for 8 days and was confirmed by a reduction in hypotensive responses to intravenous NTG [14]. All animals were randomized into the five groups: Control group—s.c. injection of 0.1 ml normal saline 3 times daily for 8 days; II—were given 0.1 ml 0.9% NaCl in the same frequency and period of administration and then NTG (in form of NITRO 5 mg/ml[2], Orion Corporation, Finland, 150 mcg/kg) i.v. injection; III—received NTG (10 mg/kg s.c) three times a day for 8 days and then NTG (150 mcg/kg) i.v. injection; IV—received NTG (10 mg/kg s.c.) three times a day for 8 days and NADCIN®, 8.0 mg/kg of body weight resolved in 0.1 ml of water for injection i.v. from the 4th days of NTG treatment and once daily 20 min after the NTG (150 mcg/kg) i.v. injection; V—were given s.c. injection of 0.1 ml 0.9% NaCl three times a day for 8 days and then received MB −2.5 mg/kg i.v. 20 minute before i.v. injection of NTG (150 mcg/kg). After 8 days the rats were anaesthetized with pentobarbital (60 mg/kg intraperitoneally).

2.2. Hemodynamics, Baroreflex Sensitivity and Splanchnic Sympathetic Nerve Activity Study

Polyethylene catheter was placed into the right femoral artery and connected to blood pressure transducer for measuring blood pressure (BP) with electromanometer and heart period (HP) with cardiotachometer. Intravenous injections were given via catheter inserted into the rigor ht femoral vein. Baroreflex sensitivity (BRS) was defined by measuring HP in response to rises BP 30 - 50 mm Hg above control after i.v. injection of phenylephrine (3 - 10 mcg/kg). The slope of relationship between BP and HP was used as an index of BRS according to [15]. Splanchnic sympathetic nerve activity (SSNA) was recorded according to [16]. A thin bipolar silver electrode was placed around a branch of the splanchnic nerve and isolated carefully with silicone rubber. Nerve activity was recorded via a cable connected to an adaptor. The nerve signal was amplified and rectified and the mean nerve activity was displayed on a polygraph. BRS was assessed with respect to control of SSNA as percentage of nerve inhibition from control per mmHg of BP rise (% mmHg) and with respect to control of heart rate (HR) as HR decrease per mmHg of BP rise (beats min^{-1} mmHg^{-1}).

2.3. Biochemical Markers of Functioning of Thoracic Aorta

Thoracic aorta was frozen and homogenized in liquid nitrogen, before the experiments homogenate was rapidly placed in modified Krebs' solution [17]. The powdered tissue was dispersed in 5 vol ice-cold aqueous 30 mM potassium phosphate buffer, pH 7.5, vortexed, sonicated, and centrifuged at 10.000 g for 10 min. Isolation of mitochondria was performed using "Mitochondria isolation kit" (BioChain Institute, Inc.) according to the manufacturer's instructions. ALDH activity in the supernatant was determined by monitoring NADH formation from NAD$^+$. The assay mixture (0.5 mL) contained 100 mM Tris-HCl (pH 8.5), 1 mM NAD$^+$, 1 mM 4-methylpyrazole, and 100 µg protein. The reaction was started by addition of 1 mM propionaldehyde to the cuvette, and absorbance changes at 340 nm as a result of NADH formation were recorded for 10 min. The mean rate of absorbance change was taken as a measure of ALDH activity (0.0125 A340 was equivalent to 1 nmol/mg/min). The ALDH-2 inhibitor benomyl (10 - 5 mol/L) was used as a negative control. The content of pyridine nucleotide in aortic mitochondries was measured using sspectrofluorimetric methods [13] [18]. The protein concentration was determined with BSA protein assay kit. Superoxide anion generation in isolated rat heart mitochondria was determined immediately following the isolation procedure. Briefly, mitochondria (0.5 mg/ml) were incubated with buffer (6 mM succinate, 70 mM sucrose, 220 mM mannitol, 2 mM, Hepes, 25 mM KH$_2$PO$_4$, 2.5 mM MgCl$_2$, 0.5 mM EDTA, 5 µg/ml catalase, pH 7.4) at 37°C. At the indicated time points, 40 mM acetylated cytochrome c was added and the change in absorbance at 550 nm was measured for 1 min at 37°C. Background absorbance for all groups was determined by the addition of SOD (1000 units/ml). Endothelin-1 (ET$_1$) in aortic homogenate concentration (pg/ml) was measures by R & D Systems for Human endothelin-1 Immunoassay (Great Britain).

2.4. Statistical Analysis.

All values are expressed as the mean ± standard error deviation of at least 6 experiments. Statistical analysis for comparison between different groups of animals was assessed by two-way unpaired Student t-test. Significance was defined as $p < 0.05$ or less.

---

[2]Each ml of concentrate for solution preparation containing: nitroglycerin saline 10% 52.5 mg (equivalent of 5.0 mg of nitroglycerin).

3. Results

3.1. Hemodynamics, Baroreflex Sensitivity and Splanchnic Sympathetic Nerve Activity

In anaesthetized rats the baseline values of BP and HP did not show any significant differences in all groups of animals (**Table 1**). The study of BRS revealed great attenuation of its cardiochronotropic vagal component in rats with NTGT (0.62 ± 0.08 ms/Hg mm^{-1}) vs. control animals (0.98 ± 0.1 ms/Hg mm^{-1}, $p < 0.05$) that correlated with the decreasing the ability to cause bradycardia reflex (1.9 ± 0.09 beats min^{-1} Hg $mm^{-1)}$) and an inhibition of SSNA (**Table 1**). The concomitant use of NADCIN® in NTGT rats markedly increased the reduced BRS (+39%, $p < 0.001$) and its ability with respect to heart rate (HR) control (+65%, $p < 0.001$) and inhibition of SSNA (+38.2%, $p < 0.01$) resulting from NTGT animals. Treatment with guanylyl cyclase inhibitor, MB, similarly to NTGT, but in less degree, caused reduction in BRS (0.72 ± 0.4 ms Hg mm^{-1}) and its properties with respect to control SSNA (1.7 ± 0.1 Hg mm^{-1}) vs control group of rats. Acute single dose of NTG (150 mcg/kg i.v) administration was accompanied with significant hypotensive reactions in non-tolerance normal rats and in group treated with NADCIN®. BRS after NTG i.v. injection was more deeply blunted in MB treated group (0.68 ± 0.15 ms Hg mm^{-1}) and especially NTGT rats (0.51 ± 0.09 ms Hg mm^{-1}) vs. in group after single i.v. treatment with NTG. NADCIN® significantly inhibits tolerance-inducing properties of the prolonged nitroglycerin infusion (BP_{max}, nitroglycerin response in % of normal controls: NTGT 51.2%, NADCIN®-91.6, MB-55.8%). NADCIN® in NTGT rats after NTG i.v. administration increased reduced BRS (+37.8%, $p < 0.05$), reflex control of SSNA (+29.4%, $p < 0.05$).

3.2. Deterioration in Biochemical Markers of Redox State, Aldehyde Dehydrogenase System and Endothelial Function

Acute action of NTG did not induce significant changes in redox-potential of mitochondria of thoracic aortic tissue and did not change the rate of superoxide anion generation, with the tendency to decrease of ALDH-2 activity (**Table 2**). In NTGT rats after the i.v. injection of NTG the changes in BRS and SSNA was accompanied with significantly decrease of redox-potential NAD/NADH by 20% in thoracic aorta tissue (**Table 2**) without changes in total pyridine nucleotide pool (**Table 2**) and in the level of vasoconstrictor cytokine (ET-1) production in vessels. The decrease in redox-potential even without changes in the total pool of pyridine nucleotide was accompanied with increased of the rate of superoxide anion generation in 1.5 times vs NTG non tolerated group. Cellular redox status is an important regulator of energy fuel metabolism, and many enzymes are under regulation of $NAD^+/NADH$ and $NADP^+/NADPH$ ratios not only in normal condition but under various pathological states [19]-[21]. No change in NADP/NADPH redox-potential of mitochondria was observed under acute single-dose treatment with NTG in normal rats which accompanied with normal rate of superoxide generation and ALDH activity (**Table 2**). Under continue administration of NTG the reaction of following i/v injection of high

Table 1. The influence of nitroglycerine treatment on the hemodynamics reaction, baroreflex sensitivity and splanchnic sympathetic nerve activity in NTG tolerant rats.

Parameters	Control n = 12	C + NTG N = 10	NTGT +NTG	NTGT +NADCIN® N = 9	NTGT NTG + NADCIN® N = 9	NTGT +MB N = 9	NTGT +NTG + MB N = 9
BP, mmHg	126 ± 8	$82 \pm 7^{***}$	$117 \pm 6^{\#\#}$	$96 \pm 7^{*\#}$	$122 \pm 5^{\#\#}$	$83 \pm 4^{***+}$	$118 \pm 6^{\#\#}$	$95 \pm 3^{***\#+}$
HP, ms	159 ± 8	$116 \pm 9^{***}$	$148 \pm 11^{\#\#}$	$125 \pm 8^{**}$	$160 \pm 8^{\#\#}$	$126 \pm 8^{**\#\#}$	$153 \pm 11^{\#\#\#}$	$134 \pm 8^{*\#\#+}$
BRS ms/ Hg mm^{-1}	0.98 ± 0.10	0.94 ± 0.1	$0.62 \pm 0.08^{*}$	$0.51 \pm 0.09^{**}$	$0.86 \pm 0.06^{***}$	$0.82 \pm 0.1^{***}$	$0.72 \pm 0.4^{*}$	$0.68 \pm 0.15^{**}$
HR beats min^{-1} Hg mm^{-1}	3.6 ± 0.2	3.5 ± 0.2	$1.90 \pm 0.09^{*}$	$1.7 \pm 0.2^{**}$	$2.9 \pm 0.2^{***}$	$2.8 \pm 0.2^{***}$	$3.2 \pm 0.3^{***}$	$3.0 \pm 0.4^{***}$
SSNA% Hg mm^{-1}	2.2 ± 0.2	2.0 ± 0.2	$1.64 \pm 0.11^{*}$	$1.23 \pm 0.08^{**}$	1.94 ± 0.07	$1.7 \pm 0.2^{***}$	$1.7 \pm 0.1^{*}$	$1.4 \pm 0.1^{**}$

Notes: BP: blood pressure; HP: heart period; HR: heart rate (upon baroreflex activation); MB: methylene blue; n: number of animals in each group; *Comparison with control group; #With control +NTG 150 mcg group; +: With III(NTGT) group. One symbol: $p < 0.05$, two: $p < 0.01$, three: $p < 0.001$.

Table 2. Influence of NADCIN® on the redox-potential, ALDH-2 activity and superoxide anion generation in aortic rings of rats with nitroglycerin tolerance.

Group	Control	NTG, 150 mcg/kg	NTG tolerance	NTG tolerance + NADCIN®	NTG tolerance + MB
NAD, nmol/mg wet tissue	6.75 ± 0.23	6.54 ± 0.37	$6.10 \pm 0.27^*$	$6.80 \pm 0.22^\#$	$6.09 \pm 0.14^*$
NADH, nmol/mg wet tissue	6.28 ± 0.39	6.55 ± 0.27	$7.05 \pm 0.17^*$	$6.25 \pm 0.17^\#$	$6.98 \pm 0.12^*$
Redox-potential, NAD/NADH	1.08 ± 0.08	1.0 ± 0.1	$0.86 \pm 0.06^{**}$	$1.09 \pm 0.09^\#$	$0.87 \pm 0.07^*$
NADP, nmol/mg wet tissue	5.70 ± 0.14	5.54 ± 0.17	5.40 ± 0.20	5.80 ± 0.20	5.39 ± 0.24
NADPH, nmol/mg wet tissue	4.67 ± 0.33	4.55 ± 0.19	4.65 ± 0.20	4.65 ± 0.15	4.68 ± 0.22
Redox-potential, NADP/NADPH	1.22 ± 0.08	1.21 ± 0.10	1.16 ± 0.08	1.24 ± 0.10	1.15 ± 0.08
Total pool of pyridine nucleotide	23.4 ± 0.5	23.2 ± 0.4	23.2 ± 0.4	23.5 ± 0.4	23.1 ± 0.3
ALDH-2, NADH nmol/mg/min	2.25 ± 0.38	$1.98 \pm 0.27^\#$	$0.65 \pm 0.07^{***}$	$2.32 \pm 0.23^{\#\#}$	$1.75 \pm 0.24^*$
Superoxide anion, µmol/mg protein/min	28 ± 4	30 ± 7	45 ± 10	27 ± 5	46 ± 6
ET-1, µg/mg protein	2.34 ± 0.21	2.14 ± 0.23	2.76 ± 0.21	2.03 ± 0.13	2.57 ± 0.18

dose of NTG disturbed: occurs decreasing in NAD/NADH redox state (without significantly decrease in NADP/NADPH potential) that leads to a increasing of generation of superoxide anion and to decrease of ALDH2 activity (**Table 2**) and give grounds to suggest that major source of oxidative stress in normal animals under NTG-tolerance formation is the mitochondrial complex 1 functioning disturbances [11]. Activity of mitochondrial ALDH significantly decrease (by 71%, p < 0.001 in comparison to normal animals and by 67% vs level after single i/v injection of 150 mcg/kg NTG) after the continue administration of NTG in normal animals and fully reverse under treatment with NADCIN® and increased up to level obtained during acute NTG injection under treatment with guanyl cyclase inhibitor, MB. Our data confirmed early hypothesis that mitochondrial complex 1 is one of the targets at which the initial oxidative stress responsible for GTN tolerance takes place. In according with this the treatment with oxidized form NAD-containing drug, NADCIN®, is a new strategy for prevention and therapy of NTG-tolerance formation, strategy of replacement therapy.

4. Discussion

Experimental and clinical investigations have provided evidence that prolonged exposure to organic nitrates during cardiovascular disease induces tolerance and endothelial dysfunction [16] [22]. However there is controversial data suggesting the development of tolerance related to long-term continues nitrate therapy [1] [8] [11] [22] [23]. It was demonstrated that a nonvasodilated concentration of NTG exerts a direct myocardial anti-ischemic effect independent of its vascular actions in isolated rat hearts and conscious rabbits [21] [24]. In addition, this effect is not diminished by the development of vascular tolerance to NTG [22] [23]. In the state of nitrate tolerance well known that the enzymatic bioconversion of NTG to NO and the consequent increase is cGMP level is responsible for the vascular effects of NTG is impaired [6] [9] [25] and administration of NTG does not affect cardiac cGMP content in the rat heart *in vivo* [16] [25]. In other investigations long-term continuous NTG therapy has been associated with endothelium dysfunction and altered autonomic neural function, including impaired baroreflex activity and prevalence of sympathetic to parasympathetic tone in the regulation of heart rate [26] with increased sensitivity to receptor-dependent vasoconstrictors such as serotonin, phenylephrine, angiotensin II and thromboxane [16] [22]. BRS proved to be highly effective for correct identification the animals at high risk of developing ventricular fibrillation during transient ischemia. Vasodilator effects of nitrates on large arterial conductance vessels are, in general, preserved even in the presence of neurohormonal activation, while tolerance to NTG-induced changes in coronary flow is usually established [16]. These observations indicate that increased levels of vasoconstrictive agents encountered with the initiation of NTG therapy cannot override the vasodilator effects of NTG on large arterial vessels but may induce vascular constriction at the arteriolar level. Our experiments showed that in NTG tolerant rats BRS was greatly attenuated with reduction of its cardiochronotropic vagal component that correlated with decreased ability to cause reflex bradycardia and an inhibition of SSNA. Such alterations in this group of animals were associated with increased of the level of redox-potential, NAD/NADH, but not NADP/NADPH, that more markedly was expressed after NTG intravenous administration. Thus, even in normal animals without significant increase in vasoconstrictor and proinflammatory cytokine, ET-1 production (**Table 2**), in a response to continue NTG infusion occurs decreased in the redox-potential of mitochondria of thoracic aortic tissue that leads to the overproduction of superoxide anion in aortic (vessels) tissue and as a result the risk of superoxide scavenging by NO with the generation of the strong oxidant peroxynitrite ($ONOO^-$) increased under continue treatment with the NTG and could be one of the intime mechanism of NTG tolerance formation. We showed that mitochondria isolated from aorta after the NTG tolerance developed in normal animals the content of ET-1 does not significantly rise (increased only for 18%, N.S.) and about 1, 6 fold greater amount of superoxide anion production compared to untreated animals.

It was demonstrated that is NTG-induced tolerance the decreased release of CGRP is associated with the decrease in aldehyde dehydrogenase (ALDH-2) activity [11] [24] [27]. NTG produced a depressor effect concomitantly with an increase in plasma CGRP concentration, which may be prevented by the pretreatment with ALDH-2 inhibitors. These results correlate with our previous investigation where CGRP receptors antagonist reduced NTG hemodynamic effects in NTG tolerant rats and increased mortality in these animals during acute myocardial infarction [3] [7] [14]. The oxidative stress concept could be compatible with the multiple different observations associated with long-term nitrate therapy [28].

5. Conclusion

NADCIN®, unlike MB, has ability to restored hemodynamic reaction and BRS in NTG tolerant rats that were associated with improved control of the SSNA throughout restoration of NAD/NADH redox-potential sate and decreased oxidative stress under NTG continue treatment. Because cellular level of NAD can modulate the SIRT1 activity (enzymatic activity of SIRT1 depends on the cellular level of NAD [11] [12]) and expression. Decreasing of the redox-potential and enhancing of oxidized state of endothelium of vessels and shear-stress deterioration may be one of the possible mechanisms by which laminar/pulsatile flow is disturbed and deteriorated vascular homeostasis. Restoring of the NAD/NADH potential with following normalization the activity SIRT1 functioning could prevent endothelium cell dysfunction [29] and counteract with the prevention of atherosclerosis development and NTG-tolerance formation. In the clinical study it was shown that NAD containing drug in patients with ischemic heart disease restored the redox-potential, decreased the superoxide production and E_1 plasma level improving clinical symptoms of ischemia-reperfusion injury in patients with chronic form [25]. Thus, the reduction of redox-potential NAD/NADH is the target-point in the development of tolerance to NTG in normal animals which accompanied by unadequate functioning of the ALDH and inducer of oxidative stress formation even without significant deterioration in endothelin-1 system functioning. Course treatment of NADCIN®, first original reduced form of NAD-containing drug, leads to complete normalization in sensitivity to NTG and to restoration of the redox-potential NAD/NADH in aortic tissue and to elimination of the overexpression of superoxide anion and to the changes in ALDH functioning.

Conflict of Interest

The authors report no conflict of interest. The authors alone are responsible for the conduct and writing of this manuscript.

Authorship Contributions

Participated in research design: Gongadze N, Sukoyan G, Kezeli T. Conducted experiments: Sukoyan G, Dolidze N, Mirziashvili M, Chipashvili M. Contributed new reagents or analytical tools: Sukoyan G, Gongadze N, Chapichadze Z. Performed data analysis: Gongadze N, Sukoyan G, Kezeli T, Dolidze N. Wrote or contributed to the writing of the manuscript: Gongadze N, Sukoyan G, Kezeli T, Dolidze N.

References

[1] Munzel, T., Daiber, A. and Gori, T. (2013) More Answers to the Still Unresolved Question of Nitrate Tolerance. *European Heart Journal*, **34**, 2666-2673. http://dx.doi.org/10.1093/eurheartj/eht249

[2] Mangione, N.J. and Glasser, S.P. (1994) Phenomenon of Nitrate Tolerance. *American Heart Journal*, **128**, 137.

http://dx.doi.org/10.1016/0002-8703(94)90020-5

[3] Munzel, T., Giaid, A., Kurz, S., et al. (1995) Evidence for a Role of Endothelin 1 and Protein Kinase C in Nitroglyce- rin Tolerance. Proceedings of the National Academy of Sciences of the United States of America, 92, 5244-5248. http://dx.doi.org/10.1073/pnas.92.11.5244

[4] Munzel, T., Daiber, A. and Mülsch, A. (2005) Explaining the Phenomenon of Nitrate Tolerance. Circulation Research, 97, 618-628. http://dx.doi.org/10.1161/01.RES.0000184694.03262.6d

[5] Thomas, G.R., Difabio, J.M., Gori, T. and Parker, J.D. (2007) Once Daily Therapy with Isosorbide-5-Mononitrate Causes Endothelial Dysfunction in Humans: Evidence of a Free Radical-Mediated Mechanism. Journal of the Ameri- can College of Cardiology, 49, 1289-1295. http://dx.doi.org/10.1016/j.jacc.2006.10.074

[6] Axelsson, K.L. and Ahlner, J. (1987) Nitrate Tolerance from a Biochemical Point of View. Drugs, 33, 63-68. http://dx.doi.org/10.2165/00003495-198700334-00013

[7] Munzel, T., Daiber, A. and Gori, T. (2011) Nitrate Therapy: New Aspects Concerning Molecular Action and Tolerance. Circulation, 123, 2132-2144. http://dx.doi.org/10.1161/CIRCULATIONAHA.110.981407

[8] Chen, C.-H., Ferreira, J.C.B., Gross, E.R. and Mochly-Rosen, D. (2014) Targeting Aldehyde Dehydrogenase 2: New Therapeutic Opportunities. Physiological Reviews, 94, 1-34. http://dx.doi.org/10.1152/physrev.00017.2013

[9] Chen, Z., Zhang, J. and Stamler, J.S. (2002) Identification of the Enzymatic Mechanism of Nitroglycerin Bioactivation. Proceedings of the National Academy of Sciences of the United States of America, 99, 8306-8311. http://dx.doi.org/10.1073/pnas.122225199

[10] Neubauer, R., Neubauer, A., Wolkart, G., et al. (2013) Potent Inhibition of Aldehyde Dehydrogenase-2 by Diphenyle- neiodonium: Focus on Nitroglycerin Bioactivation. Molecular Pharmacology, 84, 407-414. http://dx.doi.org/10.1124/mol.113.086835

[11] Garcia-Bou, R., Rocha, M., Apostolova, N., Herance, R., Hernandez-Mijares, A. and Victor, V.M. (2012) Evidence for a Relationship between Mitochondrial Complex I Activity and Mitochondrial Aldehyde Dehydrogenase during Ni- troglycerin Tolerance: Effects of Mitochondrial Antioxidants. Biochimica et Biophysica Acta (BBA)—Bioenergetics, 1817, 828-837. http://dx.doi.org/10.1016/j.bbabio.2012.02.013

[12] Koppaka, V., Thompson, D.C., Chen, Y., Ellermann, M., Nicolaou, K.C., Juvonen, R.O., Petersen, D., Deitrich, R.A., Hurley, T.D. and Vasiliou, V. (2012) Aldehyde Dehydrogenase Inhibitors: A Comprehensive Review of the Pharma- cology, Mechanism of Action, Substrate Specificity, and Clinical Application. Pharmacological Reviews, 64, 520-539. http://dx.doi.org/10.1124/pr.111.005538

[13] Sukoyan, G.V. and Kavadze, I.K. (2008) Effect of Nadcin on Energy Supply and Apoptosis in Ischemia-Reperfusion Injury to the Myocardium. Bulletin of Experimental Biology and Medicine, 146, 321-324. http://dx.doi.org/10.1007/s10517-008-0268-2

[14] Chen, Y.R., Nie, S.D., Shan, W., Jiang, D.J., Shi, R.Z., Zhou, Z., et al. (2007) Decrease in Endogenous CGRP Release in Nitroglycerin Tolerance: Role of ALDH-2. European Journal of Pharmacology, 571, 44-50. http://dx.doi.org/10.1016/j.ejphar.2007.05.042

[15] Smyth, O.A., Sleight, P. and Pickering, G. (1962) Reflex Regulation of Arterial Pressure during Sleep in Man. A Quantitative Method of Assessing Baroreflex Sensivity. Circulation Research, 24, 109-121. http://dx.doi.org/10.1161/01.RES.24.1.109

[16] Ricksten, S.E. and Thoren, P. (1981) Reflex Control of Sympathetic Nerve Activity and Heart Rate from Arterial Ba- roreceptors in Conscious Spontaneously Hypertensive Rats. Clinical Science, 61, 169s-172s. http://dx.doi.org/10.1042/cs061169s

[17] Rahimian, R., Laher, I., Dube, G. and Breemen, C.V. (1997) Estrogen and Selective Estrogen Receptor Modulator LY117018 Enhance Release of Nitric Oxide in Rat Aorta. Journal of Pharmacology and Experimental Therapeutics, 283, 116-122.

[18] Bessho, M., Tajima, T., Hori, S., Satoh, T., Fukuda, K., Kyotani, S., Ohnishi, Y. and Nakamura, Y. (1989) NAD and NADH Values in Rapidly Sampled Dog Heart Tissues by Two Different Extraction Methods. Analytical Biochemistry, 182, 304-308. http://dx.doi.org/10.1016/0003-2697(89)90599-X

[19] Baron, J.T., Sasse, M.F. and Nair, A. (2004) Effect of Angiotensin II on Energetic, Glucose Metabolism and Cytosolic NADH/NAD and NADPH/NADP Redox in Vascular Smooth Muscle. Molecular and Cellular Biochemistry, 262, 91-99. http://dx.doi.org/10.1023/B:MCBI.0000038221.44904.a1

[20] Sukoyan, G.V., Andriadze, N.A., Guchua, E.I. and Karsanov, N.V. (2005) Effect of NAD on Recovery of Adenine Nucleotide Pool, Phosphorylation Potential, a Stimulation of Apoptosis during Late Period of Reperfusion Damage to Myocardium. Bulletin of Experimental Biology and Medicine, 139, 53-56. http://dx.doi.org/10.1007/s10517-005-0208-3

[21] Ying, W. (2008) NAD$^+$/NADH and NADP$^+$/NADPH in Cellular Functions and Cell Death: Regulation and Biological

Consequences. *Antioxidants and Redox Signaling*, **10**, 179-206. http://dx.doi.org/10.1089/ars.2007.1672

[22] Milone, S.D., Pace Asciak, C.R., Reynaud, D., Azevedo, E.R., Newton, G.E. and Parker, J.D. (1999) Biochemical, Hemodynamic, and Vascular Evidence Concerning the Free Radical Hypothesis of Nitrate Tolerance. *Journal of Cardiovascular Pharmacology*, **33**, 685-690. http://dx.doi.org/10.1097/00005344-199905000-00002

[23] Kezeli, T., Rukhadze, T., Gongadze, N., Sukoyan, G., Dolidze, N., Chipashvili, M. and Mirsiashvili, M. (2014) Effect of Calcitonin Gene-Related Peptide Antagonist on the Mortality by Nitrate Induced Tolerance Rats with Acute Myocardial Infarction. *EPMA Journal*, **5**, A85. http://dx.doi.org/10.1186/1878-5085-5-S1-A85

[24] Gori, T. and Parker, J.D. (2008) Nitrate-Induced Toxicity and Preconditioning: A Rationale for Reconsidering the Use of These Drugs. *Journal of the American College of Cardiology*, **52**, 251-254. http://dx.doi.org/10.1016/j.jacc.2008.04.019

[25] Bokeria, L.A., Malikov, V.E., Arzumanyan, M.A., *et al.* (2008) Pharmacological Correction of Endothelial Dysfunction and Disturbance of Structured Organization of Thrombocyte Membranes in Ischemic Heart Disease. *Clinical Physiology of Circulation*, **1**, 39-44.

[26] Sayed, N., Kim, D.D., Fioramonti, X., Iwahashi, T., Durán, W.N. and Beuve, A. (2008) Nitroglycerin-Induced S-Nitrosylation and Desensitization of Soluble Guanylyl Cyclase Contribute to Nitrate Tolerance. *Circulation Research*, **103**, 606-614. http://dx.doi.org/10.1161/CIRCRESAHA.108.175133

[27] Hink, U., Daiber, A., Kayhan, N., Trischler, J., Kraatz, C., Oelze, M., *et al.* (2007) Oxidative Inhibition of the Mitochondrial Aldehyde Dehydrogenase Promotes Nitroglycerin Tolerance in Human Blood Vessels. *Journal of the American College of Cardiology*, **50**, 2226-2232. http://dx.doi.org/10.1016/j.jacc.2007.08.031

[28] Gupta, D., Georgiopoulou, V.V., Kalogeropoulos, A.P., Marti, C.N., Yancy, C.W., Gheorghiade, M., *et al.* (2013) Nitrate Therapy for Heart Failure. *JACC: Heart Failure*, **1**, 183-191. http://dx.doi.org/10.1016/j.jchf.2013.03.003

[29] Chen, Z., Peng, I-C., Cui, X., Li, Y.-S., Chien, S. and Shyy, J.Y.-J. (2010) Shear Stress, SIRT1, and Vascular Homeostasis. *Proceedings of the National Academy of Sciences of the United States of America*, **107**, 10268-10273. http://dx.doi.org/10.1073/pnas.1003833107

19

Solid Dose Form of Metformin with Ethyl Eicosapentaenoic Acid Does Not Improve Metformin Plasma Availability

Jeffrey H. Burton, William D. Johnson, Frank L. Greenway

Pennington Biomedical Research Center, Baton Rouge, USA
Email: Jeffrey.burton@pbrc.edu

Abstract

Background: The purpose of the study was to investigate effects of ethyl eicosapentaenoic acid on pharmacokinetics of metformin. Pharmacokinetic profiles of metformin and ethyl eicosapentaenoic acid when delivered separately or together in solid dose form were investigated and compared to determine whether the solid dose resulted in an altered metforminpharmacokinetics when given with or without food. Methods: A single-center, open-label, repeated dose study investigated the pharmacokinetic (PK) profile of metformin when administered in solid dose form with ethyl eicosapentaenoic acid compared to co-administration with icosapent ethyl, an ester of eicosapentaenoic acid and ethyl alcohol used to treat severe hypertriglyceridemia with metformin hydrochloride. Non-compartmental PK methods were used to compare area under the plasma concentration curve (AUC) and maximum plasma concentration (C_{max}) between patients randomized to either the ester or separate medications group under both fasting and fed conditions. Results: Using these two PK parameters, results showed that metformin availability was higher under fasting conditions when delivered separately from icosapent ethyl. There were no group differences in the fed condition. Conclusions: The solid dose form of metformin and ethyl eicosapentaenoic acid did not improve the pharmacokinetics of metformin in terms of plasma availability, suggesting that little is to be gained over the separate administration of ethyl eicosapentaenoic acid and metformin hydrochloride.

Keywords

AUC, Bioavailability, Eicosapentaenoic Acid, Metformin, Pharmacokinetics

1. Introduction

Metformin has been recommended as first line therapy for the treatment of type 2 diabetes due to its low cost, proven safety record, lack of weight gain and possible benefits for cardiovascular outcomes [1]. Type 2 diabetes is associated with triglyceride elevation, coronary heart disease and stroke [2]. The Nurse's Health Study found an inverse association of fish intake and omega-3 fatty acids to cardiovascular death [3]. Women in the National Health and Nutrition Examination Survey (NHANES) who consumed fish more than once a week had half the age related risk of stroke compared to women who did not eat fish [4]. Based on this and other data, the American Heart Association recommended supplementary eicosapentaenoic acid for people who need to reduce their cardiovascular risk and are not successful through diet alone [5]. Icosapent ethyl is an ester of eicosapentaenoic acid (EPA) and ethyl alcohol. This ester is converted to its components in the body. Icosapent ethyl is approved by the FDA as a medication to reduce triglyceride levels in patients with severe hypertriglyceridemia over 500 mg/dL [6].

A metformin ester of the amino acid glycine has been created and tested in drug-naïve adults with type-2 diabetes. Metformin glycinate decreased haemoglobin A1c to a significantly greater degree than placebo [7]. Metformin glycinate also had a greater maximum concentration and area under the curve at equimolar doses compared to metformin hydrochloride [8] [9]. This observation suggested the possibility that the development of a single drug (metformin eicosapentaenoate) containing both metformin and EPA might also give greater metformin bioavailability. Metformin eicosapentaenoate would presumably not only treat the diabetes, but also decrease the elevation of triglycerides which are so often elevated in patients with diabetes. As described by the manufacturer, metformin eicosapentaenoate is an ionic salt that quickly separates into metformin base and eicosapentaenoate free fatty acid in an aqueous environment. It was hypothesized that, viathis solid dose form of delivery, the plasma availability of metformin would be improved and the gastrointestinal side effects would be reduced when compared to the separate co-administration of metformin and EPA. This study describes the pharmacokinetics of metformin when given with icosapent ethyl compared to the pharmacokinetics of metformin eicosapentaenoate in a fasted and fed state.

2. Methods

2.1. Study Design

Sixteen subjects were enrolled in the trial and were randomized 5:3 to either metformin eicosapentaenoateor to metformin plus icosapent ethyl, respectively. To be included, participants in the study had to be men or women (sterile, >1 year menopausal, or practicing adequate contraception) aged 18 to 65 years with: no history of chronic diseases, a BMI ≤ 30 kg/m^2, no significant medical history including diabetes, hypertension or hyperlipidemia, negative urine alcohol and drug screening, and no usage of metformin or omega-3 fatty acid products within 2 months.

The first dose of the assigned drug therapy was given on day 1 of the study in the clinic after fasting for 10 - 12 hours. Plasma samples for PK analysis were taken at the time of drug consumption and at 0.5, 1, 2, 4, 8, and 12 hours following administration. Participants returned to the clinic 7 days later and were given the same dosage following a standardized meal. Again, plasma samples were drawn in an identical manner for subsequent PK analysis.

Metformin PK profiles were examined in a single-center, open-label, repeated dose study in which metformin was administered with icosapent ethyl or as metformin eicosapentaenoate in fasted and fed states. Metformin was delivered under the brand name Glucophage® and icosapent ethyl under the brand name Vascepa®. The dosages for each were as follows: metformin eicosapentaenoate1500 mg (via four 375 mg capsules), metformin 500 mg (via one 500 mg tablet), and icosapent ethyl 1000 mg (via one 1000 mg gel cap).

2.2. Pharmacokinetic Parameters

The pharmacokinetic (PK) analysis of metformin used non-compartmental methodologies. Specifically, three measures were estimated from the data: area under the PK curve (AUC), maximum plasma concentration (C_{max}) and time of maximum plasma concentration (t_{max}). These measures were used to compare the processing of metformin when administered as metformin eicosapentaenoate or separately with icosapent ethyl. AUC was calculated using the trapezoidal rule. The notation AUC_{last} will be used to indicate that AUC was estimated only up to the last observed concentration at 12 hours post-administration and not extrapolated to infinity.

2.3. Statistical Analysis

The primary aim of the research described here was to compare PK profiles of metformin under fasting and fed conditions when administered as metformin eicosapentaenoate versus separately as metformin and icosapent ethyl. The profiles were compared via non-compartmental PK parameters as area under the curve AUC_{last} and C_{max}. The analysis consisted of fitting two linear mixed effects models, each using one of the primary outcomes as the response variable. The models both contained fixed effects for treatment group, study condition (fasting/fed), and the interaction of these two variables. In addition, a random participant effect was included to account for within-subject correlation between repeated measurements taken under the fasting and fed conditions. Least squares means (LSM) were obtained from the models in order to compare the effects of the drug treatment groups under each study condition and to compare the effects of the study conditions within each treatment group. LSM were compared using two-sample t-tests. Since this study was exploratory in nature, two-sided t-tests were performed for each pair-wise comparison. All analyses were carried out using SAS/STAT® software, Version 9.4 of the SAS System for Windows (Cary, NC, USA), and all tests were evaluated using significance level $\alpha = 0.05$. A result was considered statistically significant if $p < \alpha$.

3. Results

See **Figure 1** for plots of individual metformin concentrations for participants in both drug treatment groups. For all analyses described here, plasma concentrations below the lower limit of quantification (BLQ) were treated as zero. Additionally, a participant missing any blood draw data at a given study visit had their complete data from that study visit excluded from the analysis. This was the case for two participants in the metformin eicosapentaenoate group at the second study visit.

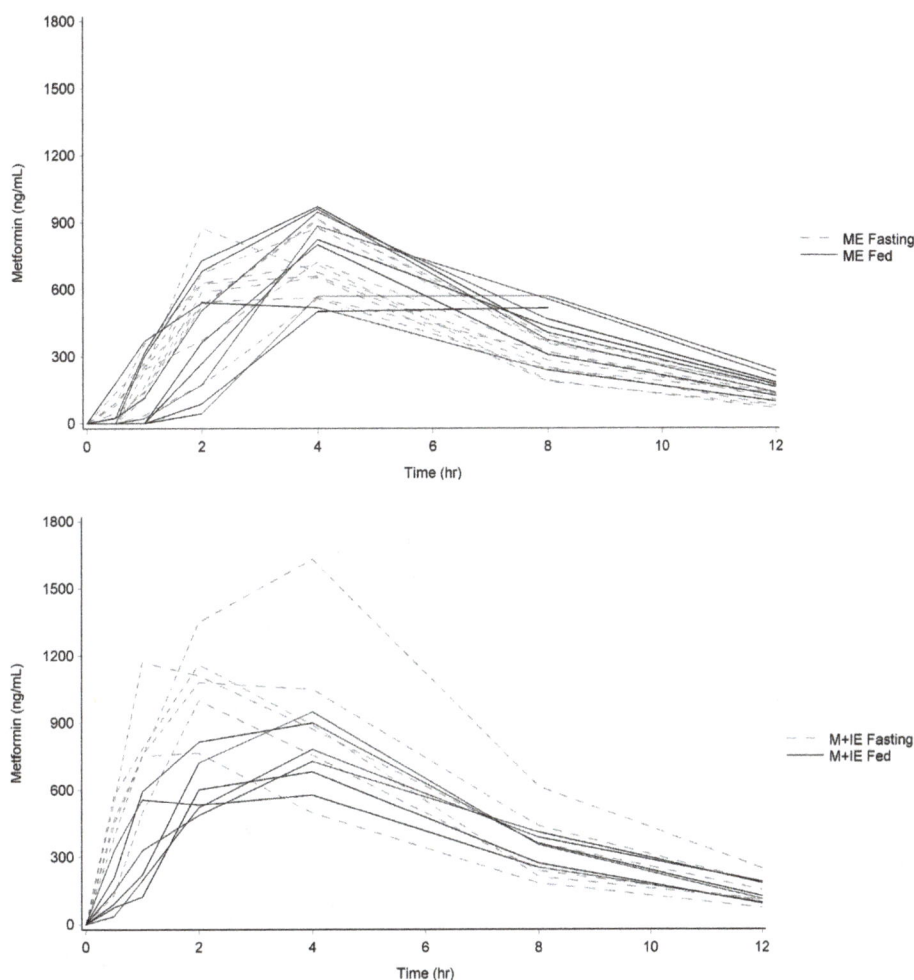

Figure 1. Individual metformin plasma concentration curves under each drug group and study condition; ME = metformin eicosapentaenoate, M + IE = metformin plus icosapent ethyl.

Summary measures of metformin plasma concentrations for each blood draw under both study conditions (fasting and fed) are summarized by treatment group in **Table 1** and presented visually in **Figure 2**. Summary statistics of the PK parameters are presented in **Table 2**.

The specific comparisons that were carried out and the results are summarized in **Table 3**. The ratio of LSM is presented as a percentage along with 90% confidence intervals and p-values. The ratios are used to show relative differences rather than absolute; however, the associated p-values are from tests of the differences of LSM. For the calculation of each ratio, the numerator was the test group mean and the denominator was the reference group mean. Thus, a ratio greater than 100 indicates a larger mean in the test group.

The results comparing AUC_{last} demonstrated that the LSM of AUC_{last} for metformin under metformin eicosapentaenoate was lower than that for metformin in the metformin plus icosapent ethyl group under both fasting and fed conditions. This difference was only statistically significant, however, in the fasting condition ($p = 0.001$). This indicates that the average plasma concentration of metformin over the 12 hour period was significantly

Table 1. Summary statistics of metformin concentrations.

Group[a]	Time (hr)	N	Mean (ng/mL)	SD (ng/mL)	Min (ng/mL)	Median (ng/mL)	Max (ng/mL)
ME Fasting	0	10	0	0	0	0	0
	0.5	10	47.1	50.3	0	34.9	138.0
	1	10	194.8	93.2	36.7	199.5	356.0
	2	10	552.4	184.7	174.0	566.0	874.0
	4	10	723.7	133.5	557.0	692.5	916.0
	8	10	290.5	71.3	187.0	300.5	391.0
	12	10	121.1	37.1	66.3	130.0	164.0
ME Fed	0	8	0	0	0	0	0
	0.5	8	29.1	62.8	0	0	182.0
	1	8	140.2	161.1	0	68.0	368.0
	2	8	412.9	242.4	44.4	434.0	728.0
	4	8	808.5	175.4	518.0	853.0	970.0
	8	8	417.8	113.8	238.0	418.5	569.0
	12	8	164.0	44.8	98.1	165.5	234.0
M + IE Fasting	0	6	0	0	0	0	0
	0.5	6	425.3	158.8	132.0	456.5	574.0
	1	6	785.0	216.0	499.0	754.0	1170.0
	2	6	1077.3	192.8	765.0	1095.0	1350.0
	4	6	949.3	380.7	497.0	881.5	1630.0
	8	6	341.3	165.5	183.0	300.0	615.0
	12	6	145.0	63.9	71.9	129.5	248.0
M + IE Fed	0	6	0	0	0	0	0
	0.5	6	148.6	106.8	37.1	120.1	329.0
	1	6	337.0	196.7	123.0	276.0	594.0
	2	6	613.2	129.5	486.0	567.5	815.0
	4	6	769.5	138.3	578.0	754.5	949.0
	8	6	339.2	63.0	253.0	356.5	410.0
	12	6	132.4	42.4	91.6	118.0	188.0

[a]ME = metformin eicosapentaenoate, M + IE = metformin plus icosapent ethyl.

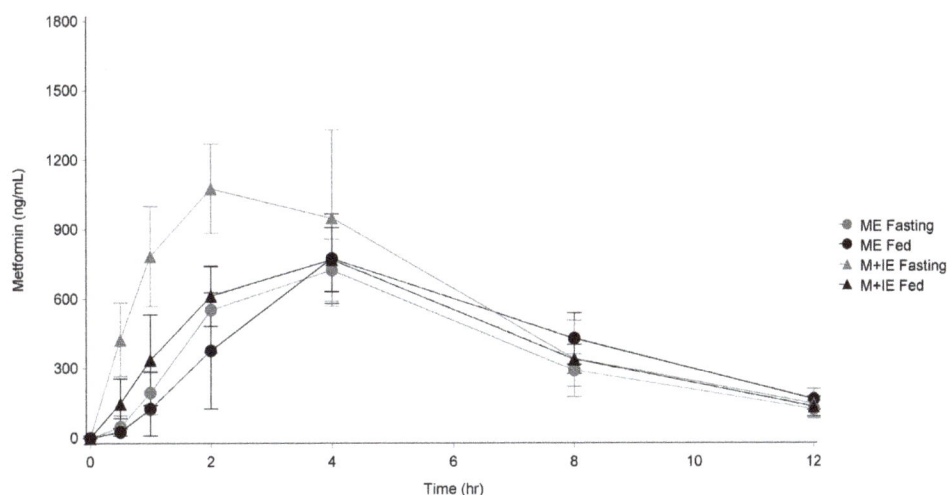

Figure 2. Group metformin plasma concenrations under each study condition (Mean ± SD); ME = metformin eicosapentaenoate, M + IE = metformin plus icosapent ethyl.

Table 2. Summary statistics of non-compartmental pharmacokinetic parameters.

Group[a]	Parameter	N	Mean	SD	Min	Median	Max
ME Fasting	Cmax (ng/mL)	10	743.6	140.1	557.0	715.5	916.0
	Tmax (hr)	10	3.8	0.6	2.1	4.0	4.0
	AUC (hr*ng/mL)	10	4573.1	778.1	3208.0	4396.2	5634.5
ME Fed	Cmax (ng/mL)	8	711.3	170.2	540.0	583.0	970.0
	Tmax (hr)	8	3.8	0.7	2.0	4.0	4.1
	AUC (hr*ng/mL)	8	5163.0	842.3	3879.2	5250.7	5187.1
M + IE Fasting	Cmax (ng/mL)	6	1134.0	284.7	765.0	1120.0	1630.0
	Tmax (hr)	6	2.2	1.0	1.0	2.0	4.0
	AUC (hr*ng/mL)	6	6925.1	2191.6	4320.1	6771.2	10655.3
M + IE Fed	Cmax (ng/mL)	6	769.5	138.3	578.0	754.5	949.0
	Tmax (hr)	6	4.0	0.0	4.0	4.0	4.1
	AUC (hr*ng/mL)	6	5179.9	739.2	4334.9	5227.5	6158.2

[a]ME = metformin eicosapentaenoate, M + IE = metformin plus icosapent ethyl.

Table 3. Results of hypothesis tests comparing non-compartmental pharmacokinetic parameters.

Outcome	Test[a]	Reference[a]	Ratio	90% LCL	90% UCL	p-value
AUC (hr*ng/mL)	ME Fasting	M + IE Fasting	67.8	56.8	81.0	0.0010
	ME Fed	M + IE Fed	99.3	82.3	119.7	0.9483
	ME Fasting	ME Fed	88.5	74.9	104.5	0.2175
	M + IE Fasting	M + IE Fed	129.5	105.8	158.6	0.0414
Cmax (ng/mL)	ME Fasting	M + IE Fasting	66.2	54.8	79.8	0.0009
	ME Fed	M + IE Fed	104.4	85.7	127.1	0.7148
	ME Fasting	ME Fed	92.4	75.9	112.4	0.4879
	M + IE Fasting	M + IE Fed	145.7	114.3	185.6	0.0164

[a]ME = metformin eicosapentaenoate, M + IE = metformin plus icosapent ethyl.

lower in subjects taking metformin eicosapentaenoate when the drugs were administered without food. The same result was observed for C_{max} in the fasting condition. The C_{max} of metformin under metformin eicosapentaenoate while fasting was significantly lower than the C_{max} under the reference drug ($p = 0.0009$), meaning that metformin had a higher average maximum plasma concentration in subjects taking metformin plus icosapent ethyl. In contrast to the results observed for AUC_{last} under the fed condition, however, the LSM for C_{max} under metformin eicosapentaenoate was slightly higher than for the reference drugs when taken with a meal. This difference was not statistically significant.

When comparing the PK parameters under the different conditions within each drug treatment group, there were no differences in either parameter for metformin eicosapentaenoate, meaning that the PK profiles defined by AUC_{last} and C_{max} were not different when the drug was taken with or without food. For the metformin plus icosapent ethyl group, on the other hand, both AUC_{last} and C_{max} were significantly higher when taking the drugs while fasting ($p = 0.0414$ and $p = 0.0164$, respectively).

4. Discussion

The primary findings from this study are that metformin has lower plasma availability when administered via metformin eicosapentaenoate than when given separately with icosapent ethyl under fasting conditions and that the availability of metformin is not different between the two delivery methods following a meal.

The hope was that AUC_{last} and C_{max} for the metformin PK curves would be larger for metformin eicosapentaenoate than for metformin plus icosapent ethyl under both study conditions, mirroring the greater bioavailability of metformin when esterified to glycine compared to metformin hydrochloride [8] [9]. Had metformin delivered through metformin eicosapentaenoate been more bioavailable, it might have resulted in a greater percentage of the metformin being absorbed and higher PK curves. Since metformin is only 60% absorbed and the unabsorbed portion of the metformin is thought to alter the gut microbiome inducing the gastrointestinal side effects of metformin, better absorption of metformin would be expected to improve the side effect profile associated with the drug [10] [11]. Due to the unanticipated results of this pharmacokinetic study, it appears that metformin eicosapentaenoate has limited advantages over giving the metformin and icosapent ethyl alone. In addition to a lack of improvement in pharmacokinetics, metformin eicosapentaenoate increases the number of required pills from two to four per dose.

One major weakness of this study was that the terminal phase of the metformin PK profile was not sufficiently long to estimate the elimination rate constant k_e. As a consequence, other PK parameters that are functions of k_e could not be estimated. These include half-life ($t_{1/2}$), clearance (Cl), volume of distribution (Vd/F), and area under the plasma concentration curve extrapolated to infinity ($AUC_{0-\infty}$). Estimates of these parameters would have allowed for a more comprehensive description and understanding of the metformin PK profile for metformin eicosapentaenoate and subsequent comparison with the reference drugs. On the other hand, an important conclusion is drawn from the analyses just utilizing parameters AUC_{last} and C_{max}, which is that the single drug containing metformin and EPA does not appear to improve the availability of metformin in the blood. Metformin eicosapentaenoate actually seems to result in less availability of metformin when taken while in a fasted state.

Based on the results and conclusions, if a similar future study is to be conducted, the number of blood draws following drug administration should be increased in a manner that provides a sufficient number of recorded plasma concentrations in the terminal elimination phase to allow for estimation of all PK parameters. Such a trial is unlikely to be done, since there seems to be little advantage gained from metformin eicosapentaenoate in terms of the pharmacokinetics of metformin.

Acknowledgements

This study was funded by Thetis Pharmaceuticals LLC. Drs. Burton and Johnson were additionally supported by 1 U54 GM104940 from the National Institute of General Medical Sciences of the NIH, which funds the Louisiana Clinical and Translational Science Center. The content of this manuscript is solely the responsibility of the authors and does not necessarily represent the official views of the National Institutes of Health. The Pennington Biomedical Research Center Institutional Review Board approved the study protocol, all participants provided written informed consent, the study complied with the Declaration of Helsinki, the trial was registered on clinicaltrials.gov (NCT02113163), and all conflicts of interest were declared.

References

[1] Inzucchi, S.E., Bergenstal, R.M., Buse, J.B., *et al.* (2015) Management of Hyperglycaemia in Type 2 Diabetes, 2015: A Patient-Centered Approach. Update to a Position Statement of the American Diabetes Association (ADA) and the European Association for the Study of Diabetes (EASD). *Diabetes Care*, **38**, 140-149. http://dx.doi.org/10.2337/dc14-2441

[2] National Institutes of Health, National Institute of Diabetes and Digestive and Kidney Diseases (2013) Diabetes, Heart Disease, and Stroke. NIH Publication No. 13-5094.

[3] Hu, F.B., Bronner, L., Willett, W.C., *et al.* (2002) Fish and Omega-3 Fatty Acid Intake and Risk of Coronary Heart Disease in Women. *JAMA*, **287**, 1815-1821. http://dx.doi.org/10.1001/jama.287.14.1815

[4] Gillum, R.F., Mussolino, M.E. and Madans, J.H. (1996) The Relationship between Fish Consumption and Stroke Incidence: The NHANES Epidemiologic Follow-Up Study (National Health and Nutrition Examination Survey). *Archives of Internal Medicine*, **156**, 537-542. http://dx.doi.org/10.1001/archinte.1996.00440050091010

[5] Kris-Etherton, P.M., Harris, W.S. and Appel, L.J., for the Nutrition Committee (2002) AHA Scientific Statement: Fish Condumption, Fish Oil, Omega-3 Fatty Acids and Cardiovascular Disease. *Circulation*, **106**, 2747-2757. http://dx.doi.org/10.1161/01.CIR.0000038493.65177.94

[6] (2012) Vascepa (Icosapen Ethyl) Package Insert. http://www.vascepa.com/full-prescribing-information.pdf

[7] Gonzalez-Ortiz, M., Martinez-Abundis, E., Robles-Cervantes, J.A., Ramos-Zavala, M.G., Barrera-Druan, C. and Gonzalez-Canudas, J. (2012) Effect of Metformin Glycinate on Glycated Hemoglobin A1c Concentration and Insulin Sensitivity in Drug-Naïve Adult Patients with Type 2 Diabetes Mellitus. *Diabetes Technology and Therapeutics*, **14**, 1140-1144. http://dx.doi.org/10.1089/dia.2012.0097

[8] Garza-Ocañas, L., Tamez-de la, O.E., Lujan-Rangel, R., Iglesias-Chiesa, J., González-Canudas, J. and Rivas-Ruiz, R. (2011) Bioavailability of Metformin Glycinate in Healthy Mexican Volunteers: An Open-Label, Single-Dose Clinical Trial. *Journal of Diabetes*, **3**, 358.

[9] Garza-Ocañas, L., Tamez-de la, O.E., Iglesias-Chiesa, J., González-Canudas, J. and Rivas-Ruiz, R. (2009) Pharmacokinetics and Gastrointestinal Tolerability of DMMET 01 (Glycinate of Metformin): Results of a Prospective Randomized Trial in Healthy Volunteers. *Diabetes*, **58**, A533.

[10] Greenway, F., Wang, S. and Heiman, M. (2014) A Novel Cobiotic Containing a Prebiotic and an Antioxidant Agments the Glucose Control and Gastrointestinal Tolerability of Metformin: A Case Report. *Beneficial Microbes*, **5**, 29-32. http://dx.doi.org/10.3920/BM2012.0063

[11] Burton, J.H., Johnson, M., Johnson, J., Hsia, D.S., Greenway, F.L. and Heiman, M.L. (2015) Addition of a Gastrointestinal Microbiome Modulator to Metformin Improves Metformin Tolerance and Fasting Glucose Levels. *Journal of Diabetes Science and Technology*, **9**, 808-814. http://dx.doi.org/10.1177/1932296815577425

20

Evaluation of Toxicological Profile of a Polyherbal Formulation

Rafeeq Alam Khan*, Maryam Aslam, Shadab Ahmed

Department of Pharmacology, Faculty of Pharmacy and Pharmaceutical Sciences, University of Karachi, Karachi, Pakistan

Email: *rkhan1959@gmail.com

Abstract

In current study toxicological profile of a commonly used herbal formulation was evaluated that is used extensively for gynecological disorders like menorrhagia, metrorrhagia, leucorrhea, irregular menstrual cycle, pre-menstrual syndrome and post-menopausal bleeding. It was also claimed to strengthen endometrium and ovaries. Since this herbal formulation was been used by a large number of population hence there was a need to assess acute and sub-chronic toxicity. Acute oral toxicity (LD_{50}) was observed in albino mice using standard protocols whereas sub-chronic, hematological and histopathological studies were assessed on 24 albino rabbits after giving herbal formulation for 60 days in two doses (20 and 60 mg/kg) against control groups. The outcomes of present study showed that the drug is safe up to 5000 mg/kg following acute oral toxicity test and no mortality was observed during sub chronic toxicity studies. Results of sub-chronic toxicity did not show any significant changes in biochemical, hematological and histopathological parameters. However, some indicators such as urea, creatinine, hemoglobin, and RBC count were altered, but these changes do not correlate with the histopathological results and may be associated to intra individual variations. Despite the safety of the drug in few animals, clinical trials and more investigations on a large number of animals are essentially needed to establish safety and efficacy of the herbal formulation.

Keywords

Acute Oral Toxicity, Sub-Chronic Toxicity, Biochemical Evaluation, Histopathological Examination, Herbal Formulation

1. Introduction

Herbal drugs often referred as traditional medicines are used to describe ancient and culture-bound health prac-

*Corresponding author.

tices existed before the development of research based modern or allopathic medicines [1] [2]. Herbal drugs form a major component of alternative system of healthcare like ayurvedic, homeopathic, naturopathic and Native American Indian medicine. They have made great contributions in the development of modern drugs as around thirty percent of all modern medicines have been derived from higher plants [3] [4]. Among the first active principles to be isolated from plants were morphine, papaverine, atropine and colchicine, which are still used widely for the treatment of various disorders [5] [6]. Herbal medicines are an essential part of traditional health care system in many cultures [7].

Herbs are products of natural origin most often used as self-treatment of diseased states or less than optimal health conditions. Many are without therapeutic effects and some are toxic [8]. Herbal medicines are usually thought to be safe due to its natural origin however several reviews summarize their significant side effects and interactions [9]-[13].

Mostly integrated research focusing the developments of commercially viable and useful herbal medicines, has not been carried out *i.e.* herbal products is not tested with the scientific rigor required for modern conventional drugs [14]. Various drug interactions are associated with the intake of some herbal medicines that may result in many adverse reactions [15]. Experts suggest that natural does not mean completely safe and high-risk groups like elderly, pediatrics, pregnant and lactating woman, patients with co-morbidities and organ failures should use herbal products with extreme caution; hence toxicological studies are essentially required before their use by general public [8] [16] [17].

The herbal formulation under study consists of *Saraca indica*, *Symplocos racemosa*, *Valeriana wallichii*, *Matricaria chamomilla*, *Vitex agnuscastus* and *Areca catechu*. It is indicated for gynecological disorders like menorrhagia, metrorrhagia, leucorrhea, irregular menstrual cycle, pre-menstrual syndrome and post-menopausal bleeding. It is also claimed to be beneficial for strengthening endometrium and ovaries.

Saraca indica has been used for its astringent and uterine sedative actions. It acts directly on the muscle fibers of uterus and stimulates the endometrium and ovarian tissue. It has oxytocic activity and historically used for the treatment of excessive endometrial bleeding and dysmenorrhea. It is also used for depression in women and for bleeding in Piles [18] [19].

Symplocos racemosa is useful in bowel complaints, Dropsy, liver complaints, fevers, ulcers and scorpion-sting. It also resolves inflammation and relaxes uterine tissues, and thus is used for menorrhagia. It is also recommended for skin and eye infections and in cases of hemorrhage [20] [21].

Valeriana wallichii is used for restlessness, sleeping disorders, lack of concentration, stress, headache, epilepsy, menstrual states of agitation, menopause, stomach cramps, colic and uterine spasticity. It is a powerful nerve tonic, stimulant, carminative, antispasmodic, calmative and analeptic [22] [23].

Matricaria chamomilla is a pleasant aromatic plant with a bitter taste. It possesses antispasmodic, expectorant, carminative, anthelmintic, sedative and diuretic properties. It is principally used as a nerve tonic, in false labor pains, dysmenorrhea, metrorrhagia and cramps in the leg [24].

Vitex agnuscastus is a deciduous tree indigenous to the Mediterranean region as far as western Asia. In folk medicine, it has been used to treat infertility, amenorrhea and hormonal imbalance in both sexes, and also to prevent pre-menstrual mastodynia [25] [26].

Areca catechu has intoxicant, stimulant, astringent, vermifuge, taenifuge, nerve tonic and emmenagogue properties. It is used in the treatment of cholera, colitis, diarrhea, dysentery, fatigue, fever, gastrosis, gonorrhea, leucorrhea, hematuria, herpes, hysteria, malaria, small pox, and tapeworm [27] [28].

Since no legal guidelines exist for regulating the manufacturing, packaging, marketing and use of herbal drugs in Pakistan, these drugs are freely available in the market to be used through self-guidance or untrained advise. Hence pharmacological and toxicological evaluation of such drugs is very important, where large populations are exposed to such preparations without prescription from a licensed or trained medical practitioner.

2. Material and Method

2.1. Selection of Animals

Two different animal species mice and rabbits were selected for present investigation acute toxicity studies were done on mice and sub-chronic studies were performed on rabbits.

2.2. Acute Toxicity Testing (LD$_{50}$)

Acute oral toxicity (LD$_{50}$) was performed by the method of Lorke [29]. Albino mice of either sex; weighing 20 - 25 gm, were maintained under persistent environmental conditions 25°C ± 2°C and were provided standard diet and water *ad libitum*. Three groups of mice each comprising of 3 animals was administered with 10, 100 and 1000 mg/kg of herbal formulation by mouth and examined for mortality within 24 hours. Following the results of mortality in each group, another set of 3 groups of mice were administered higher doses of the test drug, to achieve the least and most toxic value and LD$_{50}$ was calculated by geometric mean of the values.

2.3. Sub-Chronic Toxicity

This test was performed on 24 healthy white rabbits of either sex from 1200 to 1800 grams. All animals were equally separated into three groups, one group regarded as control and other two received 20 and 60 mg/kg doses of herbal formulation for consecutive 60 days through oral intubation tube. Doses were prepared in DMSO however control group received DMSO orally equal to the volume of individual doses according to their body weight. Before administration of drug, physical health of these animals was observed during the conditioning period under the laboratory environment for a week explicitly seeing loss of hair, diarrhea, edema, ulceration and lack of activity.

2.4. Sample Collection

Blood sample of around 6 ml were collected from these animals by cardiac puncture at the completion of dosing on 61st day to determine various biochemical and hematological parameters.

2.5. Assessment of Toxicities

2.5.1. Physical Examination

Gross toxicities were perceived every one-week after giving herbal formulation for 60 days explicitly noticing skin ulceration, average weight variation, loss of hair, loss of appetite, loss of activity, hematuria, vomiting, diarrhea, edema, lacrimation, salivation, muscle tone, tremor and aggressive behavior. Autopsy was performed after random selection, at the completion of dosage and sample collection for biochemical tests.

2.5.2. Biochemical Evaluation

Blood samples were collected from fasted animals prior to necropsy. Approximately 7 ml of blood samples were collected by cardio puncture. Serum were immediately separated by centrifugation for 10 min at 4000 rpm and was examined for the following parameters within 3 hours of sample collection on Humalyzer 3000 (GmBH Germany) at 37°C utilizing reagents supplied by Human Gmbh Germany.

   1) Cardiac parameters: CK-NAC, LDH, AST.
   2) Renal parameters: Total protein, urea, creatinine, uric acid.
   3) Hepatic parameters: Alkaline phosphatase, ALT, γ-GT, total and direct bilirubin.
   4) Lipid profile: cholesterol and triglycerides.
   5) Blood glucose level.
   6) Calcium and phosphorus.

2.5.3. Hematological Evaluation

Blood samples were collected under 10% EDTA at 7.2 pH and hematological parameters *i.e.* RBC, WBC, PLT, Hematocrit, & hemoglobin were explored using Humacount hematology analyzer GmbH 17400, a fully automated cell counter with a built-in veterinary software module.

2.5.4. Microscopic Examination

Representative blocks from different areas of heart, liver and kidney were cut from each sample after separating all fat from respective organs. The blocks were processed through Gilford 101 s automatic tissue processor.

   Tissue slices of 3 - 4 micron were taken from the wax blocks by rotary microtome. The tissue slices were mounted on slides and dehydrated softly by pressing with filter paper. The mounted slides were placed primarily for drying on a hot plate (45°C) for 90 minutes and then left in an incubator at 37°C overnight to dry before microscopic examination.

2.6. Statistical Analysis

All the values for biochemical tests were stated as the mean and standard error to the mean (S.E.M.) and were analyzed by using one way unstacked ANOVA and p values were observed [30]. Results were considered significant if p value was less than 0.05 and highly significant if p value was less than 0.005.

3. Results

3.1. Physical Examination

Apparent physical health of the animals was observed in various groups on different doses of herbal formulation during the entire period of experiment.

Skin ulceration, average weight variation, loss of hair, loss of appetite, loss of activity, hematuria, vomiting, diarrhea, edema, lacrimation, salivation, respiratory rate, muscle tone, exophthalmia, tremor, and aggressive behavior. Animals of no group exhibited gross toxicities at any time during the entire period of experiment and none of the animals expired.

3.2. Biochemical Evaluation

Table 1 reveals the comparison of biochemical markers e.g. CK-NAC, LDH, AST, Total protein, urea, creatinine, uric acid, ALP, ALT, γ-GT, Total and Direct Bilirubin, cholesterol, triglycerides, calcium, phosphorus and glucose following 20 and 60 mg/kg dose administration of herbal formulation for 60 days.

Generally results did not reveal any significant toxicity. Herbal formulation had elevated serum urea highly significantly at 20 mg/kg however at 60 mg/kg the increase was significant, as compared to control. Serum creatinine was also reduced significantly at 60 mg/kg as compared to control. Rest of the biochemical parameter appears to be in normal ranges with respect to control group animals.

Table 1. Effect of herbal formulation after 60 days on biochemical markers.

Parameters	Animal groups		
	Control	Herbal formulation	
		20 mg/kg	60 mg/kg
CK-NAC (U/I)	470 ± 58	479 ± 102	494 ± 48
LDH (U/l)	236 ± 33	216 ± 33	252 ± 33
AST (U/l)	95 ± 21	66.7 ± 16.7	59 ± 7.4
Tot. Protein (gm/dl)	7.94 ± 0.65	6.74 ± 0.68	8.1 ± 1.86
Urea (mg/dl)	20.35 ± 3.18	59.69 ± 4.6**	33.3 ± 1.93*
Creatinine (mg/dl)	1.67 ± 0.132	1.95 ± 0.13	1.21 ± 0.11*
Uric Acid (mg/dl)	1.34 ± 0.295	0.76 ± 0.24	1.08 ± 0.18
ALP (U/I)	86.4 ± 16.85	86.5 ± 21.9	75.14 ± 17.67
ALT (U/l)	75.3 ± 8.5	86.6 ± 19.6	57.14 ± 5.89
γ GT (U/l)	6.43 ± 0.428	7.7 ± 0.92	6.57 ± 0.84
Tot. Bilirubin (mg/dl)	0.34 ± 0.02	0.3 ± 0.08	0.4 ± 0.07
Dir. Bilirubin (mg/dl)	0.08 ± 0.02	0.09 ± 0.01	0.09 ± 0.01
Cholesterol (mg/dl)	14.40 ± 2.6	15.7 ± 3.53	9.7 ± 2.86
Triglycerides (mg/dl)	59.43 ± 13.89	38.43 ± 8.9	52.6 ± 17
Calcium (mg/dl)	7.5 ± 1.5	8.68 ± 1.39	8.86 ± 0.99
Phosphorus (mg/dl)	6.56 ± 0.51	6.82 ± 0.88	6.22 ± 0.43
Glucose (mg/dl)	178 ± 27.65	173.9 ± 29.78	133.3 ± 2.18

n = 8. Average values ± S.E.M. *p < 0.05 significant as compared to control. **p < 0.005 highly significant as compared to control.

3.3. Hematological Evaluation

Table 2 reveals the comparison of *Hemoglobin, Hematocrit, RBC, WBC, and Platelet* following 20 and 60 mg/kg dose of herbal formulation for 60 days. There was highly significant decrease in hemoglobin hematocrit and significant decrease in RBC count at 60 mg/kg dose of herbal formulation, in comparison to control group, while there was no significant change in WBCs and platelet count, in comparison to control group animals.

3.4. Microscopic Examination

Gross examination of various vital organs such as heart, liver and kidney showed no significant macroscopic changes in any group. However, on microscopic examination, one animal at 60 mg/kg revealed congestion and mild focal interstitial inflammation in renal tissue (**Figure 1**). Similarly one animal at 60 mg/kg also showed congestion with mild portal inflammation in hepatic tissue (**Figure 2**) but rest of the animals did not revealed any cellular changes (**Figure 3** & **Figure 4**).

4. Discussion

Herbal medicine is the oldest form of healthcare and had been used by all cultures throughout history. The WHO has assessed that 80% of the world's population stays to use traditional therapies, a main part of which are obtained from plants, as their primary health care tools [4] [31].

Table 2. Effects of herbal formulation after 60 days on hematological parameters.

Parameters	Animal groups		
	Control	Herbal formulation	
		20 mg/kg	60 mg/kg
Hemoglobin (gm/dl)	10.6 ± 0.25	9.5 ± 0.77	$9 \pm 0.382^{**}$
Hematocrit (%)	33.93 ± 0.73	30.28 ± 2.22	$29.69 \pm 0.85^{**}$
RBC $\times 10^6/\mu l$	5.49 ± 0.21	5.03 ± 0.43	$4.87 \pm 0.13^{*}$
WBC $\times 10^3/\mu l$	5.44 ± 0.51	3.98 ± 0.45	4.25 ± 0.32
Platelet $\times 10^3/\mu l$	306 ± 49	324 ± 44.4	433 ± 62

n = 8. Average values ± S.E.M. $^{*}p < 0.05$ significant as compared to control. $^{**}p < 0.005$ highly significant as compared to control.

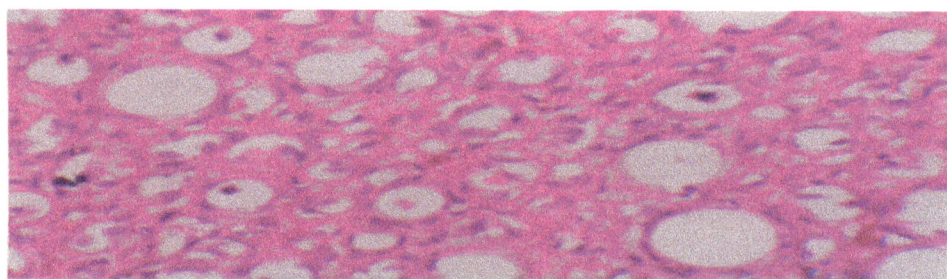

Figure 1. Renal tissue showing congestion and mild focal interstitial inflammation.

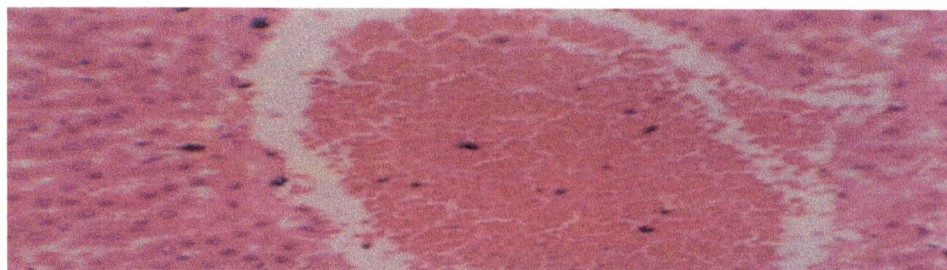

Figure 2. Hepatic tissue showing congestion and mild portal inflammation.

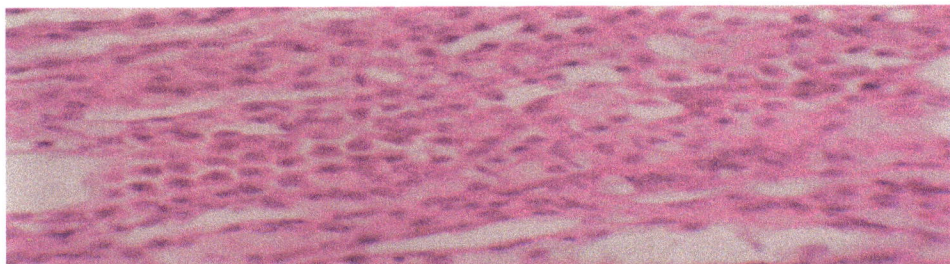

Figure 3. Hepatic tissue showing no microscopic changes.

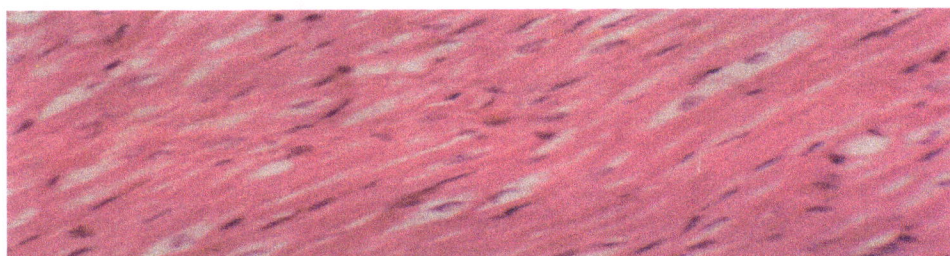

Figure 4. Cardiac tissue showing no microscopic changes.

Herbal medicines are usually regarded as safe, but case reports indicate that serious side effects and pertinent interactions with other drugs can arise altering physiology and these changes can be reflected in abnormal test results [32] [33]. Hence plants should be evaluated by modern scientific methods in order to demonstrate their usefulness and to avoid the use of useless and toxic herbs. Thus, herbal formulation was evaluated for its safety against gross toxicities and toxic effects on biochemical, hematological and histopathological parameters in rabbits.

The overall physiology of rabbits is comparable to humans, thus rabbits have been used as a model for human diseases. Rabbits are large enough to provide suitable amounts of tissue for experimental work without pooling of samples but are small enough to be economical for most studies.

Moreover rabbits were selected since biochemical and histopathological changes made are comparatively similar as observed in humans [34]. Secondly, sufficient amount of blood samples can be obtained at different stages of experiment and thirdly, rabbits are not only easily available but are also easy to handle.

The result of acute toxicity (LD_{50}) after oral administration reveals that herbal formulation has LD_{50} greater than 5000 mg/kg. Moreover, there was no death reported at any dose following administration of herbal formulation for 60 days. These findings suggest that this preparation possesses wide therapeutic range and is relatively safe.

In present study, comparison of gross toxicities e.g. skin ulceration, weight variation, loss of hair, loss of activity, hematuria, loss of interest in food, vomiting, diarrhea, edema, salivation, and aggressive behavior etc., were seen after the administration of herbal formulation during the entire period of experiment. The results showed no significant toxicities, however, average weight loss was observed during the course of experimentation in animals of all three groups.

Study of the renal profile such as total protein, urea, creatinine, and uric acid levels give useful information about the drug-induced renal toxicities. Animals which received herbal formulation in 20 and 60 mg/kg doses did not show any significant changes in total protein and uric acid levels. However, animals at 20 mg/kg dose showed highly significant increase in urea, while, animals at 60 mg/kg showed less significant increase in urea and significant decrease in creatinine. The decrease in urea was not consistent with the dose and might be due to increased protein metabolism also indicated by weight loss in all animal groups.

Liver damage tempted by drugs may consist of hepatocellular necrosis, cholestasis, or a mixture of biochemical and histopathological patterns [35]. The estimation of AST and ALP is suitable in the early diagnosis of viral or toxic hepatitis and thus patients exposed to hepatotoxic drugs [36]. Hence animals were tested for ALP, AST, γ-GT and Bilirubin levels to check for hepatic toxicity. There were no significant changes ALP, AST, γ-GT and Bilirubin (Total and Direct) in animals of either group received herbal formulation.

Animals received 20 and 60 mg/kg doses of herbal formulation did not show any significant changes in Cardiac enzymes such as LDH, CK and GOT. Moreover, microscopic examination of cardiac tissue also did not reveal any Cardiac damage.

Animals received 20 and 60 mg/kg doses of herbal formulation showed no significant changes in lipid profile (triglycerides and cholesterol) and other biochemical parameters (glucose, calcium and phosphorus).

Study of the hematological parameters like hemoglobin concentration, hematocrit, RBC, WBC, and platelet count gives valuable information about the drug-induced hematological toxicities. Animals received 60 mg/kg doses of herbal formulation showed highly significant decrease in hemoglobin and hematocrit, and significant decrease in RBC count.

The herbal formulation did not revealed any macroscopic changes at 20 mg as well as 60 mg/kg doses, similarly microscopic examination in animals received 20 and 60 mg/kg herbal formulation did not reveal any remarkable changes in heart. However, there was mild focal interstitial inflammation in kidney at 60 mg/kg, which might be due to intra individual variation, since biochemical changes do not confirm any damage in these tissues. Similarly there was mild portal inflammation in hepatic tissue of animals at 20 mg/kg which might be due to any circulating antigen, since biochemical alterations did not correlate microscopic changes and are thus insignificant.

5. Conclusion

Investigation on acute, sub-chronic, biochemical, hematological and histopathological parameters did not reveal any significant toxicity; therefore it may indeed be concluded as safe formulation; however despite safety of the drug in animals, trial in humans is the only valid way of establishing safety and efficacy of any drug prior to use in humans.

Acknowledgements

Authors are grateful to Herbion Pakistan Limited for providing herbal formulation and financial support to complete this piece of work.

References

[1]   Farnsworth, N.R. (1988) Screening of Plants for New Medicines. In: Wilson, E.O., Ed., Chapter 9 in Biodiversity, National Academy Press, Washington DC.

[2]   Gurib-Fakim, A. (2006) Medicinal Plants: Traditions of Yesterday and Drugs of Tomorrow. *Molecular Aspects of Medicine*, **27**, 1-93. http://dx.doi.org/10.1016/j.mam.2005.07.008

[3]   Burns, M.M. (2000) Alternative Medicine: Herbal Preparation. *Clinical Pediatric Emergency Medicine*, **1**, 186-190. http://dx.doi.org/10.1016/S1522-8401(00)90026-0

[4]   Khan, R.A., Arif, M., Sherwani, B. and Ahmed, M. (2013) Acute and Sub Chronic Toxicity of *Mucuna pruriens, Cinnamomum zeylanicum, Myristica fragrans* and Their Effects on Hematological Parameters. *Australian Journal of Basic and Applied Sciences*, **7**, 641-647.

[5]   Drews, J. (2000) Drug Discovery: A Historical Perspective. *Science*, **287**, 1960-1964. http://dx.doi.org/10.1126/science.287.5460.1960

[6]   Newman, D.J., Cragg, G.M. and Snada, K.M. (2000) The Influence of Natural Products upon Drug Discovery. *Natural products Reports*, **17**, 215-234. http://dx.doi.org/10.1039/a902202c

[7]   Vickers, A. and Zollman, C. (1999) ABC of Complementary Medicine: Herbal Medicine. *British Medical Journal*, **319**, 1050-1053. http://dx.doi.org/10.1136/bmj.319.7216.1050

[8]   Tyler, V.E., Brady, L.R. and Robbers, J.E. (1988) Pharmacognosy. 9th Edition, Lea & Febiger, Philadelphia.

[9]   De Smet, P.A.G.M. (1997) The Role of Plant-Derived Drugs and Herbal Medicines in Healthcare. *Drugs*, **54**, 801-840. http://dx.doi.org/10.2165/00003495-199754060-00003

[10]   Miller, L.G. (1998) Hepatotoxic Herbs. *Archives of Internal Medicine*, **158**, 2200-2210. http://dx.doi.org/10.1001/archinte.158.20.2200

[11]   Ernst, E. (2000) Possible Interactions between Synthetic and Herbal Medicinal Products. Part 1: A Systematic Review of the Indirect Evidence. *Perfusion*, **13**, 4-15.

[12]   Ernst, E. (2000) Possible Interactions between Synthetic and Herbal Medicinal Products. Part 2: A Systematic Review of the Direct Evidence. *Perfusion*, **13**, 60-70.

[13]   Skalli, S., Zaid, A. and Soulaymani, R. (2007) Drug Interactions with Herbal Medicines. *Therapeutic Drug Monitoring*,

29, 1-7. http://dx.doi.org/10.1097/FTD.0b013e31815c17f6

[14] Subramoniam, A. (2001) The Problems and Prospects of Plant Drug Research in India: Pharmacological Evaluation of Ecotypes in Herbal Drug Development. *Indian Journal of Pharmacology*, **33**, 145-146.

[15] Kistorp, T.K. and Laursen, S.B. (2002) Herbal Medicines—Evidence and Drug Interactions in Clinical Practice. *Ugeskr Laeger*, **164**, 4161-4165.

[16] World Health Organization (1991) Guidelines for the Assessment of Herbal Medicines. Program on Traditional Medicines, Geneva, 1-4.

[17] World Health Organization (2005) WHO Global Atlas of Traditional, Complementary and Alternative Medicine. World Health Organization, Geneva, 1-2.

[18] Venugopal, S. (1998) Effect of Eve Care in Oligomenorrhoea. *Antiseptic*, **95**, 329-330.

[19] Pradhan, P., Joseph, L., Gupta, V., Chulet, R., Arya, H., Verma, R. and Bajpai, A. (2009) Saraca Asoca (Ashoka): A Review. *Journal of Chemical and Pharmaceutical Research*, **1**, 62-71.

[20] Bhutani, K.K., Jadhav, A.N. and Kalia, V. (2004) Effect of *Symplocos racemosa* Roxb. on Gonadotropin Release in Immature Female Rats and Ovarian Histology. *Journal of Ethnopharmacology*, **94**, 197-200. http://dx.doi.org/10.1016/j.jep.2004.04.022

[21] Jadhav, A.N. and Bhutani, K.K. (2005) Ayurveda and Gynecological Disorders. *Journal of Ethnopharmacology*, **97**, 151-159. http://dx.doi.org/10.1016/j.jep.2004.10.020

[22] Gilani, A.H., Khan, A.U., Jabeen, Q., Subhan, F. and Ghafar, R. (2005) Antispasmodic and Blood Pressure Lowering Effects of *Valeriana wallichii* Are Mediated through K+ Channel Activation. *Journal of Ethnopharmacology*, **100**, 347-352. http://dx.doi.org/10.1016/j.jep.2005.05.010

[23] Sahu, S., Ray, K., Yogendra, K.M.S., Gupta, S., Kauser, H., Kumar, S., Mishra, K. and Panjwani, U. (2012) *Valeriana wallichii* Root Extract Improves Sleep Quality and Modulates Brain Monoamine Level in Rats. *Phytomedicine*, **19**, 924-929. http://dx.doi.org/10.1016/j.phymed.2012.05.005

[24] Avallone, R., Zanoli, P., Corsi, L., Cannazza, G. and Baraldi, M. (1996) Benzodiazepine-Like Compounds and GABA in Flower Head of *Matricaria chamomilla*. *Phytotherapy Research*, **10**, s177-s179.

[25] Christoffel, V., Spengler, B., Jarry, H. and Wuttke, W. (1999) Prolactin Inhibiting Dopaminergic Activity of Diterpenes from Vitex Agnus Castus. In: Loew, D., Blume, H. and Dingermann, T., Eds., *Phytopharmaka V*, Springer-Verlag, Berlin Heidelberg, 209-214. http://dx.doi.org/10.1007/978-3-642-58709-2_25

[26] van Diana, D., Burger, H.G., Teede, H. and Bone, K. (2012) Vitex Agnus-Castus Extracts for Female Reproductive Disorders: A Systematic Review of Clinical Trials. *Planta Medica*, **79**, 562-575.

[27] Gilani, A.H., Ghayur, M.N., Saify, Z.S., Ahmed, S.P., Choudhary, M.I. and Khalid, A. (2004) Presence of Cholinomimetic and Acetylcholinesterase Inhibitory Constituents in Betel Nut. *Life Science*, **75**, 2377-2389. http://dx.doi.org/10.1016/j.lfs.2004.03.035

[28] Peng, W., Liu, Y.-J., Wu, N., Sun, T., He, X.-Y. and Gao, Y.-X. (2015) *Areca catechu* L. (Arecaceae): A Review of Its Traditional Uses, Botany, Phytochemistry, Pharmacology and Toxicology. *Journal of Ethnopharmacology*, **164**, 340-356. http://dx.doi.org/10.1016/j.jep.2015.02.010

[29] Lorke, D. (1983) A New Approach to Practical Acute Toxicity Testing. *Archives of Toxicology*, **54**, 275-287. http://dx.doi.org/10.1007/BF01234480

[30] Larson, D.A. (1992) Analysis of Variance with Just Summary Statistics as Input. *The American Statistician*, **46**, 151-152.

[31] Akerele, O. (1993) Summary of WHO Guidelines for the Assessment of Herbal Medicines. *Herbal Gram*, **28**, 13-19.

[32] Barnes, J., Anderson, L.A. and Phillipson, J.D. (2007) Herbal Medicine. 3rd Edition, Pharmaceutical Press, London, 1-23.

[33] Tsai, H.H., Lin, H.W., Simon, A.P. and Mahady, G.B. (2012) Evaluation of Documented Drug Interactions and Contraindications Associated with Herbs and Dietary Supplements: A Systematic Literature Review. *International Journal of Clinical Practice*, **66**, 1056-1078. http://dx.doi.org/10.1111/j.1742-1241.2012.03008.x

[34] Chojnowska, I., Kucharczyk, K., Myszkowski, L., Radzikowski, A. and Szymańska, K. (1979) Blood Serum Proteins in Experimental Chronic Liver Injury in Rabbit. *Patologia Polska*, **30**, 71-88.

[35] Bonadonna, G. (1988) Chemotherapy Induced Complications. In: Bonadonna, G. and Robustelli-Della-Cuna, G., Eds., *Handbook of Medical Oncology*, 3rd Edition, Masson, Milano, Parigi, Barecellona and Mexico, 963-975.

[36] Zimmerman, H.J. (1984) Function and Integrity of the Liver. In: Henry, J.B., Ed., *Clinical Diagnosis and Management by Laboratory Methods*, 17th Edition, W. B. Saunders, Philadelphia, 217-250.

21

Evaluation of the Management of Hyperlipidemia and Hypertension in an Outpatient Cardiac Transplant Clinic

Jane J. Xu[1], Ilene Burton[2], Wayne J. Tymchak[3,4], Glen J. Pearson[3,4]

[1]Alberta Health Services, Pharmacy Services, Edmonton, Canada
[2]Alberta Health Services, Transplant Services, Edmonton, Canada
[3]University of Alberta, Division of Cardiology, Edmonton, Canada
[4]Mazankowski Alberta Heart Institute, Edmonton, Canada
Email: Glen.Pearson@ualberta.ca

Abstract

Background: Allograft coronary artery disease (ACAD) is a common cause of morbidity and mortality post-orthotopic heart transplantation (OHT). ACAD progression may be reduced by modifying cardiovascular risk factors, such as hyperlipidemia and hypertension. We sought to evaluate the management of hyperlipidemia and hypertension among OHT recipients followed in an outpatient cardiac transplant clinic. Objective: The primary objective was to assess the proportion of OHT patients achieving both the recommended LDL target of <2.0 mmol/L and BP targets of <140/90 mmHg (or <130/80 mmHg for diabetics) in an outpatient cardiac transplant clinic. Methods: A cross-sectional retrospective analysis of the medical records of all adult OHT recipients actively followed in our outpatient cardiac transplant between January-March 2009. Results: Of the 193 patients included, both the low-density lipoprotein (LDL) cholesterol and blood pressure (BP) targets were achieved in 111 (57.5%) patients. The LDL target alone was achieved by 140 (72.5%) patients and the BP target alone by 153 (79.3%) patients. Statins were prescribed in 183 (94.8%) patients with a mean LDL of 1.81 mmol/L (±0.55). Angiotensin converting enzyme-inhibitors [ACE-I] (or angiotensin receptor blockers [ARB]) were prescribed in 154 (79.8%) patients, diltiazem in 101 (52.3%) patients, and both in 85 (44.0%) patients, with a mean BP of 124.2/77.8 mmHg (±13.6/8.2). Adverse reactions related to statins, ACE-inhibitors or diltiazem were uncommon and rarely resulted in drug discontinuation. Conclusions: Guideline recommended that LDL and BP targets are achievable in a significant proportion of OHT recipients. The high utilization rates of statins for dyslipidemia and ACE-I (or ARB) and diltiazem for BP were consistent with guideline recommendations for the prevention of ACAD. Despite concerns regarding the potential for pharmacokinetic drug interactions in OHT patients, the reported rates of any drug intolerance to these medications were low in our population.

Keywords

Cardiac Transplant, Allograft Coronary Artery Disease, Graft Vaculopathy, Dyslipidemia, Hypertension

1. Introduction

Heart transplantation is a life-saving medical intervention indicated for highly selected patients with end-stage heart disease; however, <200 heart transplants are performed annually across Canada [1]. Allograft coronary artery disease (ACAD), a rapidly progressive form of atherosclerosis in orthotopic heart transplantation (OHT) recipients, is a common cause of morbidity and mortality [2]. ACAD is characterized by intimal proliferation, luminal stenosis of epicardial branches, and occlusion of smaller arteries [3]. By 10 years post-transplant, >50% of surviving recipients have angiographic ACAD [4]. Both immunologic risk factors and non-immunologic risk factors are reported to be implicated [3]. It has been reported that 93% of surviving recipients have hyper-lipidemia and 99% have hypertension by 10 years post-OHT [4]. The only definitive treatment for ACAD is re-transplantation, but this not only poses risks for the patient but also causes ethical dilemmas for clinicians because of the scarcity of donor organs [3]. Because of the significant influence ACAD has on morbidity and mortality, it is important to focus on preventing this silent progressive disease, rather than treating its consequences.

Hyperlipidemia is the most consistently associated metabolic risk factor for the development of ACAD in the OHT recipient and can be caused by factors such as pre-transplant hyperlipidemia, immunosuppressant medications, obesity, and diabetes [2] [5] [6]. Low-density lipoprotein (LDL) is significantly associated with coronary intimal thickening and graft dysfunction [3] [7]. Prospective, randomized studies have demonstrated that statins reduce all-cause mortality at 1-year post-OHT [5] [8]. Kobashigawa concluded that the early use of pravastatin safely lowered cholesterol levels, decreased the incidence of major rejection, improved 1-year survival, and reduced the development of ACAD [9]. Follow-up studies have shown that these benefits were maintained for 10 years [10]. Similar findings are reported with use of simvastatin [11]-[13]. Other statins have shown benefit in smaller studies and appear to be safe and effective in aggressively lowering low-density lipoprotein (LDL) cholesterol in OHT recipients where other statins failed to reach therapeutic goals [14]-[16].

Based on this evidence, the Canadian Cardiovascular Society (CCS) consensus on cardiac transplantation recommends all patients receive a statin after cardiac transplantation regardless of their baseline LDL [2]. Since OHT recipients are at significant risk of ACAD, it is reasonable to adopt the LDL targets currently recommended for high risk CAD patients [6]. The current recommended goal for high-risk patients is LDL < 2.0 mmol/L [17].

Non-statin lipid-lowering agents are not commonly used in OHT recipients due to interactions with calcineurin inhibitors (CNIs) and statins, or adverse effects [5] [6] [18]. Patients who are intolerant of statins or who do not reach target lipid levels may require the addition of a second agent such as ezetimibe [19] [20]. However, lower initial doses and close monitoring are needed due to reports of supra-therapeutic response to ezetimibe when taken with cyclosporine [21].

The adverse drug reactions associated with statins that generate the greatest apprehension among patients are myotoxicity (myopathy and myositis) and increased liver enzymes. However, many of the statin trials have failed to demonstrate severe adverse effects or showed reversible creatine kinase (CK) elevations, suggesting that statins are safe [9] [11] [14]-[16]. Statin safety trials concluded that since the incidence of severe complications is low, statins are safe in this population if closely monitored [22] [23].

Hypertension in OHT patients can occur within days of transplantation as a consequence of immunosuppressive therapy and the denervation of cardiac volume receptors [24] [25]. The CNIs increase endothelin-1, decrease nitric oxide (NO), and activate the renin-angiotensinaldosterone system (RAAS), resulting in vasoconstriction and elevation in blood pressure (BP) [25]. Additionally, due to the denervation of cardiac volume receptors, volume expansion from salt loading fails to suppress the RAAS, therefore producing hypertension [26].

Angiotensin-converting enzyme-inhibitors (ACE-Is) can blunt the effects of the neurohormonal systems that fail to respond to volume expansion and can enhance the activation of NO [27]. Calcium channel blockers (CCBs), particularly diltiazem, inhibit the vasoconstriction associated with cyclosporine by blocking the calcium channels [25]. The benefits of ACE-Is and CCBs may extend beyond their antihypertensive effects [25] [27]-[30].

Canadian guidelines for cardiac transplantation recommend that if an antihypertensive is required, diltiazem or an ACE-I should be considered first-line due to the potential benefits in reducing ACAD [2]. For OHT patients who have concurrent diabetes, it is appropriate to target a BP goal of <130/80 mmHg adopted from the Canadian Hypertension Education Program (CHEP) guidelines. For OHT patients without diabetes, the recommended BP goal of <140/90 mmHg from CHEP is endorsed [31]. Commonly reported adverse effects of ACE-Is in the studies included hypotension and increased serum creatinine [24]. Diltiazem has been reported to cause sinus bradycardia [29] and peripheral edema [24]. Concomitant use of diltiazem and cyclosporine may result in increased cyclosporine levels secondary to CYP 450 interactions; however, this is an exploitable drug interaction [29].

A survey of 59 American heart transplant centers revealed that statin therapy was included in the post-OHT protocol in 85% of centers [32]. Despite proportion of patients on statins and the low rate of adverse drug reactions, only 58.5% of adult cardiac transplant patients achieve an institutional LDL target of <2.6 mmol/L [32]. Since ACAD is a significant contributor to morbidity and mortality, it is essential to reduce the progression by treating modifiable risk factors, such as hyperlipidemia and hypertension.

The purpose of this study was to evaluate the management of hyperlipidemia and hypertension among OHT recipients followed in the outpatient cardiac transplant clinic at the University of Alberta. Characterizing the proportion of patients achieving LDL and BP targets and the current patterns of use of lipid-lowering and antihypertensive agents will assist in improving the medical management of heart transplant recipients.

The primary objective was to assess the proportion of OHT patients achieving both the LDL target of <2.0 mmol/L and BP targets of <140/90 mmHg or <130/80 mmHg for diabetics in an outpatient cardiac transplant clinic. Secondary objectives included the assessment of: 1) the proportion of patients achieving the LDL target of <2.0 mmol/L; 2) the proportion of patients currently achieving the BP targets of <130/80 mmHg for diabetics (patients taking anti-diabetic agents or with a fasting plasma glucose > 7 mmol/L) or <140/90 mmHg for all others; and 3) the current usage patterns and intolerance to lipid-lowering and antihypertensive agents among OHT recipients.

2. Methods

2.1. Design and Patient Population

This study was a cross-sectional, retrospective analysis of all post-OHT patients being actively followed and collaboratively managed in the outpatient cardiac transplant clinic at the University of Alberta. Patients were included if they had undergone OHT and were >18 years old. Patients who received OHT at the University of Alberta Hospital but were actively being followed in another transplant clinic were excluded from the analysis.

2.2. Data Collection

A standardized case report form was used to extract information from the patients' clinic charts. Information was collected between January to March 2009 from the charts by a single investigator and included: 1) demographic data; 2) most recent fasting lipid profile; 3) BP readings taken during the last three clinic visits; 4) description of statins, ACE-Is, and diltiazem therapies; 5) documented intolerances or adverse effects associated with statins, ACE-Is, and diltiazem. Elevated ALT and AST was defined as >3 times the upper limit of normal (ULN), myalgia as muscle ache or weakness without CK elevation, myositis as CK elevation of >3 times but <10 times the ULN, and rhabdomyolysis as muscle symptoms with CK elevation of >10 times the ULN. Elevated creatinine was defined as >30% increase from baseline and hyperkalemia was defined as >5.0 mmol/L.

2.3. Sample Size and Data Analysis

The sample size was based on the 209 post-OHT patients currently followed in the cardiac transplant clinic at the University of Alberta. Descriptive statistical analysis was performed using Microsoft Access and Excel. Documented intolerances associated with statins, ACE-Is, and diltiazem were described using the Naranjo algorithm [33]. The study was approved by the Health Research Ethics Board of the University of Alberta.

3. Results

3.1. Patient Characteristics

Between 1985 and January 2009, 613 patients received heart transplants at the University of Alberta. Of those, 404 patients were excluded from the study (deceased, combined heart and lung transplants, orpediatric transplant). From 209 eligible patients, 16 patients were excluded due to being either lost to follow-up or being routinely followed by another clinic. A total of 193 patients were included (**Figure 1**). Demographic characteristics of included patients are summarized in **Table 1**. The patient population consisted of 76.7% maleswith a mean age of 59.2 ± 13.0 years, who were a mean 8.2 ± 4.8 years post-OHT. ACAD was diagnosed by coronary angiography with or without myocardial scintigraphy in 43 (22.3%) patients.

3.2. Primary Objective

A total of 111 (57.5%) patients achieved both the LDL target of <2.0 mmol/L and the BP target of <140/90 mmHg (or <130/80 mmHg for diabetics).

3.3. Secondary Objectives

Of the 193 patients, 140 (72.5%) patients achieved the LDL target of <2.0 mmol/L. Patients who were prescribed a statin were more likely to reach this goal (**Table 1**). The mean LDL was 1.81 ± 0.55 mmol/L for the entire cohort, 1.78 ± 0.49 mmol/L for patients prescribed a statin and 2.43 ± 1.09 mmol/L for those who were not (**Table 1**). For patients who did not achieve the LDL target, the mean LDL was 2.43 ± 0.57 mmol/L.

The BP target of either <140/90 mmHg or <130/80 mmHg was achieved by 153 (79.3%) patients. The mean SBP of all patients was 124.2 ± 13.6 mmHg, and the DBP was 77.8 ± 8.2 mmHg (**Table 2**). These numbers did not differ greatly for patients who were or were not prescribed an ACE-I (or ARB) or diltiazem. For patients who did not achieve the <140/90 mmHg or the <130/80 mmHg target, their mean BP was 144.4 ± 11.3 mmHg (SBP) and 87.9 ± 11.4 mmHg (DBP) and 136.5 ± 11.9 mmHg (SBP) and 81.4 ± 5.2 mmHg (DBP) respectively.

Statins were prescribed in 183 (94.8%) patients with an atorvastatin-equivalent dose of 27.7 ± 23.8 mg once daily (**Table 2**). Atorvastatin (88.1%) was the most commonly prescribed statin, followed by pravastatin (3.1%) and simvastatin (2.6%) (**Table 2**). The next two commonly used lipid-lowering agents were ezetimibe (12.4%) and fish oil (2.1%). Of 193 patients, 81.9% were on one lipid-lowering agent and 14.0% were on two lipid-lowering agents.

For the use of antihypertensive agents, 88.1% of patients were on either or both an ACE-I (or ARB) and diltiazem. ACE-Is (or ARBs) were prescribed in 154 (79.8%) patients, diltiazem in 101 (52.3%) patients, and both in 85 (44.0%) patients. The rates of prescribing for additional classes of antihypertensive agents were low, except for thiazide diuretics (**Figure 2**). Of the 193 patients, 22.3% were on one antihypertensive agent, 32.1% were on two, 22.8% were on three, 10.9% were on four, and 2.1% were on five.

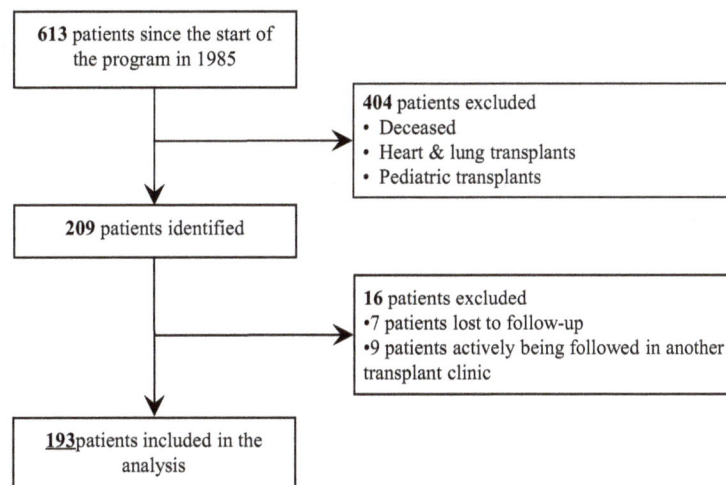

Figure 1. Flow diagram of patient selection.

Table 1. Patient demographics.

Characteristic	Patients				
	All (n = 193)	Prescribed statin (n = 183)	Not prescribed statin (n = 10)	Prescribed ACEI/ARB or CCB (n = 170)	Not prescribed ACEI/ARB or CCB (n = 23)
Age (y)					
Mean ± SD	59.2 ± 13	59.6 ± 12.6	52.7 ± 11.4	59.4 ± 12.4	57.8 ± 16.9
Range	19.8 - 88.9	19.8 - 88.9	21.7 - 72.8	22.4 - 88.9	19.8 - 75.6
Gender, male (%)	148 (76.7)	142 (77.6)	6 (60)	129 (75.9)	19 (82.6)
Height (cm)					
Mean ± SD	171.8 ± 9.0	171.8 ± 9.0	171.8 ± 9.8	172.0 ± 8.9	170.4 ± 9.3
Range	147.5 - 193	147.5 - 193	157 - 186	147.5 - 193	152 - 183
Weight (kg)					
Mean ± SD	84.2 ± 19	84.0 ± 18.5	87.4 ± 28	84.9 ± 19.4	78.3 ± 15.4
Range	31.4 - 151.6	48.2 - 151.6	31.4 - 131.8	31.4 - 151.6	48.8 - 113.2
Time since transplant (y)					
Mean ± SD	8.2 ± 4.8	8.2 ± 4.9	8.2 ± 2.2	8.2 ± 4.7	8.2 ± 5.3
Range	0.1 - 22.6	0.1 - 22.6	4.7 - 12.1	0.5 - 22.6	0.1 - 19.5
Indication for transplant, n (%)					
CAD	92 (50.3)	87 (47.5)	5 (50)	81 (47.6)	11 (47.8)
CM	75 (38.9)	71 (38.8)	4 (40)	67 (39.4)	8 (34.8)
Dilated CM	42 (21.8)	39 (21.3)	3 (30)	38 (22.4)	4 (17.4)
Idiopathic CM	23 (11.9)	23 (12.6)	0	20 (11.8)	3 (13)
Hypertrophic CM	5 (2.6)	5 (2.7)	0	4 (2.4)	1 (4.3)
ACAD-repeat OHT	7 (3.6)	7 (3.8)	0	6 (3.5)	1 (4.3)
Others	19 (9.8)	18 (9.8)	1 (10)	16 (9.4)	3 (13)
Immunosuppressive regimen, n (%)					
Cyclosporine	119 (61.7)	114 (62.3)	5 (50)	105 (61.8)	14 (60.9)
Tacrolimus	73 (37.8)	69 (37.7)	4 (40)	64 (37.6)	9 (39.1)
MMF	135 (69.9)	126 (68.9)	9 (90)	120 (70.6)	15 (65.2)
Azathioprine	27 (14)	27 (14.8)	0	24 (15.1)	3 (13.0)
Corticosteroid	40 (20.7)	36 (19.7)	4 (40)	32 (18.8)	8 (34.8)
Sirolimus	21 (10.9)	19 (9.8)	2 (20)	18 (10.6)	3 (13)
Everolimus	3 (1.6)	3 (1.6)	0	2 (1.3)	1 (4.3)
ACAD, n (%)	43 (22.3)	40 (21.9)	3 (30)	36 (21.2)	7 (30.4)
Lipid (mmol/L); mean ± SD					
TC	3.67 ± 0.77	3.63 ± 0.69	4.35 ± 1.57	-	-
TG	1.61 ± 1.04	1.63 ± 1.03	1.48 ± 1.27	-	
HDL-C	1.12 ± 0.39	1.11 ± 0.37	1.24 ± 0.62	-	-
LDL-C	1.81 ± 0.55	1.78 ± 0.49	2.43 ± 1.09	-	-
TC:HDL-C	3.53 ± 1.05	3.49 ± 1.00	4.05 ± 1.75	-	-
BP (mmHg)					
SBP[a]	124.2 ± 13.6	-	-	124.6 ± 13.9	121.7 ± 11.1
DBP[a]	77.8 ± 8.2	-	-	77.8 ± 8.1	77.9 ± 8.3

ACEI = angiotensin converting enzyme inhibitor, ARB = angiotensin receptor blocker, CAD = coronary artery disease, ACAD = allograft coronary artery disease, CCB = calcium channel blocker, CM = cardiomyopathy, DBP = diastolic blood pressure, HDL-C = high-density lipoprotein, LDL-C = low-density lipoprotein, MMF = mycophenolate mofetil, OHT = orthotopic heart transplant, SBP = systolic blood pressure, TC = total cholesterol, TG = triglyceride.

Table 2. Pattern of use of statins, ACE-inhibitors, and non-dihydropyridine calcium channel blockers.

Medications	No. of patients, n = 193 (%)	Strength[a] (mg)	Route	Directions
Statins				
Atorvastatin	170 (88.1)	28.9 ± 24.0	PO	QD (x167) & Q2D (x3)
Pravastatin	6 (3.1)	31.3 ± 28.9	PO	QD
Simvastatin	5 (2.6)	26.0 ± 13.4	PO	QD
Rosuvastatin	1 (0.5)	20	PO	QD
Lovastatin	1 (0.5)	5	PO	QD
Fluvastatin	0	-	-	-
None	10 (5.2)	-	-	-
Atorvastatin-equivalent[b]	183 (94.8)	27.7 ± 23.8	PO	QD (x180) & Q2D (x3)
ACE-inhibitors				
Quinapril	102 (52.8)	29.5 ± 15.3	PO	QD
Ramipril	16 (8.3)	7.1 ± 3.6	PO	QD (x15) & BID (x1)
Lisinopril	6 (3.1)	17.5 ± 8.8	PO	QD
Enalapril	3 (1.6)	7.5 ± 4.3	PO	QD (x2) & BID (x1)
Non-dihydropyridine CCB				
Diltiazem	101 (52.3)	218.3 ± 93.9	PO	QD

ACE = angiotensin converting enzyme, BID = twice daily, CCB = calcium channel blocker, PO = per os (by mouth), QD = once daily, Q2D = every two days. [a]Mean ± SD. [b]Atorvastatin 10 mg = rosuvastatin 5 mg = simvastatin 20 mg = pravastatin 40 mg = lovastatin 40 mg = fluvastatin 80 mg.

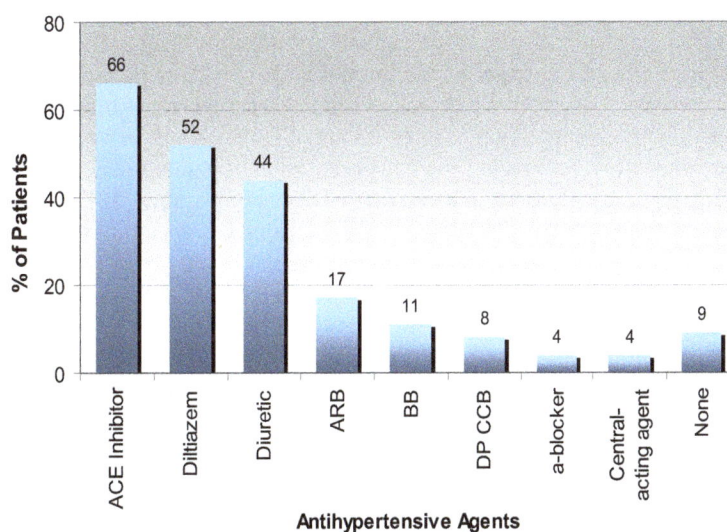

Figure 2. Proportion of patients taking antihypertensive agents by class.

Among the 183 patients prescribed a statin, a total of 27 (14.8%) patients had some statin-related intolerance, of which 20 (10.9%) had slightly elevated CK (<3 times the ULN) and 11 (6.0%) reported myalgia (**Table 3**). Of the 127 patients who were prescribed an ACE-I, 37 (29.1%) patients had ACE-I-related intolerance, of which 27 (21.3%) had minor elevations in serum creatinine and 7 (5.5%) had hyperkalemia. Of the 101 patients who were prescribed diltiazem, 11 (10.9%) patients had diltiazem-related intolerances, of which 8 (7.9%) had lower leg edema. Using the Naranjo algorithm, it was determined that none of the intolerances were classified as "definite" adverse drug reactions; rather, most were determined to be either "probable" or "possible" reactions.

4. Discussion

In our cardiac transplant clinic, 58% of OHT patients achieved both an LDL target of <2.0 mmol/L and a BP

Table 3. Reported drug-related intolerances.

Patient reported intolerances on therapy	N (%)
Statins (n = 183)	**27 (14.8)**
Elevated CK*	20 (10.9)
Myalgia	11 (6.0)
Elevated ALT	2 (1.1)
Hip pain	1 (0.5)
ACE-inhibitors (n = 127)	**37 (29.1)**
Elevated serum creatinine**	27 (21.3)
Hyperkalemia	7 (5.5)
Dry cough	3 (2.4)
Dizziness or lightheadedness	2 (1.6)
Diltiazem (n = 101)	**11 (10.9)**
Lower leg edema	8 (7.9)
Dizziness	1 (1.0)
Bradycardia	1 (1.0)
Stool incontinence	1 (1.0)

*All elevated CK levels were between 250 - 750 U/L. **Defined as >30% increase from baseline serum creatinine.

target of <140/90 mmHg (or <130/80 mmHg for patients with diabetes). When separately assessing the proportion of patients achieving the LDL target, 73% of patients achieved the target. This proportion is much higher than that reported for non-cardiac transplantation patients with cardiovascular disease in general practices (30.5 - 51.2%) [34] [35]. If the higher LDL target of <2.5 mmol/L was used, as previously recommended in the 2003 CCS guidelines, the proportion of patients who achieved this target increases to 93.8%. Remarkably, the proportion of patients achieving this higher target LDL (<2.5 mmol/L) has been very consistent (93.3%) since we first evaluated this in our patients > 5 years ago [36]. This proportion of patients successfully treated to target is 35% higher than previously been reported, when the target LDL is comparable [32]. Even for patients who did not achieve the aggressive LDL target of <2.0 mmol/L, their mean LDL was only slightly (mean of 0.43 mmol/L) above target. Similarly, the proportion of patients achieving the blood pressure goal (79%) is higher than that reported for the general population (57% - 58%) [35] [37]. For those who did not achieve the goal, their BP readings were only 1 - 6 mmHg above their target.

The successful attainment of these treatment goals may be due to the close patient monitoring and the collaborative interdisciplinary team approach operational in our outpatient cardiac transplant clinic. Consistent with the recommendations regarding dyslipidemia management, the majority of our patients were prescribed a statin (95%). While published data supports the efficacy of pravastatin and simvastatin [9]-[13], our results expand the evidence with atorvastatin, as it was the most commonly prescribed agent in the class. In combination with or in place of statins, ezetimibe was the most common agent. Since 82% of our patients were on a regimen with only one lipid-lowering agent, our results suggest that most patients can achieve the LDL target with monotherapy. Also, consistent with the CCS recommendation regarding hypertension management, 88% of our patients were managed with either one or both an ACE-I (or ARB) and diltiazem. Two or more antihypertensive agents were used in 78% of patients, demonstrating that multiple antihypertensive agents are often required for the management of hypertension in OHT recipients.

Previous studies have reported up to 20% of OHT recipients may suffer adverse effects of initial statin therapy; however, problems resolve with close monitoring and severe adverse events are rare [9] [11] [14]-[16] [22] [23]. Our data is consistent with these findings and demonstrates a similar low incidence of medication intolerance. Although 15% of patients had statin-related intolerances including minor CK or ALT elevations and myalgias, none were classified as definite, rather as possible or probable reactions. Furthermore, there were no documented cases of either myositis or rhabdomyolysis among patients on statin therapy. Only 7 patients had documented intolerances or contraindications that were severe enough to warrant discontinuation of statin therapy. Elevated serum creatinine was a common intolerance of ACE-Is; however, all of these were determined to be either possible or doubtful reactions. This can be explained by the fact that, independent of ACE-Is, renal insufficiency is often a co-morbidity among cardiac transplantation recipients caused by concurrent long-term therapy with CNIs. Similarly, immunosuppressant agents also promote fluid retention, and in combination with diltiazem, can lead to a worsening of lower extremity edema. Although the incidences of the intolerances may seem more common than the general population, they are not attributable to single agents. This reinforces the need for close follow-up monitoring in this patient population.

This study was a cross-sectional retrospective analysis; therefore, it has several limitations. Firstly, cholesterol and serum creatinine levels were collected from the most recent clinic follow-up laboratory results; therefore, trends or fluctuations were not captured or evaluated. Secondly, the BP readings were taken from clinic readings, and discrepancies may exist from home readings if patients had white coat syndrome. In attempt to control for this possible discrepancy, three BP readings from the last 3 clinic visits were used to calculate the average BP for each patient. Thirdly, we made no attempt to evaluate or ensure compliance to medications directly. However, compliance is routinely assessed at each follow-up clinic visit, and any evidence of non-adherence is documented. Fourthly, the appropriateness of a patient not being prescribed drug therapy was not evaluated. The avoidance of lipid-lowering or antihypertensive therapy may have been appropriate if there was an absolute contraindication. And finally, since this was a cross-sectional evaluation of the management of hyperlipidemia and hypertension, we cannot draw conclusions regarding how successful treatments to guideline targets have impacted clinical outcomes such as ACAD. Nevertheless, the rate of ACAD diagnosed in our study population (22.3%) appears to be significantly lower than reported in the literature (53% by 10-year), which may be the result of our high degree of success in modifying these risk factors.

5. Conclusion

It is possible to successfully achieve the guideline recommended LDL-cholesterol target of <2 mmol/L and the recommended BP target of <140/90 mmHg (or <130/80 mmHg for diabetic patients) in a significant proportion of OHT recipients. The high utilization rates of statins for dyslipidemia and ACE-Is (or ARBs) and diltiazem for hypertension were consistent with the CCS consensus recommendations for the prevention of ACAD. Despite concerns regarding the potential for pharmacokinetic drug interactions due to complex poly-pharmacy in OHT patients, the reported rates of any drug intolerance to the medications were low in our population.

References

[1]   (2012) E-Statistics Report on Organ Transplants, Waiting Lists and Donor Statistics, 2012 Summary Statistics. Ottawa (ON): Canadian Institute for Health Information.
http://www.cihi.ca/CIHI-ext-portal/pdf/internet/REPORT_STATS2012_PDF_EN

[2]   Ross, H., Hendry, P., Dipchand, A., Giannetti, N., Hirsch, G., Isaac, D., *et al.* (2003) Canadian Cardiovascular Society Consensus Conference on Cardiac Transplantation. *Canadian Journal of Cardiology*, **19**, 620-654.

[3]   Valantine, H. (2004) Cardiac Allograft Vasculopathy after Heart Transplantation: Risk Factors and Management. *Journal of Heart and Lung Transplantation*, **23**, S187-S193. http://dx.doi.org/10.1016/j.healun.2004.03.009

[4]   Taylor, D.O., Edwards, L.B., Aurora, P., Christie, J.D., Dobbels, F., Kirk, R., *et al.* (2008) Registry of the International Society for Heart and Lung Transplantation: Twenty-Fifth Official Adult Heart Transplant Report—2008. *Journal of Heart and Lung Transplantation*, **27**, 943-956. http://dx.doi.org/10.1016/j.healun.2008.06.017

[5]   Wenke, K. (2004) Management of Hyperlipidaemia Associated with Heart Transplantation. *Drugs*, **64**, 1053-1068. http://dx.doi.org/10.2165/00003495-200464100-00003

[6]   Bilchick, K.C., Henrikson, C.A., Skojec, D., Kasper, E.K. and Blumenthal, R.S. (2004) Treatment of Hyperlipidemia in Cardiac Transplant Recipients. *American Heart Journal*, **148**, 200-210.
http://dx.doi.org/10.1016/j.ahj.2004.03.050

[7]   Kobashigawa, J.A., Starling, R.C., Mehra, M.R., Kormos, R.L., Bhat, G., Barr, M.L., *et al.* (2006) Multicenter Retrospective Analysis of Cardiovascular Risk Factors Affecting Long-Term Outcome of *de Novo* Cardiac Transplant Recipients. *Journal of Heart and Lung Transplantation*, **25**, 1063-1069. http://dx.doi.org/10.1016/j.healun.2006.05.001

[8]   Mehra, M.R. and Raval, N.Y. (2004) Metaanalysis of Statins and Survival in *de Novo* Cardiac Transplantation. *Transplantation Proceedings*, **36**, 1539-1541. http://dx.doi.org/10.1016/j.transproceed.2004.05.036

[9]   Kobashigawa, J.A., Katznelson, S., Laks, H., Johnson, J.A., Yeatman, L., Wang, X.M., *et al.* (1995) Effect of Pravastatin on Outcomes after Cardiac Transplantation. *New England Journal of Medicine*, **333**, 621-627.
http://dx.doi.org/10.1056/NEJM199509073331003

[10] Kobashigawa, J.A., Moriguchi, J.D., Laks, H., Wener, L., Hage, A., Hamilton, M.A., *et al.* (2005) Ten-Year Follow-Up of a Randomized Trial of Pravastatin in Heart Transplant Patients. *Journal of Heart and Lung Transplantation*, **24**, 1736-1740. http://dx.doi.org/10.1016/j.healun.2005.02.009

[11] Wenke, K., Meiser, B., Thiery, J., Nagel, D., von Scheidt, W., Steinbeck, G., *et al.* (1997) Simvastatin Reduces Graft Vessel Disease and Mortality after Heart Transplantation: A Four-Year Randomized Trial. *Circulation*, **96**, 1398-1402. http://dx.doi.org/10.1161/01.CIR.96.5.1398

[12] Wenke, K., Meiser, B., Thiery, J., Nagel, D., von Scheidt, W., Krobot, K., *et al.* (2003) Simvastatin Initiated Early after Heart Transplantation: 8-Year Prospective Experience. *Circulation*, **107**, 93-97. http://dx.doi.org/10.1161/01.CIR.0000043241.32523.EE

[13] Wenke, K., Meiser, B., Thiery, J. and Reichart, B. (2005) Impact of Simvastatin Therapy after Heart Transplantation an 11-Year Prospective Evaluation. *Herz*, **30**, 431-432. http://dx.doi.org/10.1007/s00059-005-2685-6

[14] Patel, D.N., Pagani, F.D., Koelling, T.M., Dyke, D.B., Baliga, R.R., Cody, R.J., *et al.* (2002) Safety and Efficacy of Atorvastatin in Heart Transplant Recipients. *The Journal of Heart and Lung Transplantation*, **21**, 204-210. http://dx.doi.org/10.1016/S1053-2498(01)00369-2

[15] Samman, A., Imai, C., Straatman, L., Frolich, J., Humphries, K. and Ignaszewski, A. (2005) Safety and Efficacy of Rosuvastatin Therapy for the Prevention of Hyperlipidemia in Adult Cardiac Transplant Recipients. *The Journal of Heart and Lung Transplantation*, **24**, 1008-1013. http://dx.doi.org/10.1016/j.healun.2004.07.016

[16] O'Rourke, B., Barbir, M., Mitchell, A.G., Yacoub, M.H. and Banner, N.R. (2004) Efficacy and Safety of Fluvastatin Therapy for Hypercholesterolemia after Heart Transplantation: Results of a Randomised Double Blind Placebo Controlled Study. *International Journal of Cardiology*, **94**, 235-240. http://dx.doi.org/10.1016/j.ijcard.2003.04.009

[17] Genest, J., McPherson, R., Frohlich, J., Anderson, T., Campbell, N., Carpentier, A., *et al.* (2009) Canadian Cardiovascular Society/Canadian Guidelines for the Diagnosis and Treatment of Dyslipidemia and Prevention of Cardiovascular Disease in the Adult—2009 Recommendations. *Canadian Journal of Cardiology*, **25**, 567-579. http://dx.doi.org/10.1016/S0828-282X(09)70715-9

[18] Page II, R.L., Miller, G.G. and Lindenfeld, J. (2005) Drug Therapy in the Heart Transplant Recipient: Part IV: Drug-Drug Interactions. *Circulation*, **111**, 230-239. http://dx.doi.org/10.1161/01.CIR.0000151805.86933.35

[19] Patel, A.R., Ambrose, M.S., Duffy, G.A., Cote, H. and DeNofrio, D. (2007) Treatment of Hypercholesterolemia with Ezetimibe in Cardiac Transplant Recipients. *The Journal of Heart and Lung Transplantation*, **26**, 281-284. http://dx.doi.org/10.1016/j.healun.2007.01.008

[20] Shaw, S.M., Chaggar, P., Ritchie, J., Shah, M.K., Baynes, A.C., O'Neill, N., *et al.* (2009) The Efficacy and Tolerability of Ezetimibe in Cardiac Transplant Recipients Taking Cyclosporin. *Transplantation*, **87**, 771-775. http://dx.doi.org/10.1097/TP.0b013e318198d7d0

[21] Koshman, S.L., Lalonde, L.D., Burton, I., Tymchak, W.J. and Pearson, G.J. (2005) Supratherapeutic Response to Ezetimibe Administered with Cyclosporine. *Annals of Pharmacotherapy*, **39**, 1561-1565. http://dx.doi.org/10.1345/aph.1G015

[22] Marzoa-Rivas, R., Crespo-Leiro, M.G., Paniagua-Marin, M.J., Llinares-Garcia, D., Muniz-Garcia, J., Aldama-Lopez, G., *et al.* (2005) Safety of Statins When Response Is Carefully Monitored: A Study of 336 Heart Recipients. *Transplantation Proceedings*, **37**, 4071-4073. http://dx.doi.org/10.1016/j.transproceed.2005.09.163

[23] Grigioni, F., Carigi, S., Potena, L., Fabbri, F., Russo, A., Musuraca, A.C., *et al.* (2006) Long-Term Safety and Effectiveness of Statins for Heart Transplant Recipients in Routine Clinical Practice. *Transplantation Proceedings*, **38**, 1507-1510. http://dx.doi.org/10.1016/j.transproceed.2006.02.071

[24] Brozena, S.C., Johnson, M.R., Ventura, H., Hobbs, R., Miller, L., Olivari, M.T., *et al.* (1996) Effectiveness and Safety of Diltiazem or Lisinopril in Treatment of Hypertension after Heart Transplantation. Results of a Prospective Randomized Multicenter Trail. *Journal of the American College of Cardiology*, **27**, 1707-1712. http://dx.doi.org/10.1016/0735-1097(96)00057-5

[25] Rockx, M.A. and Haddad, H. (2007) Use of Calcium Channel Blockers and Angiotensin-Converting Enzyme Inhibitors after Cardiac Transplantation. *Current Opinion in Cardiology*, **22**, 128-132. http://dx.doi.org/10.1097/hco.0b013e3280210681

[26] Eisen, H.J. (2003) Hypertension in Heart Transplant Recipients: More than Just Cyclosporine. *Journal of the American College of Cardiology*, **41**, 433-434. http://dx.doi.org/10.1016/S0735-1097(02)02821-8

[27] Erinc, K., Yamani, M.H., Starling, R.C., Crowe, T., Hobbs, R., Bott-Silverman, C., *et al.* (2005) The Effect of Combined Angiotensin-Converting Enzyme Inhibition and Calcium Antagonism on Allograft Coronary Vasculopathy Validated by Intravascular Ultrasound. *The Journal of Heart and Lung Transplantation*, **24**, 1033-1038. http://dx.doi.org/10.1016/j.healun.2004.06.005

[28] Mehra, M.R., Ventura, H.O., Smart, F.W., Collins, T.J., Ramee, S.R. and Stapleton, D.D. (1995) An Intravascular Ul-

trasound Study of the Influence of Angiotensin-Converting Enzyme Inhibitors and Calcium Entry Blockers on the Development of Cardiac Allograft Vasculopathy. *American Journal of Cardiology*, **75**, 853-854. http://dx.doi.org/10.1016/S0002-9149(99)80432-9

[29] Schroeder, J.S., Gao, S.Z., Alderman, E.L., Hunt, S.A., Johnstone, I., Boothroyd, D.B., *et al.* (1993) A Preliminary Study of Diltiazem in the Prevention of Coronary Artery Disease in Heart-Transplant Recipients. *The New England Journal of Medicine*, **328**, 164-170. http://dx.doi.org/10.1056/NEJM199301213280303

[30] Leenen, F.H., Coletta, E. and Davies, R.A. (2007) Prevention of Renal Dysfunction and Hypertension by Amlodipine after Heart Transplant. *American Journal of Cardiology*, **100**, 531-535. http://dx.doi.org/10.1016/j.amjcard.2007.03.058

[31] Khan, N.A., Hemmelgarn, B., Herman, R.J., Rabkin, S.W., McAlister, F.A., Bell, C.M., *et al.* (2008) The 2008 Canadian Hypertension Education Program Recommendations for the Management of Hypertension: Part 2—Therapy. *Canadian Journal of Cardiology*, **24**, 465-475. http://dx.doi.org/10.1016/S0828-282X(08)70620-2

[32] de Denus, S., Al-Jazairi, A., Loh, E., Jessup, M., Stanek, E.J. and Spinler, S.A. (2004) Dyslipidemias and HMG-CoA Reductase Inhibitor Prescription in Heart Transplant Recipients. *Annals of Pharmacotherapy*, **38**, 1136-1141. http://dx.doi.org/10.1345/aph.1D535

[33] Naranjo, C.A., Busto, U., Sellers, E.M., Sandor, P., Ruiz, I., Roberts, E.A., *et al.* (1981) A Method for Estimating the Probability of Adverse Drug Reactions. *Clinical Pharmacology & Therapeutics*, **30**, 239-245. http://dx.doi.org/10.1038/clpt.1981.154

[34] Yan, A.T., Yan, R.T., Tan, M., Hackam, D.G., Leblanc, K.L., Kertland, H., *et al.* (2006) Contemporary Management of Dyslipidemia in High-Risk Patients: Targets Still Not Met. *American Journal of Medicine*, **119**, 676-683. http://dx.doi.org/10.1016/j.amjmed.2005.11.015

[35] Saposnik, G., Goodman, S.G., Leiter, L.A., Yan, R.T., Fitchett, D.H., Bayer, N.H., *et al.* (2009) Applying the Evidence: Do Patients with Stroke, Coronary Artery Disease, or both Achieve Similar Treatment Goals? *Stroke*, **40**, 1417-1424. http://dx.doi.org/10.1161/STROKEAHA.108.533018

[36] Pearson, G.J., Stewart, G.G., Burton, I., Chorney, S.G., Tymchak, W.J., Lalonde, L.D. and Burton, J.R. (2004) Successful Treatment to Guideline Recommended LDL Cholesterol Targets in Heart Transplant Recipients. *Canadian Journal of Cardiology*, **21**, 241C.

[37] Farahani, P. and Levine, M. (2009) Goal Attainment for Multiple Cardiovascular Risk Factors in Community-Based Clinical Practice (a Canadian Experience). *Journal of Evaluation in Clinical Practice*, **15**, 212-216. http://dx.doi.org/10.1111/j.1365-2753.2008.01002.x

22

Haemolytic Anaemia Following High Dose Intravenous Immunoglobulin Treatment for Epidermolysis Bullosa Acquisita

Sarah Madeline Brown*, Philip Jeremy Hampton

Department of Dermatology, The Newcastle upon Tyne Hospitals NHS Foundation Trust, Royal Victoria Infirmary, Newcastle, UK

Email: *sarahmadelinebrown@nhs.net

Abstract

Background: Epidermolysis bullosa aquisita (EBA) is a severe acquired blistering skin disease that is often resistant to prednisolone but can respond well to intravenous immunoglobulin infusion (IVIg). Main Observations: We describe the case of a 35 years old male patient with EBA who developed clinically significant haemolytic anaemia with a drop in Hb from 15.3 g/dL to a nadir of 8.4 g/dL within 5 days post IVIg infusion. The patient was blood group A and the IVIg batch was found to have a high titre of anti-A immunoglobulin. Conclusions: IVIg is an effective treatment for EBA. Haemolysis associated with IVIg has not previously been reported in the dermatology literature but review of data from other specialties shows that the problem is well recognised. Dermatologists using IVIg should be aware of this potential complication and patients should be consented appropriately and warned about this potential side effect.

Keywords

Haemolytic Anaemia, Haemolysis, Intravenous Immunoglobulin, Epidermolysis Bullosa Aquisita, EBA

1. Introduction

Epidermolysis bullosa acquisita (EBA) is a rare immunobullous disorder characterised by autoantibodies against collagen VII and the development of blisters which heal with scarring [1]. Treatment can be challenging and standard immunosuppressive regimes combining prednisolone plus azathioprine or mycophenolate mofetil are

---

*Corresponding author.

not always effective. Intravenous immunoglobulin (IVIg) is used as a third line agent in the management of EBA. We describe a case of a 35 years old male, blood group A patient with epidermolysis bullosa acquisita (EBA) who developed haemolytic anaemia following the administration of high dose intravenous immunoglobulin (IVIg).

2. Case Report

A 35 years old male presented with a 1 year history of a blistering eruption. He was otherwise well apart from a past history of vitiligo and at presentation was taking no medication. The distribution of blisters was highly variable with blisters developing at the oral mucosa, forehead, arms, hands and the genitals. Scarring had developed at the wrists (**Figure 1**). Indirect immunofluorescence on salt split skin showed linear IgG at the floor of the blister. A collagen VII ELISA was positive at a titre of 37 arbitrary units (upper limit of normal, 6 arbitrary units). This confirmed the diagnosis of epidermolysis bullosa acquisita (EBA).

Initial treatment over 2 years included immunosuppression with prednisolone plus azathioprine (150 mg daily), terminated following elevated ALT. He then received prednisolone plus mycophenolate mofetil (2 g per day). Over this 2-year period his cumulative prednisolone dose was 8810 mg with a mean dose of 12.5 mg/day. There were some short periods of disease remission but the blistering recurred, despite periods on higher doses of prednisolone. To regain disease control and to limit the cumulative dose of oral prednisolone, IVIg was selected as the next treatment. The first course of treatment was of IVIg, (Octagam) at a dose of 160 g over 4 days (500 mg/kg/day). There were no problems and the rate of new blisters decreased along with healing of eroded areas. Two months later a further infusion was planned. Due to a lack of availability of Octogam the next course of treatment was with a different brand of IVIg. The patient received 160 g of 10% IVIg (Privigen) in divided doses by slow IV infusion over 4 days (500 mg/kg per day). Two days following Privigen infusion he presented with symptoms of anaemia; with shortness of breath, clinically jaundiced and with skin mottling. On investigation his haemoglobin was found to have dropped from a baseline of 15.3 g/dL to a nadir of 8.4 g/dL within 5 days post IVIg infusion (**Figure 2**). Other biochemical markers of haemolysis included a raised bilirubin, raised LDH and a positive direct antiglobulin test. A blood film showed features consistent with haemolysis with spherocytes, polychromasia and a reticulocytosis.

A two unit blood transfusion was required. The episode of haemolysis was investigated by blood transfusion services and the Privigen bottle transfused was found to have a high titre of anti-A antibodies. Our patient was blood group A positive. The patient recovered quickly from the haemolysis and went on to receive further IVIg infusions with no evidence of haemolysis. Pre-infusion IVIg titres of anti-A1 IgG were checked in subsequent transfusions and given only when present at less than 1/64 dilution. The EBA blisters responded reasonably well

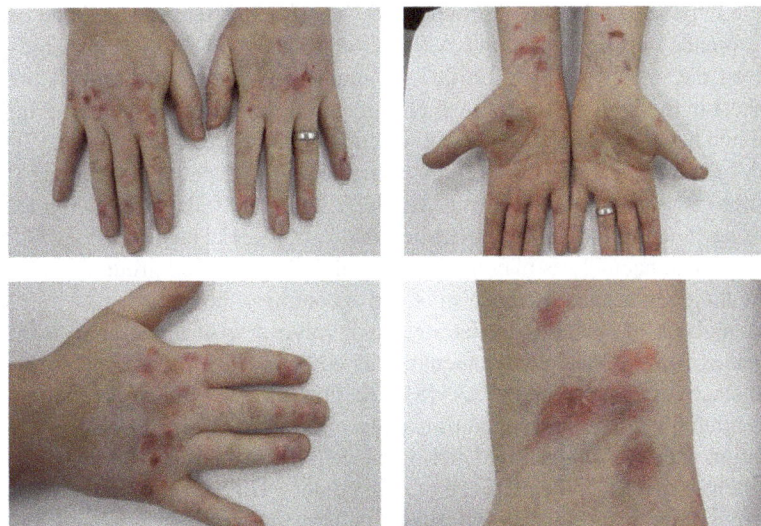

Figure 1. Clinical appearances of EBA blistering at the wrists and hands. Scarring has developed in some areas following sub basement membrane blistering secondary to anti-collagen VII antibody mediated inflammation.

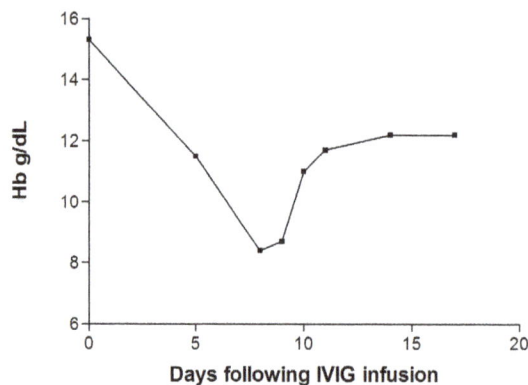

Figure 2. Levels of haemoglobin following IVIg. The haemoglobin concentration fell from 15.3 g/dL to 8.4 g/dL over 8 days.

to IVIg and the disease went into remission with maintenance treatment of mycophenolate mofetil 500 mg BD, dapsone 50 mg OD and prednisolone 5 mg OD. More recently, following a further relapse, the patient has received two infusions of rituximab 1000 mg with a 14-day interval with good benefit and is well controlled with 7.5 mg prednisolone only.

3. Discussion

Although there are no randomised controlled trials of IVIg in EBA, numerous case series and reports have demonstrated good results [2] [3]. The incidence of clinically significant haemolytic anaemia post IVIg is relatively rare [4]. This is the first reported case involving IVIg induced haemolysis when treating an immunobullous disease despite relatively widespread use of IVIg in the treatment of EBA and pemphigus. IVIg is prepared by collecting pooled immunoglobulin from blood donors and therefore the composition of different batches of IVIg does have some variation. The titres of anti-A and anti-B blood group antigens varies between different batches of IVIg. The problem has been more widely reported in the haematology literature and also in relation to patients with neurological diseases such as Guillain-Barré syndrome, multifocal motor neuropathy, chronic inflammatory demyelinating polyneuropathy, and dermatomyositis [5] [6]. The risk of haemolysis is greater in those patients receiving high dose IVIg (doses greater than or equal to 2 g/kg [7]). The risk of haemolysis is also greater when the recipient has a non-O blood type with one review finding that 81% cases of post IVIg haemolysis were found in patients with blood group-A [7]. Another risk factor which can predispose to haemolysis is the use of IVIg brands with high titre anti-A/B IgG antibodies [7]. In one case study all identified cases of haemolysis involved the use of the IVIg products Gamunex, Gammagard liquid or Privigen [7]. The risk of haemolysis is highest in the high A/B titre isosmolar preparations, however the lower titre preparations are usually hyperosmotic and have a greater risk of causing acute renal failure or thrombosis [7]. One case series identified 16 cases of IVIg induced haemolysis out of approximately 1000 patients receiving IVIg over a 2.5-year period. It was identified that haemolysis occurred within 12 hours to 10 days following IVIg administration, with the lowest level of haemoglobin identified between 1 day and 2 weeks post infusion [8]. Mild cases of clinically insignificant IVIg induced haemolysis may occur relatively often in blood group A and B patients. Post infusion full blood count in clinically healthy patients is not carried out in all hospitals.

IVIg-related haemolysis has been demonstrated to involve anti-A and anti-B haemagglutinin in the IVIg preparations as well as both IgG and complement mediated hemolysis. It has been proposed that the haemolysis takes place in two stages or as a two hit process [8]. The first hit is felt to be related to passive transfer of anti-A and anti-B haemagglutinin. These haemagglutinins cause red cell aggregation. The second hit is related to the increased degradation and loss of sensitised red blood cells in an individual with an underlying inflammatory state due to erythrophagocytosis in the presence of complement. High dose IVIg fixes complement onto red cells resulting in haemolysis and also binds to red bloods cells which are then removed by the spleen [7] [9]. The current European Pharmacopoeia have suggested guidelines such that the titre of anti-A and anti-B haemagglutinins should not be detected at the 1:64 dilution, however there are reports in literature of haemolysis occurring regardless of these limits [7] [9].

4. Conclusion

EBA can be a difficult disease to control and IVIg is a useful treatment option. We report the first described case of clinically significant IVIg induced haemolysis in a patient with EBA. Dermatologists need to be aware of the possibility of haemolysis and vigilance is important as patients can become symptomatic requiring prompt assessment and monitoring. A rational approach to monitoring for post IVIg haemolytic anaemia would be to monitor full blood count and bilirubin 24 to 48 hours post infusion and again 1 week later. Patients must be fully informed and consented regarding this potential complication. In order to reduce the risk of occurrence of IVIg associated haemolysis, pre-infusion isohaemagglutinin titres can be measured and given only when present at less than 1/64 dilution (European Pharmacopeia Recommendation). Alternatively a direct antiglobulin test between IVIg product and recipients blood could be performed [7]. These are especially relevant in patients with non-O blood groups. Since most patients receive IVIg without complication the need for these extra tests as part of routine management would need to be discussed with the patient. In many cases blood monitoring will be adequate.

Conflict of Interest

None of the authors have any conflicts of interest to declare.

References

[1] Kim, J.H., Kim, Y.H., *et al.* (2013) Serum Levels of Anti-Type VII Collagen Antibodies Detected by Enzyme-Linked Immunosorbent Assay in Patients with Epidermolysis Bullosa Acquista Are Correlated with the Severity of Skin Lesions. *Journal of the European Academy of Dermatology and Venereology*, **27**, e224-e230. http://dx.doi.org/10.1111/j.1468-3083.2012.04617.x

[2] Intong, L.R. and Murrell, D.F. (2011) Management of Epidermolysis Bullosa Acquista. *Dermatologic Clinics*, **29**, 643-647. http://dx.doi.org/10.1016/j.det.2011.06.020

[3] Czernik, A., Toosi, S., *et al.* (2012) Intravenous Immunoglobulin in the Treatment of Autoimmune Bullous Dermatoses: An Update. *Autoimmunity*, **45**, 111-118. http://dx.doi.org/10.3109/08916934.2011.606452

[4] Berard, R., Whittemore, B., *et al.* (2012) Hemolytic Anaemia Following Intravenous Immunoglobulin Therapy in Patients Treated for Kawasaki Disease: A Report of 4 Cases. *Pediatric Rheumatology Online Journal*, **10**, 10. http://dx.doi.org/10.1186/1546-0096-10-10

[5] Hughes, R.A., Dalakas, M.C., *et al.* (2009) Clinical Applications of Intravenous Immunoglobulins in Neurology. *Clinical & Experimental Immunology*, **158**, 34-42. http://dx.doi.org/10.1111/j.1365-2249.2009.04025.x

[6] Markvardsen, L.H., Christiansen, I., *et al.* (2014) Hemolytic Anaemia Following High Dose Intravenous Immunoglobulin in Patients with Chronic Neurological Disorders. *European Journal of Neurology*, **21**, 147-152. http://dx.doi.org/10.1111/ene.12287

[7] Kahwaji, J., Barker, E., *et al.* (2009) Acute Hemolysis after High-Dose Intravenous Immunoglobulin Therapy in Highly HLA Sensitized Patients. *Clinical Journal of the American Society of Nephrology*, **4**, 1993-1997. http://dx.doi.org/10.2215/CJN.04540709

[8] Daw, Z., Padmore, R., *et al.* (2008) Hemolytic Transfusion Reactions after Administration of Intravenous Immune (Gamma) Globulin: A Case Series Analysis. *Transfusion*, **48**, 1598-1601. http://dx.doi.org/10.1111/j.1537-2995.2008.01721.x

[9] Padmore, R.F. (2012) Hemolysis upon Intravenous Immunoglobulin Transfusion. *Transfusion and Apheresis Science*, **46**, 93-96. http://dx.doi.org/10.1016/j.transci.2011.11.004

23

Clinical Medication Review and Falls in Older People—What Is the Evidence Base?

N. Tanna[1,2], T. Tatla[1], T. Winn[1], S. Chita[1], K. Ramdoo[1], C. Batten[1], J. Pitkin[1,2]

[1]London North West Healthcare NHS Trust, London, UK
[2]School of Science & Medicine, Imperial College, London, UK
Email: nuttantanna@nhs.net

Abstract

Background: This paper reports findings from a literature review undertaken to assess the current evidence base for clinical medication review and falls in older people. This forms part of a larger, organisational supported project design work-stream, where the objectives are to define the operational details for clinical medication review as part of multi-factorial assessment for elderly fallers in the community. Patients will be identified and targeted through an integrated care pathway mapping and elderly patient care screening service. Objective: A review of national and best practice guidance to help our understanding of how clinical medication review could be optimised. Methods: A PubMed database search was undertaken with search terms including "elderly" and "falls" and "medicines" followed by study of relevant publications in English and including cited referenced publications within selected papers. Results: Our findings were that both medication over-use and under-use in the elderly occur frequently and can be harmful. Many drugs commonly used by older persons have not been systematically studied as risk factors for falls. The screening tool of older people's prescriptions (STOPP) and screening tool to alert to right treatment (START), validated for assessment of potentially inappropriate prescribing in the elderly, offer the possibility of provision of a structured clinical medication review to patients, with a need for more research on the impact of the STOPP START interventions on both the rates of falls and risk of falls in the elderly.

Keywords

Clinical Medication Review, Falls, Elderly, Medicines, Multi-Factorial Interventions

1. Introduction

Falls are a common, costly and preventable consequence of ageing [1] [2]. Older people are susceptible to falling due to an age-related decline in the sensory and neuromuscular systems that contribute to postural stability. A fall occurs when the physical ability of the individual is unable to match the immediate demands of the environment and/or of the activity being undertaken and is defined as an event which results in a person coming to rest inadvertently on the ground or floor or other lower levels [2]. Around 30% of people aged 65 and over living in the community and more than 50% of those living in residential care facilities or nursing homes fall every year, and about half of those who fall do so repeatedly [2]-[6].

Factors increasing an older person's risk of falling include advanced age, reduced leg strength, balance deficits, history of falling, culprit medication use, and visual and cognitive impairment [5]. Lin and Ferrucci [7] have also noted that people with hearing loss and balance problems experience problems with walking and mobility. Sensory impairment and age related hearing loss (presbyacusis) may add to the number of falls sustained [8] [9]. In addition, symptoms of hearing loss and dementia maybe confused, with a combination likely to increase the number and severity of symptoms experienced by patients [10].

In 2012 the World Health Organisation reported *"falls"* as the second leading cause of accidental or unintentional injury deaths worldwide [2]. Injuries received from unintentional falls result in death, disability, nursing-home admission and direct medical costs [4]. Although certain interventions can reduce falls (e.g., exercising regularly or having medicines reviewed to reduce side effects and interactions), implementation at the community level remains limited and additional measures are needed to promote widespread adoption [4] [11] [12]. Recent guidance to support the care of older people living with frailty in the community or outpatient settings [13] stated that *"falls"* and *"susceptibility to side effects of medicines"* are two presentations that should raise suspicion that an individual has frailty that may mask more serious underlying disease.

2. Objectives

The objectives for this paper are to assess what the current evidence base is to support a clinical medication review service to reduce falls risk and falls related injuries in older people in the community setting. The evidence base will be utilised in the next phase of this work-stream to help define the operational details for providing a clinical medication review service to elderly fallers as part of an integrated care pathway mapping and multi-disciplinary elderly patient care screening service. The pathway will also include assessment for early cognitive impairment, hearing loss, vision and balance as part of a Falls Care Bundle implementation approach [14] to ensure a high standard of quality health care delivery.

Background: Optimising Clinical Medication Review

Care facilities and hospitals setting: A recent Cochrane Database review [6] assessed the effectiveness of interventions designed to reduce falls by older people in care facilities and hospitals. 43 randomised controlled trials with 30,373 participants in care facilities were included in this systematic review with the authors noting that despite the large number of trials there was limited evidence to support any one intervention. Rate of falls were calculated as falls per person year with risk of falling classified as the number of people falling (fallers) in each group.

Results from 13 trials testing exercise interventions in care facilities were inconsistent; exercise programmes seem to increase falls in frail residents in nursing homes, but reduce falls in people in intermediate care facilities. For multi-factorial interventions in care facilities, both the rate of falls and risk of falls showed a trend towards possible benefit. Multi-factorial interventions [15] usually include medication review, but current published literature does not define a process for a structured clinical medication review. The British Geriatric Society in their recent guidance [13] recommend that evidence based medication reviews should be conducted for older people with frailty, and cite the use of STOPP START criteria [6] [17] as an example.

Considering trials for specific medicines, Cameron *et al.* [6] noted that Vitamin D supplementation was effective in reducing the rate of falls, but not the risk of falling. Bjelakovic *et al.* [18] have reported findings from their updated Cochrane Database review where the objective was to assess the beneficial and harmful effects of Vitamin D supplementation for prevention of mortality in healthy adults and adults in a stable phase of disease. Including 56 trials with 95,286 participants providing usable data on mortality, the authors noted that Vitamin D3 may decrease mortality in elderly people living independently or in institutionalised care, but there was a need for further evidence from placebo controlled randomised trials in this area.

Community setting: Community dwelling older individuals are a large group identified as at high risk of future falls and injuries [1]. Many are subsequently admitted into intermediate care facilities.

Gillespie *et al.* [19] reviewed the interventions for preventing falls in older people living in the community, with this review including 159 trials with 79,193 participants. The most common interventions tested were exercise as a single intervention (59 trials) and multi-factorial programmes (40 trials). Kannus *et al.* [3] suggest that a multi-factorial intervention for elderly people is more effective than its single intervention counterpart since "*causes and risk factors of falling are usually multiple with striking intra-individual (fall to fall) and inter-individual variation*". The Cochrane review [19] found that multi-factorial interventions which included individualised risk assessment reduced rate of falls but not risk of falling. Trials looking at medication review did not demonstrate benefit but a prescribing modification programme also involving primary care physicians and their patients significantly reduced risk of falling. The Cochrane review [19] also found that gradual withdrawal of psychotropic medication reduced rate of falls but not risk of falling.

3. Methods

A PubMed database literature review was undertaken. Search strategy terms used were "elderly" and "falls" and "medicines", with the search undertaken in and to July 2014, with selection criteria including review of all abstracts (NT), followed by review of selected publications in English and any relevant cited references within selected publications, critiqued by three members of the research group (TT, JP and CB). Including the search term "older" in the search strategy did not elicit any further publications of relevance.

4. Results with Discussion

An observational study in older men living in the community [20] found that a self-reported history of falls in the previous 12 months was independently associated with number of medicines taken (odds ratio [OR] = 1.06, 95% confidence interval [CI] 1.02, 1.09) and use of one or more potentially inappropriate medicines (PIMs) (OR = 1.23, 95% CI 1.04, 1.45). Use of one or more PIMs had a correlation with hospital admission (hazard ration [HR] = 1.16, 95% CI 1.08, 1.24), whilst potential under-utilization was associated with cardiovascular events (HR = 1.20, 95% CI 1.03, 1.40), with the authors concluding that both medication over-use and under-use occur frequently among older men and may be harmful.

Gnjidic *et al.* [21] studied the optimal discriminating number of concomitant medications that were associated with geriatric syndromes, functional outcomes, and mortality in their study population of community-dwelling older men. They validated this as the use of five or more medications, accepted as the current definition of polypharmacy, and found this to be helpful in estimating the medication-related adverse effects for frailty, disability, mortality, and falls.

The aims for a 2007 critical systematic review [22] were to include all original articles examining medication use as a risk factor for falls or fall-related fractures in people aged 60 years or older with findings reported after the research group had assessed 28 observational studies and one randomized controlled trial. The number of participants in the trials ranged from 70 to 132,873. The outcome measure was a fall in 22 studies and a fracture in 7 studies. The authors found that the main group of drugs associated with an increased risk of falling were psychotropics, including benzodiazepines, antidepressants, and antipsychotics (**Table 1**). Antiepileptics and drugs that lower blood pressure were weakly associated with falls. However limitations included a need for improvement in the quality of observational studies, as many did not have a clear definition of a fall or target medicines, or prospective follow-up. The researchers concluded that many drugs commonly used by older persons are not systematically studied as risk factors for falls.

A recent Australian study [23] undertook a retrospective analysis of the management of pain control and reported that over 90% of residents in aged care facilities (ACF) were prescribed analgesics. Of those, 2057 residents were taking regular opioids (28.1%). Only 50% of those taking regular opioids received regular paracetamol at doses of 3 - 4 g/day. The concurrent use of sedatives was high, with 48.4% of those taking regular opioids also taking an anxiolytic/hypnotic. With the risk of falls and fractures increased by concurrent use of opioids and sedatives, the widespread use of these drugs in a population already at high risk was concerning. The researchers commented on the need to optimise the prescribing and administration of regular paracetamol as a first line and continuing therapy for pain management in ACF residents, to potentially improve pain management and reduce opioid requirements.

Nishtala *et al.* [24] reported findings from a large multi-database study that assessed the impact of polypharmacy

Table 1. Medicines optimisation.

- Psychotropics and cardiovascular drugs associated with increased risk of falling.
  - o Risk of falls and fractures increases with concurrent use of opioids and sedatives.
  - o Poly-pharmacy and cumulative exposure to anticholinergic and sedative medicines associated with fall related hospitalizations.
- Need to optimise prescribing and administration of regular Paracetamol as first line and continuing therapy for pain management.
- Recent changes in psychotropic and cardiovascular medications associated with substantial increase in risk of hospital admission for falls and fractures.
- Use of psychotropic medication in females associated with increased risk of falls and fractures, and body mass index (BMI) is a confounding variable.

and exposure to Drug Burden Index (DBI) medicines, with exposure defined by the researchers as quantification of each individual's cumulative exposure to anticholinergic and sedative medicines. Both criteria were independently associated with fall-related hospitalisations, frequency of GP visits, and risk of mortality. DBI drugs were associated with fall-related hospitalisations with an incidence rate ratio (IRR) of 1.56 (95% CI = 1.47 - 1.65) and greater number of GP visits (IRR 1.13, 95% CI = 1.12 - 1.13).

Another study [25] evaluated the prevalence of adverse drug events in an acute geriatric setting over a 6 month period and reported a rate of 12.7% (n = 313; mean age 84.8). Cardiovascular (39%), psychotropic (36.6%) and opiate (7.3%) medicines were the most frequently involved. The adverse events that occurred most frequently were bleeding (28.6%), falls (14.3%), and sleepiness (9.5%), with the authors noting that these could have been "*prevented*" in 31% of cases. Preventability by the research group was determined by assessment of inadequacy with standards of care, medication-related factors (excluding contra-indication) and use of standard lists of harmful medication in the elderly.

A French retrospective case control study [26] reported that 50% of falls occurred in patients in their first week after hospital admission, with these classified as severe in 16% cases. The characteristics of the two groups under study (patients who fell and those who did not) were similar: there were no significant differences in variables such as age, sex, number of medicines or prevalence of hypertension or Parkinson's disease. Probability of falls increased when the patients used zolpidem (adjusted odds ratio [AOR] 2.59; 95% CI 1.16, 5.81; p = 0.02), meprobamate (AOR 3.01; 95% CI 1.36, 6.64; p = 0.01) or calcium channel antagonists (AOR 2.45; 95% CI 1.16, 4.74; p = 0.02).

Payne *et al.* reported data from a larger Scottish retrospective case-cohort study [27] which included over 39,000 patients aged over 65 years. They found that the period with recent changes in psychotropic and cardiovascular medications was associated with a substantial increase in risk of hospital admission for falls and fractures; with an odds ratio of 1.54 (95% CI 1.17 - 2.03) and 1.68 (95% CI 1.28 - 2.22) respectively (**Table 1**). These findings are in line with work reported by Beer *et al.* [20] with correlation both for falls risk and hospital admission with use of potentially inappropriate medicines. Notably Payne *et al.* (27) found evidence (p = 0.003) for variation in the association between change in different psychotropic medications and admission, with the strongest associations for changes with selective serotonin reuptake inhibitor (SSRI) antidepressants (OR 1.99 [95% CI 1.29 - 3.08]), non-SSRI/tricyclic antidepressants (OR 4.39 [95% CI 2.21 - 8.71]) and combination psychotropic medication (OR 3.05 [95% CI 1.66 - 5.63]).

The Australian Longitudinal Study of Ageing [28] specifically looked at the risk of falls with use of psychotropic medicines. Interestingly, use was associated with increased risk of falls in females (IRR = 1.47, 95% CI = 1.31 - 1.64) but not in males (IRR = 1.03, 95% CI = 0.85 - 1.26). Use of psychotropic medications was also associated with an increased risk of a fracture in females (relative risk [RR] 2.54; CI 1.57 - 4.11; p < 0.0001) but not in males (RR = 0.66; p = 0.584; CI 0.15 - 2.86). In both analyses, body mass index (BMI) was found to be the only confounding variable. After adjusting for BMI, the IRR in females decreased to 1.22 (95% CI 1.02 - 1.45; p < 0.015) for falls and the RR decreased to 1.92 (p < 0.015, CI 1.13 - 3.24) for fractures.

Gallagher *et al.* [16] have validated a comprehensive screening tool that enables the prescribing physician to assess an older patient's prescription drugs in the context of his/her concurrent diagnoses. Inter-rater reliability is favourable [17] with a kappa-coefficient of 0.75 for STOPP and 0.68 for START (**Table 2**).

STOPP (Screening Tool of Older Person's Prescriptions) encompasses 65 clinically significant criteria for potentially inappropriate prescribing in older people. Each criterion is linked with a concise explanation as to why the prescribing practice is potentially inappropriate. START (Screening Tool to Alert doctors to Right

Table 2. STOPP START tool criteria.

- The Screening Tool of Older Persons' potentially inappropriate prescriptions (STOPP) classifies 65 common drug issues that contribute to inappropriate prescribing in the elderly.
- International studies using STOPP criteria indicate high potentially inappropriate medication prevalence rates.
- START (Screening Tool to Alert doctors to Right Treatment) consists of 22 evidence-based prescribing indicators for commonly encountered diseases in older people.

Treatment) consists of 22 evidence-based prescribing indicators for commonly encountered diseases in older people.

International studies using STOPP criteria worryingly indicate high potentially inappropriate medication (PIM) prevalence rates. A PIM index is calculated by dividing the total number of PIMs by the total number of medications. A UK study [29] carried out within an acute hospital setting found that the admission PIM prevalence was 26.7% (95% CI 20.5 - 32.9; 52 patients, 74 PIMs). The most common PIM categories on admission were central nervous system and psychotropic drugs, drugs adversely affecting patients at risk of falls and drugs acting on the urogenital system. The likelihood of having a PIM on admission was doubled in patients receiving more than ten medications compared with those taking fewer (odds ratio 2.3 [95% CI 1.2 - 4.4]; p = 0.01). The study reported a discharge PIM prevalence of 22.6% (95% CI 16.7 - 28.5; 44 patients, 51 PIMs), with a significant reduction of PIMs on discharge (p = 0.005).

Wahab et al. [30] assessed the prevalence and nature of pre-admission inappropriate prescribing by using the STOPP criteria amongst a sample of hospitalised elderly inpatients in South Australia. The total number of pre-admission medications screened during the study period was 949 and the median number of medicines per patient was nine (range 2 - 28). Overall the STOPP criteria identified 138 PIMs in 60% patients. The most frequent PIM was for opiates prescribed in patients with recurrent falls (12.3%). The other two culprit medicines were benzodiazepines in fallers (10.1%) and proton pump inhibitors prescribed for peptic ulcer disease for long-term at maximum doses (9.4%). The number of medications being taken had a positive correlation with pre-admission PIM use (r(s) = 0.49, p < 0.01).

Medication review for patients may be undertaken by various health professionals. A randomised control trial [31] assessed the effect of clinical medication review undertaken by a pharmacist for elderly people living in care homes. This included 661 residents aged 65 years and over, on one or more medicines. The study found that general practitioners did not review most care home patients' medication. Medication changes initiated and proposed by the pharmacist were usually accepted, with a reduction in number of falls, but without any changes to overall drug costs. In addition, there were no significant changes in consultations, hospitalisations, mortality, standardised mini mental state examination or Barthel scores (Barthel Index consists of 10 items that measure a person's daily functioning, specifically the activities of daily living).

Wilcock et al. [32] utilised community pharmacists to collate data for their cross sectional survey which included a study population of 581 residents recruited from eighteen UK residential homes. They found that the use of psychotropic drugs was common, and observed a trend for increase in prescribing rates as compared to data from a previous survey in 2001. There was limited use of Calcium and Vitamin D supplements, which have the potential for reducing morbidity associated with falls. Although use of both calcium and vitamin D had increased significantly (8.3% in 2005 vs. 2.1% in 2001), overall this was relatively low with an eight percentage usage level in this at risk population (**Table 3**).

In their paper on prevention of falls and consequent injuries in elderly people, Kannus et al. [3] discuss the traditional approach often used for prevention of bone fracture injury with focus on prevention and treatment of osteoporosis. The aims are to maximise peak bone mass and prevent ongoing bone loss with regular exercise, calcium and vitamin D and treatment of osteoporosis with pharmacological medicines [15]. Service development in the UK NHS has included pharmacist-led, multidisciplinary team-supported, medication management clinics that focus on osteoporosis, falls and fracture prevention [33]. The pharmaceutical care approach [34] [35] utilised in these clinics within the secondary care setting, provide a structured framework to help identify polypharmacy issues and ensure safe and efficacious medication usage by patients. Assessment of compliance and adherence with medication taking [36] is undertaken by the pharmacist, with patients encouraged to raise their medication and health related concerns, and where the aims are to agree to an ongoing management plan [37] [38].

Table 3. Medication review.

- Medication review for patients may be undertaken by various health professionals.
- Clinical medication review by a pharmacist for older people in care home settings is associated with reduced falls risk.
- A traditional approach often used for falls and bone fracture injury prevention is management of osteoporosis risk.

Limitations for the findings reported from this review include study of publications identified via a search utilising only the PubMed database. Our work was undertaken as a quick, time-limited, preliminary fact finding exercise to understand what the current evidence base is for clinical medication review and falls in older people. Readers may find that the findings reported in this paper provides useful knowledge, and that our work helps inform wider database searches and helps inform more research activity in this area.

Tables 1-3 highlight the main knowledge generated from this review. These data will help inform our work as we move forward with the designing of a pharmacist delivered clinical medication review service for elderly fallers. This service would be part of the larger multi-disciplinary team supported integrated care pathway. In clinical practice elderly fallers often have numerous co-morbidities and are on multiple medicines. We aim to develop a research and evaluation strategy incorporating improvement science methodology [39], that generates more knowledge for medication related falls risk, with use of the STOPP/START tools as a starting point. It will be important also to remember that for delivery of effective pharmaceutical care, elderly people with age related deficits may benefit more from discontinuation and de-prescribing of some of their medications. This decision needs to be made considering all the medicines taken, and where the elderly patient reports side effects, and not only for medicines that are already defined as causing adverse events and therefore on the STOPP list.

5. Conclusion

This paper reports the current knowledge from the evidence base for clinical medication review and falls in the elderly. Both medication over-use and under-use occur frequently and may be harmful; many drugs commonly used by older persons have not been systematically studied as risk factors for falls. The STOPP START tools, validated for assessment of potentially inappropriate prescribing in the elderly, offer the possibility of provision of a structured clinical medication review to patients. There is a need for more research on the impact of these interventions on both the rates of falls and risk of falls in the elderly.

Acknowledgements

Research & Development Department, Academic Directorate, London North West Healthcare NHS Trust for supporting this work.

Financial Support

This research received no specific grant from any funding agency, commercial or not-for-profit sectors.

Conflict of Interest

None.

References

[1]   Department of Health (2009) The Prevention Package for Older People. http://webarchive.nationalarchives.gov.uk/20130107105354/http:/www.dh.gov.uk/en/Publicationsandstatistics/Publications/dh_103146

[2]   World Health Organisation (2012) Falls. WHO Factsheet No 344. http://www.who.int/mediacentre/factsheets/fs344/en/

[3]   Kannus, P., Sievänen, H., Palvanen, M., Järvinen, T. and Parkkari, J. (2005) Prevention of Falls and Consequent Injuries in Elderly People. *Lancet*, **366**, 1885-1893. http://dx.doi.org/10.1016/S0140-6736(05)67604-0

[4]   Centers for Disease Control and Prevention (CDC) (2006) Fatalities and Injuries from Falls among Older Adults—United States, 1993-2003 and 2001-2005. *Morbidity and Mortality Weekly Report*, **55**, 1221-1224.

[5]   Rubenstein, L.Z. (2006) Falls in Older People: Epidemiology, Risk Factors and Strategies for Prevention. *Age and*

Ageing, **35**, 37-41. http://dx.doi.org/10.1093/ageing/afl084

[6]   Cameron, I.D., Gillespie, L.D., Robertson, M.C., Murray, G.R., Hill, K.D., Cumming, R.G. and Kerse, N. (2012) Interventions for Preventing Falls in Older People in Care Facilities and Hospitals. *Cochrane Database of Systematic Reviews*, No. 12, Article No.: CD005465. http://dx.doi.org/10.1002/14651858.CD005465.pub3

[7]   Lin, F.R. and Ferrucci, L. (2012) Hearing Loss and Falls among Older Adults in the United States. *Archives of Internal Medicine*, **172**, 369-371. http://dx.doi.org/10.1001/archinternmed.2011.728

[8]   Viljanen, A., Kaprio, J., Pyykkö, I., Sorri, M., Koskenvuo, M. and Rantanen, T. (2009) Hearing Acuity as a Predictor of Walking Difficulties in Older Women. *Journal of the American Geriatrics Society*, **57**, 2282-2286. http://dx.doi.org/10.1111/j.1532-5415.2009.02553.x

[9]   Skalska, A., Wizner, B., Piotrowicz, K., Klich-Rączka, A., Klimek, E., Mossakowska, M., *et al.* (2013) The Prevalence of Falls and Their Relation to Visual and Hearing Impairments among a Nation-Wide Cohort of Older Poles. *Experimental Gerontology*, **48**, 140-146. http://dx.doi.org/10.1016/j.exger.2012.12.003

[10]   Crowe, K. (2013) Increasing Isolation in a Confusing World: Dementia with Age Related Hearing Impairment. *Old Age Psychiatrist*, **55**.

[11]   Department of Health (2009) Hip Fracture including the Secondary Prevention of Further Fractures Related to Falls and Bone Fragility.
        http://www.pathwaysforhealth.org/application/render08.asp?reference=E866CB3073EF4E0CA4289A3A0C20407E

[12]   Laybourne, A.H., Martin, F.C., Whiting, D.G. and Lowton, K. (2011) Could Fire and Rescue Services Identify Older People at Risk of Falls? *Primary Health Care Research & Development*, **12**, 395-399.
        http://dx.doi.org/10.1017/S1463423611000120

[13]   British Geriatrics Society (2014) Fit for Frailty. Consensus Best Practice Guidance for the Care of Older People Living with Frailty in Community and Outpatient Settings. British Geriatrics Society in Association with the Royal College of General Practitioners and Age UK. http://www.bgs.org.uk/campaigns/fff/fff_full.pdf

[14]   Robb, E., Jarman, B., Suntharalingam, G., Higgens, C., Tennant, R. and Elcock, K. (2010) Using Care Bundles to Reduce In-Hospital Mortality: Quantitative Survey. *BMJ*, **340**, c1234. http://dx.doi.org/10.1136/bmj.c1234

[15]   NICE (2013) Falls in Older People: Assessing Risk and Prevention. Guidelines CG161.
        http://www.nice.org.uk/guidance/cg161/chapter/recommendations

[16]   Gallagher, P., Ryan, C., Byrne, S., Kennedy, J., O'Mahony, D., STOPP (Screening Tool of Older Person's Prescriptions) and START (Screening Tool to Alert Doctors to Right Treatment) (2008) Consensus Validation. *International Journal of Clinical Pharmacology and Therapeutics*, **46**, 72-83. http://dx.doi.org/10.5414/CPP46072

[17]   Gallagher, P., Baeyens, J.P., Topinkova, E., Madlova, P., Cherubini, A., Gasperini, B., *et al.* (2009) Inter-Rater Reliability of STOPP (Screening Tool of Older Persons' Prescriptions) and START (Screening Tool to Alert Doctors to Right Treatment) Criteria amongst Physicians in Six European Countries. *Age and Ageing*, **38**, 603-606. http://dx.doi.org/10.1093/ageing/afp058

[18]   Bjelakovic, G., Gluud, L.L., Nikolova, D., Whitfield, K., Wetterslev, J., Simonetti, R.G., *et al.* (2014) Vitamin D Supplementation for Prevention of Mortality in Adults. *Cochrane Database of Systematic Reviews*, No. 1, Article ID: CD007470.

[19]   Gillespie, L.D., Robertson, M.C., Gillespie, W.J., Sherrington, C., Gates, S., Clemson, L.M. and Lamb, S.E. (2012) Interventions for Preventing Falls in Older People Living in the Community. *Cochrane Database of Systematic Reviews*, No. 9, Article ID: CD007146. http://dx.doi.org/10.1002/14651858.CD007146.pub3

[20]   Beer, C., Hyde, Z., Almeida, O.P., Norman, P., Hankey, G.J., Yeap, B.B. and Flicker, L. (2011) Quality Use of Medicines and Health Outcomes among a Cohort of Community Dwelling Older Men: An Observational Study. *British Journal of Clinical Pharmacology*, **71**, 592-599. http://dx.doi.org/10.1111/j.1365-2125.2010.03875.x

[21]   Gnjidic, D., Hilmer, S.N., Blyth, F.M., Naganathan, V., Waite, L., Seibel, M.J., *et al.* (2012) Polypharmacy Cutoff and Outcomes: Five or More Medicines Were Used to Identify Community-Dwelling Older Men at Risk of Different Adverse Outcomes. *Journal of Clinical Epidemiology*, **65**, 989-995. http://dx.doi.org/10.1016/j.jclinepi.2012.02.018

[22]   Hartikainen, S., Lönnroos, E. and Louhivuori, K. (2007) Medication as a Risk Factor for Falls: Critical Systematic Review. *Journals of Gerontology Series A: Biological Sciences and Medical Sciences*, **62**, 1172-1181.
        http://dx.doi.org/10.1093/gerona/62.10.1172

[23]   Veal, F.C., Bereznicki, L.R., Thompson, A.J. and Peterson, G.M. (2014) Pharmacological Management of Pain in Australian Aged Care Facilities. *Age and Ageing*, **43**, 851-856. http://dx.doi.org/10.1093/ageing/afu072

[24]   Nishtala, P.S., Narayan, S.W., Wang, T. and Hilmer, S.N. (2014) Associations of Drug Burden Index with Falls, General Practitioner Visits, and Mortality in Older People. *Pharmacoepidemiology and Drug Safety*, **23**, 753-758.
        http://dx.doi.org/10.1002/pds.3624

[25] Berthoux, E., Dufour, C., Raharisondraibe, E. and Bonnefoy, M. (2013) Preventable Drug Events in Acute Geriatric Unit. *Gériatrie et Psychologie Neuropsychiatrie du Vieillissement*, **11**, 15-20.

[26] Rhalimi, M., Helou, R. and Jaeker, P. (2009) Medication Use and Increased Risk of Falls in Hospitalized Elderly Patients: A Retrospective, Case-Control Study. *Drugs & Aging*, **26**, 847-852. http://dx.doi.org/10.2165/11317610-000000000-00000

[27] Payne, R.A., Abel, G.A., Simpson, C.R. and Maxwell, S.R. (2013) Association between Prescribing of Cardiovascular and Psychotropic Medications and Hospital Admission for Falls or Fractures. *Drugs & Aging*, **30**, 247-254. http://dx.doi.org/10.1007/s40266-013-0058-z

[28] Vitry, A.I., Hoile, A.P., Gilbert, A.L., Esterman, A. and Luszcz, M.A. (2010) The Risk of Falls and Fractures Associated with Persistent Use of Psychotropic Medications in Elderly People. *Archives of Gerontology and Geriatrics*, **50**, e1-e4. http://dx.doi.org/10.1016/j.archger.2009.04.004

[29] Onatade, R., Auyeung, V., Scutt, G. and Fernando, J. (2013) Potentially Inappropriate Prescribing in Patients on Admission and Discharge from an Older Peoples' Unit of an Acute UK Hospital. *Drugs & Aging*, **30**, 729-737. http://dx.doi.org/10.1007/s40266-013-0097-5

[30] Wahab, M.S., Nyfort-Hansen, K. and Kowalski, S.R. (2012) Inappropriate Prescribing in Hospitalised Australian Elderly as Determined by the STOPP Criteria. *International Journal of Clinical Pharmacy*, **34**, 855-862. http://dx.doi.org/10.1007/s11096-012-9681-8

[31] Zermansky, A.G., Alldred, D.P., Petty, D.R., Raynor, D.K., Freemantle, N., Eastaugh, J. and Bowie, P. (2006) Clinical Medication Review by a Pharmacist of Elderly People Living in Care Homes—Randomised Controlled Trial. *Age and Ageing*, **35**, 586-591. http://dx.doi.org/10.1093/ageing/afl075

[32] Wilcock, M., MacMahon, D. and Woolf, A. (2005) Use of Medicines That Influence Falls or Fractures in a Residential Home Setting. *Pharmacy World and Science*, **27**, 220-222. http://dx.doi.org/10.1007/s11096-004-3707-9

[33] Tanna, N. (2004) Care of the Elderly—An Osteoporosis Medication Management Clinic. *Hospital Pharmacist*, **11**, 231-238.

[34] Cipolle, R.J., Strand, L.M. and Morley, P.C. (1998) Pharmaceutical Care Practice. McGraw-Hill, Health Professions Division, New York.

[35] Cipolle, R.J., Strand, L.M. and Morley, P.C. (2012) Pharmaceutical Care Practice: The Patient Centered Approach to Medication Management. 3rd Edition, McGraw-Hill, Health Professions Division, New York.

[36] NICE (2009) Guidelines CG76. Medicines Adherence. http://pathways.nice.org.uk/pathways/medicines-adherence/medicines-adherence-overview#content=view-node%3Anodes-reviewing-medicines

[37] Tanna, N., Batten, C., Pitkin, J., Rogers, P. and Kelham, C. (2005) Shared Decision Making and Care Planning with Patients. *The Journal of the British Menopause Society*, **11**, 180.

[38] Tanna, N., Batten, C., Pitkin, J., Rogers, P. and Kelham, C. (2007) Evaluation of a Medication Management Clinic Service, Using Action Research Methodology. *Osteoporosis International*, **18**, S310.

[39] Marshall, M., Pronovost, P. and Dixon-Woods, M. (2013) Promotion of Improvement as a Science. *The Lancet*, **381**, 419-421. http://dx.doi.org/10.1016/S0140-6736(12)61850-9

24

The Effect of MRP5-Expression on Human Erythroleukemia (HEL) Cell Growth and cGMP Levels

Xiaoyan Chen, Roy A. Lysaa, Ragnhild Jaeger, Emanuel Boadu, Georg Sager

Medical Pharmacology and Toxicology, Department of Medical Biology, Faculty of Health Sciences, Arctic University of Norway, Tromso, Norway
Email: georg.sager@uit.no

Abstract

Background: Previous studies of patients with acute leukemia showed that plasma cGMP levels were markedly elevated before treatment, fell after successful therapy but increased after relapse. In many cells high concentrations of GMP have an antiproliferative effect. The cellular cGMP extrusion from cancer cells may represent an acquired resistance against an endogenous antiproliferative signal molecule. Multidrug resistance associated protein 5 (MRP5) has been identified as an important cGMP transporter. Methods: A human erythroleukemia cell line (HEL) was used to study the impact of cGMP and cGMP-elevating compounds like theophylline, sodium nitroprusside (SNP) and sodium nitrite ($NaNO_2$). MRP5 was overexpressed in HEL cells by transfection. Concentrations of cGMP were determined with RIA or HPLC and cell densities were determined by cytometry. Results: The concentration ratio between extra- and intracellular cGMP concentrations was >1, meaning that HEL cells extruded cGMP against a concentration gradient and MRP5 was identified in these cells. In some cell types butyrate increases cellular cGMP levels by stimulating soluble guanylyl cyclase (sGC) and thereby the cellular efflux. This effect did not exist for HEL cells. MRP5 transfected HEL cells which were exposed to cGMP was clearly more sensitive to the antiproliferative effect than the wild type. On the other hand, exposing the transfected HEL cells to cGMP-elevating agents (theophylline, SNP and $NaNO_2$) showed less sensitivity than the wildtype. Conclusion: This study supports the idea that some cancers acquire resistance against endogenous signal molecules with antiproliferative potency.

Keywords

Cyclic GMP, MRP5, Resistance, Cancer, Growth, Regulation

1. Introduction

The observation that some cancer types were associated with increased extracellular cGMP levels during active disease forwarded the idea of an acquired resistance against an endogenous molecule with antiproliferative properties. This phenomenon has been well documented for leukemia and some gynecologic cancers. In patients with acute leukemia the plasma cGMP levels were markedly elevated before treatment, fell after successful therapy but increased after relapse [1]. In cancer of the uterine cervix, the urinary cGMP levels were elevated in untreated cancer but decreased after successful treatment [2]-[4]. In a comparison between a control group (n = 83) and women with epithelial ovariancancer (n = 92) elevated urinary cGMP levels were evident among 53% of the patients [5]. In a two-center follow-up study serial samples from 60 patients with ovarian cancer were monitored up to 2 years after the start of therapy [6]. Urine cGMP levels were significantly higher in those patients with poorly differentiated tumors. Serial measurements made it possible to predict relapse in 64% prior to other clinical signs. However, these studies showed that low sensitivity and poor specificity made extracellular cGMP as tumor marker unsuitable for screening purposes.

Efflux of cGMP from hRBC (human erythrocytes) was composed of high and low affinity transport [7] and the cGMP transporter was identified as MRP5 (the ATP-Binding-Cassette transporter ABCC5) [8]. Cyclic AMP was not able to compete with the high affinity ATP-dependent cGMP transport [9] [10] but inhibited the low affinity transport [10]. Based on the observations in hRBC and the effects of elevating cGMP levels in HEK293 cells [11] we employed a human hemopoietic cell line; human erythroleukemia cells (HEL) [12] for the present study. Since butyrate increases cGMP efflux in some cells [13] the effect on HEL cell growth and elevation of cGMP levels was characterized. In addition, HEL-cells were transfected with MRP5 to test the hypothesis whether increased cGMP efflux may represent acquired resistance against endogenous growth control.

2. Materials and Methods

2.1. Chemicals

The following chemicals were obtained from Sigma-Aldrich: Guanosine 3', 5'-cyclic monophosphate (cGMP), bromo-guanosine 3', 5'-cyclic monophosphate (Br-cGMP), sodium nitroprusside (SNP), sodium nitrite ($NaNO_2$), theophylline, butyric acid, dithiothreitol. Ethidium bromide was purchased from Biological Molecular Reagents, hygromycin B from Life Technologies Inc. All other chemicals were of analytical grade.

2.2. Cell Culture

Human erythroleukemia (HEL) wildtype (wt) cells were obtained from European Collection of Cell Cultures. The cells were seeded at $3 - 4 \times 10^4$/ml in RPMI 1640 supplemented with 10% FCS, 1% L-glutamine with daily renewal. The cell densities were determined in a cytometer and viability assessed with the trypan blue exclusion test. After seeding, a short lag phase (1 - 2 days) was observed before the HEL$_{wt}$ cells entered a logarithmic growth phase. Under these experimental conditions the doubling time of was 25.1 ± 2.5 h.

2.3. Transfection of HEL Cells with MRP5

HEL cells were stably transfected with the plasmid by liposome-mediated method [14] with Qiagen plasmid kits. The plasmid pc DNA 3.1/Hygro-MRP5 cDNA was obtained from Professor Dietrich Keppler, Heidelberg, Germany. The plasmid in *E. coli* cells were extracted and purified. The transfection experiments were performed two times (MRP5[1] and MRP5[2]). The expression of the MRP5 proteins was verified using Western Blot. ECL This method included Western blotting detection reagents from Amersham, UK with anti-MRP5 (human) MAb (M5I-1) and peroxidase conjugated anti-rat IgG and HRP-conjugated anti-biotin antibody. **Figure 1** shows a 180 kDa band of MRP5 from each lane and with clearly more MRP5 proteins in HEL-MRP5[1] and HEL-MRP5[2] than in the HEL$_{wt}$ cells. The doubling time of HEL-MRP5-cells was similar to wildtype (27.0 ± 1.6 h).

2.4. Cyclic GMP Assay

Radioimmunoassay (RIA) was used to determine intra- and extracellular concentrations of cGMP in some of the experiments. The cGMP-analysis with Amerlex-M [125I] kits was performed as recommended by the manufacturer (Amersham International plc). High extracellular cGMP concentrations were determined in a HPLC-assay

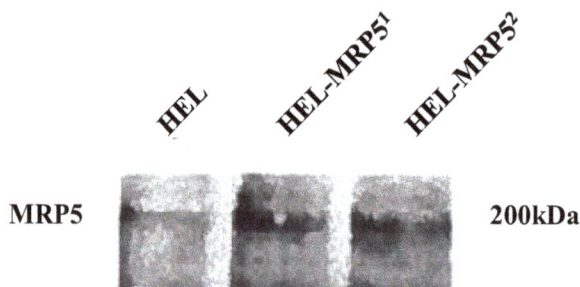

MRP5   200kDa

Figure 1. Western blot with expression of MRP5 in HEL cells. The band of 200 kDa represents MRP5 and the protein amount (from identical number cells) was higher in HEL-MRP5[1] and HEL-MRP5[2] than HEL$_{wt}$ cells. HEL-MRP5[1] and HEL-MRP5[2] represent the first and second time transfected HEL cells, respectively.

with UV detection (254 nm) as previously described [11].

2.5. Statistics and IC$_{50}$-Values

Descriptive statistics were presented as mean ± SE. The concentration inhibition curves were analyzed according to Chou [15] to obtain IC$_{50}$-values.

3. Results

3.1. Butyrate and Cell Growth

Butyrate may increase cellular cGMP efflux in some cell types [13] but also modulate cell growth; for review see [16]. In the present study, butyrate concentrations up to 100 μM had minimal effect on HEL cell growth compared to baseline. However, concentrations above 100 μM showed a marked reduction in cell densities with an estimated IC$_{50}$-value of 470 μM. The effect of butyrate on intra- and extracellular cGMP levels were determined below growth-modulating concentrations. Inhibition of PDE (cyclic nucleotide phosphodiesterase) by theophylline did not change cGMP levels markedly (**Table 1**). After sGC (soluble guanylyl cyclase) stimulation by SNP and NaNO$_2$ the intracellular cGMP levels appeared to be raised somewhat. However, the extra- to intracellular concentration ratio did not indicate any major changes in cellular cGMP efflux.

3.2. Exogenous cGMP and Cell Growth

The possibility that cGMP modulated cell growth differently was explored. The cells were cultured with exogenously added cGMP to achieve concentrations in the medium from 0 to 1000 μM. Cyclic GMP inhibited both HEL$_{wt}$ and HEL-MRP5 cell growth in a concentration-dependent manner (**Figure 2**). However, exogenous cGMP was apparently less effective as inhibitor of MRP5-transfected cell growth. The IC$_{50}$-value for HEL$_{wt}$ was estimated to be 250 μM, whereas the corresponding values for HEL-MRP5[1] and HEL-MRP5[2] were 750 μM and 3 mM, respectively. The intra- and extracellular cGMP levels were assayed by HPLC. However, the intracellular levels were below the limit of detection, and 24 h after addition the extracellular cGMP levels were reduced with 50% - 60% (100 μM) and 5% - 10% (1000 μM). It was not possible to see any effect of transfection on the extracellular levels with the methods employed.

3.3. SNP-Stimulated Soluble Guanylyl Cyclase and Cell Growth

After exposure to SNP, the HEL$_{wt}$ cell densities were reduced concentration-dependently (**Figure 3**). After seven days with 100 μM SNP the cell densities fell to 71.1% ± 13.9% for HEL$_{wt}$, 33.8% ± 9.3% and 52.2% ± 5.0% (mean ± SE) for HEL-MRP5[1] and HEL-MRP5[2], respectively. The IC$_{50}$-values were estimated to be 5 mM for the HEL$_{wt}$-cells. The transfected cell lines were more sensitive to SNP (**Figure 3**). However, even if the transfections were conducted with an identical protocol a clear difference in sensitivity was observed. The estimated IC$_{50}$-values were 20 μM and 130 μM for HEL-MRP5[1] and HEL-MRP5[2], respectively.

Table 1. The effect of butyrate on HEL-cell cGMP levels in absence or presence of theophylline, SNP, NaNO$_2$. The cells were seeded at a concentration of 4×10^5 cells/ml. They were cultured in a medium described in methods and supplemented with 1 and 100 μM butyrate, respectively. After 24 h the cells were transferred to new tubes and incubated for 36 min in the absence or in presence of 1 mM theophylline. Soluble guanylyl cyclase was stimulated with 10 μM SNP or 10 mM NaNO$_2$ for 6 min at 37˚C. Intra- and extracellular cGMP levels (given as fmol/10^4 cells) were quantified by radioimmunoassay.

Intracellular cGMP (fmol/10^4 cells)			
Butyrate	0	1 μM	100 μM
Control	8.3 ± 0.8	7.2 ± 0.8	9.8 ± 1.7
Theophylline	7.4 ± 0.7	9.4 ± 1.2	9.2 ± 0.8
Theophylline + SNP	10.5 ± 1.0	13.1 ± 1.5	12.9 ± 1.6
Theophylline + NaNO$_2$	9.0 ± 0.7	11.0 ± 0.8	13.7 ± 1.5
Extracellular (fmol/10^4 cells)			
Butyrate	0	1 μM	100 μM
Control	12.1 ± 1.9	10.0 ± 1.4	13.4 ± 2.2
Theophylline	12.1 ± 1.5	13.2 ± 2.0	13.5 ± 2.1
Theophylline + SNP	13.7 ± 1.7	13.8 ± 1.7	15.7 ± 2.0
Theophylline + NaNO$_2$	11.1 ± 1.3	12.7 ± 1.6	10.5 ± 1.2

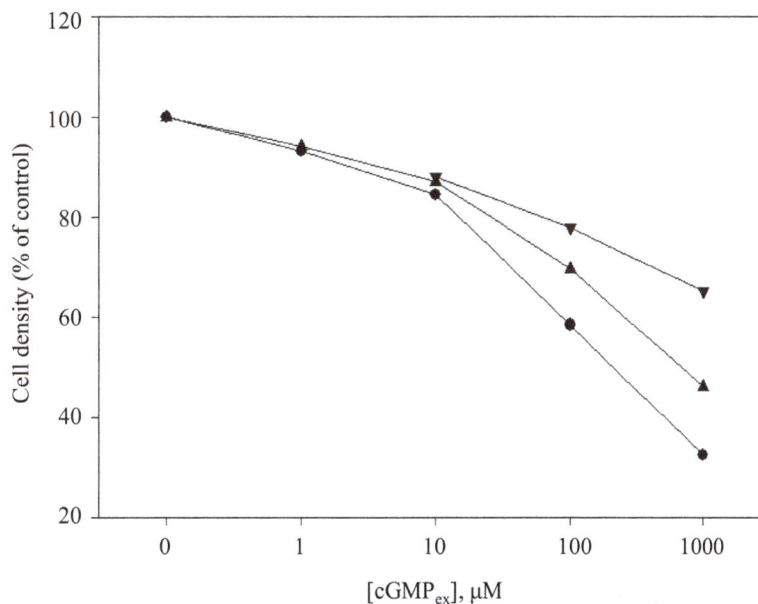

Figure 2. The effect of cGMP-supplemented culture medium on wildtype HEL (●), transfected HEL-MRP5[1] (▲) and HEL-MRP5[2] (▼) cell densities. The cells were seeded at a concentration of 4×10^4 cells/ml. The medium was changed daily and supplemented with cGMP (0, 1 μM, 10 μ, 100 μ and 1000 μM). The last part of the inhibition curves showed a steeper reduction of densities of HEL$_{wt}$ cells (slope = −26.0, r = −1.00) than the transfected cells; MRP5[1] (slope = −20.5, r = −0.996) and MRP5[2] (slope = −11.5, r = −0.998).

4. Discussion

This study with the human erythroleukemia cell line (HEL) was performed based on the consistent finding of increased cGMP plasma levels in other human leukemia [1] and based on our characterization of ATP-dependent cGMP extrusion from human erythrocytes [7] [10] [17]. The report that butyrate increased cGMP efflux from the cancer coli cells [13] attained our attention and raised the question whether this effect existed in HEL-cells. Butyrate is a short chain fatty acid with a number of biological effects and appear to protect against the development of cancer [16] [18]. In agreement, the present study showed that butyrate caused HEL cell death in concentrations above 100 μM. To avoid an interference of the antiproliferative effect of butyrate cGMP efflux

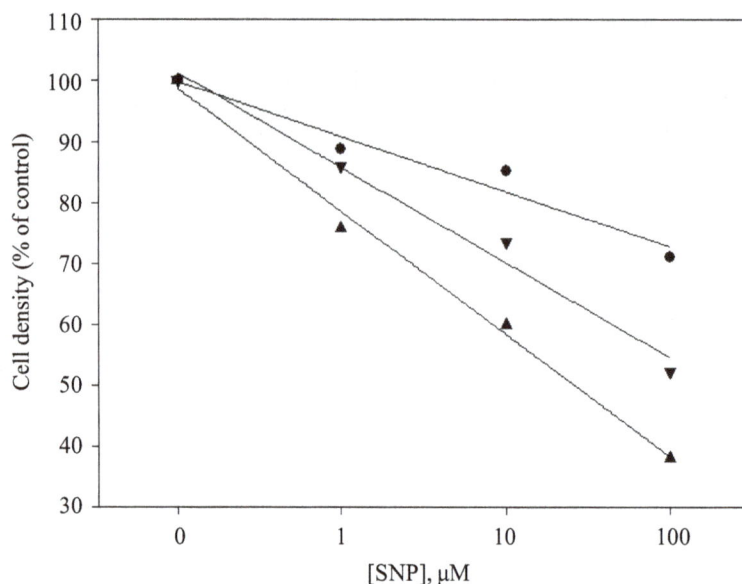

Figure 3. The effect of SNP-supplemented culture medium on wildtype HEL (●), transfected HEL-MRP5[1] (▲) and HEL-MRP5[2] (▼) cell densities. The cells were seeded at a concentration of approximately 3.0×10^4 cells/ml and the medium was changed daily and supplemented with SNP (1 μM, 10 μM and 100 μM). Linear regression showed a less steep reduction of densities of HEL_{wt} cells (slope = −8.9, r = −0.934) than observed for the transfected cells; HEL-MRP5[1] (slope = −20, r = −0.990) and HEL-MRP5[2] (slope = −16.9, r = −0.989).

was studied for concentrations below 100 μM. Under the present experimental conditions, butyrate did not affect the HEL cell distribution of cGMP between the extra- and intracellular compartment. This effect appears also to be variable among colon cancer cells. Both T84 cells and Caco-2 cells responded similar, whereas COS cells did not show any enhanced cGMP accumulation [13]. The non-specific cyclic phosphodiesterase inhibitor theophylline tended to increase cGMP levels after exposure to the highest concentrations of butyrate. The potent sCG stimulators SNP and $NaNO_2$ in the presence of theophylline gave a small but marked elevation. The peak concentration of cGMP after SNP stimulation has been reported to occur after 3 - 5 min [19]. A short incubation time was used in the present study to capture the potential concentration peak of cGMP but such peak was not observed in the HEL cells.

Western blot showed an overexpression of MRP5 in the transfected cells. Cyclic cGMP was added to the culture medium to elevate intracellular concentrations but the permeability is counteracted by the activity of MRP5 that is an effective efflux pump [8]. In agreement, low extracellular cGMP concentrations (1.0 - 10 μM) did not give detectable increase of intracellular concentrations in HEK 293 cells [11] or hRBC [20]. However, these and other studies have shown that cGMP in millimolar concentrations may permeate the membrane from the ecto-side. This is consistent with a facilitated inward transport by OAT2 (SLC27A) with a K_m-value of approximately 100 μM [21]. However, the employed methods made it unable to detect clear changes in extracellular cGMP levels between wildtype and transfected cells. On the other hand, a marked antiproliferative effect was obtained with an apparent IC_{50}-value of 250 μM. The antiproliferative potency of cGMP was lower in HEK 293 cells since cGMP concentrations above 1000 μM were needed to reduce cell density 50% [11]. The most important observation in the present study was the reduced sensitivity to cGMP after MRP5 transfection. In addition, the two series of transfection showed a clear difference in sensitivity (HEL-MRP5[1] > HEL-MRP5[2]). These results are compatible with the hypothesis that overexpression of MRP5 is a resistance mechanism in some cancer cells to avoid the antiproliferative effect of cGMP. This is also compatible with the idea that plasma cGMP may serve as a surrogate marker for treatment efficiency in leukemic patients [22]. A study of cell lines from cancers of the uterine cervix showed a limited but distinct increase of MRP5 expression during cell growth [23]. This is compatible with the reports of increased urine cGMP levels in patients with an active cancer [3] [4]. High expression of MRP5 and related transport proteins was prognostic unfavorable in acute lymphoblastic leukemia [24]. MRP8 (ABCC11) also represents a cGMP efflux system [25] and may serve as a predictive marker for treatment outcome in acute myeloid leukemia.

However, the transfected cells were less sensitive to SNP than the wildtype and the sensitivity differed between them (HEL-MRP5[1] > HEL-MRP5[2]). In a previous study [11], SNP reduced the intracellular concentration ratio between GSH and GSSG from 260 to 80. An increased expression of MRP5 may favor the export of GS-X (glutathione conjugates) and thereby reduce the cell toxic effects. If nitric oxide analogues like SNP or their cytotoxic metabolites are eliminated, it is possible that the balance between growth inhibitory and stimulatory effects is modified [26].

5. Conclusion

The present study suggests that reduced antiproliferative effect of cGMP is associated with increased expression of MRP5, but raises several questions which have to be addressed in future studies to verify the role of MRP5 in the cancer cell cGMP biokinetics.

Conflict of Interests

There are no conflicts of interests to declare.

References

[1] Peracchi, M., Bamonti-Catena, F., Lombardi, L., Toschi, V., Bareggi, B., Cortelezzi, A., Maiolo, A.T. and Polli, E.E. (1985) Plasma Cyclic Nucleotide Levels in Monitoring Acute Leukemia Patients. *Cancer Detection and Prevention*, **8**, 291-295.

[2] Turner, G.A., Ellis, R.D., Guthrie, D., Latner, A.L., Monaghan, J.M., Ross, W.M., Skillen, A.W. and Wilson, R.G. (1982) Urine Cyclic Nucleotide Concentrations in Cancer and Other Conditions; Cyclic GMP: A Potential Marker for Cancer Treatment. *Journal of Clinical Pathology*, **35**, 800-806. http://dx.doi.org/10.1136/jcp.35.8.800

[3] Orbo, A., Jaeger, R. and Sager, G. (1998) Urinary Levels of Cyclic Guanosine Monophosphate (cGMP) in Patients with Cancer of the Uterine Cervix: A Valuable Prognostic Factor of Clinical Outcome? *European Journal of Cancer*, **34**, 1460-1462. http://dx.doi.org/10.1016/S0959-8049(98)00079-3

[4] Orbo, A., Hanevik, M., Jæger, R., van Heusden, S. and Sager, G. (2007) Urinary Cyclic GMP after Treatment of Gynecological Cancer. A Prognostic Marker of Clinical Outcome. *Anticancer Research*, **27**, 2591-2596.

[5] Luesley, D.M., Blackledge, G.R., Chan, K.K. and Newton, J.R. (1986) Random Urinary Cyclic 3',5' Guanosine Monophosphate in Epithelial Ovarian Cancer: Relation to Other Prognostic Variables and to Survival. *British Journal of Obstetrics and Gynaecology*, **93**, 380-385.

[6] Turner, G.A., Greggi, S., Guthrie, D., Benedetti, P.P., Ellis, R.D., Scambia, G. and Mancuso, S. (1990) Monitoring Ovarian Cancer Using Urine Cyclic GMP. A Two-Centre Study. *European Journal of Gynaecological Oncology*, **11**, 421-427.

[7] Sager, G., Orbo, A., Pettersen, R.H. and Kjørstad, K.E. (1996) Export of Guanosine 3',5'-Cyclic Monophosphate (cGMP) from Human Erythrocytes Characterized by Inside-Out Membrane Vesicles. *Scandinavian Journal of Clinical and Laboratory Investigation*, **56**, 289-293. http://dx.doi.org/10.3109/00365519609090579

[8] Jedlitschky, G., Burchell, B. and Keppler, D. (2000) The Multidrug Resistance Protein 5 Functions as an ATP-Dependent Export Pump for Cyclic Nucleotides. *The Journal of Biological Chemistry*, **275**, 30069-30074. http://dx.doi.org/10.1074/jbc.M005463200

[9] Schultz, C., Vaskinn, S., Kildalsen, H. and Sager, G. (1998) Cyclic AMP Stimulates the Cyclic GMP Egression Pump in Human Erythrocytes: Effects of Probenecid, Verapamil, Progesterone, Theophylline, IBMX, Forskolin, and Cyclic AMP on Cyclic GMP Uptake and Association to Inside-Out Vesicles. *Biochemistry*, **37**, 1161-1166. http://dx.doi.org/10.1021/bi9713409

[10] Orvoll, E., Lysaa, R.A., Ravna, A.W. and Sager, G. (2013) Misoprostol and the Sildenafil Analog (PHAR-0099048) Modulate Cellular Efflux of cAMP and cGMP Differently. *Pharmacology & Pharmacy*, **4**, 104-109. http://dx.doi.org/10.4236/pp.2013.41015

[11] Sager, G., Sundkvist, E., Jaeger, R., Lysaa, R.A. and Fuskevaag, O.M. (2014) Sodium Nitroprusside Inhibits HEK293 Cell Growth by cGMP-Dependent and Independent Mechanisms. *Pharmacology & Pharmacy*, **5**, 262-271. http://dx.doi.org/10.4236/pp.2014.53033

[12] Martin, P. and Papayannopoulou, T. (1982) HEL Cells: A New Human Erythroleukemia Cell Line with Spontaneous and Induced Globin Expression. *Science*, **216**, 1233-1235. http://dx.doi.org/10.1126/science.6177045

[13] Crane, J.K. (2000) Redistribution of Cyclic GMP in Response to Sodium Butyrate in Colon Cells. *Archives of Biochemistry and Biophysics*, **376**, 163-170. http://dx.doi.org/10.1006/abbi.2000.1703

[14] Whitt, M., Buonocore, L. and Rose, J.K. (2001) Liposome-Mediated Transfection. *Current Protocols in Immunology*, **3**, 10.16.1-10.16.4.

[15] Chou, T.C. (1976) Derivation and Properties of Michaelis-Menten Type and Hill Type Equations for Reference Ligands. *Journal of Theoretical Biology*, **39**, 253-276. http://dx.doi.org/10.1016/0022-5193(76)90169-7

[16] Pajak, B., Orzechowski, A.F. and Gajkowska, B. (2007) Molecular Basis of Sodium Butyrate-Dependent Proapoptotic Activity in Cancer Cells. *Advances in Medical Sciences*, **52**, 83-88.

[17] Sundkvist, E., Jaeger, R. and Sager, G. (2002) Pharmacological Characterization of the ATP-Dependent Low K(m) Guanosine 3',5'-Cyclic Monophosphate (cGMP) Transporter in Human Erythrocytes. *Biochemical Pharmacology*, **63**, 945-949. http://dx.doi.org/10.1016/S0006-2952(01)00940-6

[18] Mu, D., Gao, Z.F., Guo, H.F., Zhou, G.F. and Sun, B. (2013) Sodium Butyrate Induces Growth Inhibition and Apoptosis in Human Prostate Cancer DU145 Cells by Up-Regulation of the Expression of Annexin A1. *PLoS ONE*, **8**, e74922. http://dx.doi.org/10.1371/journal.pone.0074922

[19] Schroder, H., Leitman, D.C., Bennett, B.M., Waldman, S.A. and Murad, F. (1988) Glyceryl Trinitrate-Induced Desensitization of Guanylate Cyclase in Cultured Rat Lung Fibroblasts. *Journal of Pharmacology and Experimental Therapeutics*, **245**, 413-418.

[20] Flo, K., Hansen, M., Orbo, A., Kjørstad, K.E., Maltau, J.M. and Sager, G. (1995) Effect of Probenecid, Verapamil and Progesterone on the Concentration-Dependent and Temperature-Sensitive Human Erythrocyte Uptake and Export of Guanosine 3',5' Cyclic Monophosphate (cGMP). *Scandinavian Journal of Clinical and Laboratory Investigation*, **55**, 715-721. http://dx.doi.org/10.3109/00365519509075401

[21] Cropp, C.D., Komori, T., Shima, J.E., Urban, T.J., Yee, S.W., More, S.S. and Giacomini, K.M. (2008) Organic Anion Transporter 2 (SLC22A7) Is a Facilitative Transporter of cGMP. *Molecular Pharmacology*, **73**, 1151-1158. http://dx.doi.org/10.1124/mol.107.043117

[22] Peracchi, M., Toschi, V., Bamonti-Catena, F., Lombardi, L., Bareggi, B., Cortelezzi, A., Colombi, M., Maiolo, A.T. and Polli, E.E. (1987) Plasma Cyclic Nucleotide Levels in Acute Leukemia Patients. *Blood*, **69**, 1613-1616.

[23] Eggen, T., Sager, G., Berg, T., Nergaard, B., Moe, B.T.G. and Orbo, A. (2012) Increased Gene Expression of the ABCC5 Transporter without Distinct Changes in the Expression of PDE5 in Human Cervical Cancer Cells during Growth. *Anticancer Research*, **32**, 3055-3061.

[24] Plasschaert, S.L., de Bont, E.S., Boezen, M., vander Kolk, D.M., Daenen, S.M., Faber, K.N., Kamps, W.A., de Vries, E.G. and Vellenga, E. (2005) Expression of Multidrug Resistance-Associated Proteins Predicts Prognosis in Childhood and Adult Acute Lymphoblastic Leukemia. *Clinical Cancer Research*, **11**, 8661-8668. http://dx.doi.org/10.1158/1078-0432.CCR-05-1096

[25] Guo, Y., Kock, K., Ritter, C.A., Chen, Z.S., Grube, M., Jedlitschky, G., Illmer, T., Ayres, M., Beck, J.F., Siegmund, W., Ehninger, G., Gandhi, V., Kroemer, H.K., Kruh, G.D. and Schaich, M. (2009) Expression of ABCC-Type Nucleotide Exporters in Blasts of Adult Acute Myeloid Leukemia: Relation to Long-Term Survival. *Clinical Cancer Research*, **15**, 1762-1769. http://dx.doi.org/10.1158/1078-0432.CCR-08-0442

[26] Napoli, C., Paolisso, G., Casamassimi, A., Al-Omran, M., Barbieri, M., Sommese, L., Infante, T. and Ignarro, L.J. (2013) Effects of Nitric Oxide on Cell Proliferation: Novel Insights. *Journal of American College of Cardiology*, **62**, 89-95. http://dx.doi.org/10.1016/j.jacc.2013.03.070

25

Establishment and Effects of Ginger and Kikyoto of a Haloperidol-Induced Dysphagia Model in Guinea Pigs

Takahiro Mizoguchi[1], Mitsue Ishisaka[1], Yui Kobatake[2], Hiroaki Kamishina[2], Yasuhiko Nishioka[3], Tsukasa Kirimoto[3], Masamitsu Shimazawa[1], Hideaki Hara[1*]

[1]Molecular Pharmacology, Department of Biofunctional Evaluation, Gifu Pharmaceutical University, Gifu, Japan
[2]Department of Veterinary Medicine, Faculty of Applied Biological Sciences, Gifu University, Gifu, Japan
[3]Taiho Pharmaceutical Co., Ltd., Tokushima, Japan
Email: *hidehara@gifu-pu.ac.jp

Abstract

Dysphagia induces aspiration and causes aspiration pneumonia. There is no treatment for dysphagia fundamentally. Haloperidol reportedly induces dysphagia. In the present study, we established a haloperidol-induced dysphagia model in guinea pigs, and evaluated the effects of ginger, kikyoto, and a mixture of ginger and kikyoto on swallowing. Swallowing ability was evaluated using behavioral tests, computed tomography (CT), and videofluoroscopic examination of swallowing. To investigate the effect of ginger and kikyoto on swallowing, ginger, kikyoto, or a mixture of ginger and kikyoto was administered orally to guinea pigs with haloperidol-induced dysphagia. Effects of these compounds were evaluated with behavioral tests. Chronic administration of haloperidol reduced the number of swallows, as evaluated by the behavioral test and videofluoroscopic examination of swallowing. In our model, these compounds improved swallowing dysfunction. Our results suggest that this model might be useful in revealing the pathogenesis of dysphagia and evaluating compounds that might improve swallowing.

Keywords

Dysphagia, Guinea Pig, Videofluoroscopic Examination of Swallowing, Haloperidol, Ginger

1. Introduction

Dysphagia is the impairment of swallowing abilities, and often causes aspiration pneumonia [1]-[3]. Because

*Corresponding author.

pneumonia is the leading cause of death in the elderly, it is necessary to improve dysphagia. Several compounds were suggested to improve dysphagia [4]-[6]; however, no available medicine treats dysphagia fundamentally. To date, few studies report about animal models of dysphagia [7]. Therefore, animal models of swallowing dysfunction are required to develop novel therapeutic drugs for the treatment of dysphagia.

It has been reported that dysphagia is induced by various diseases such as stroke, Parkinson's disease, and amyotrophic lateral sclerosis [8]-[11]. Recent studies revealed that dysphagia is present in up to 50% of patients who suffered a stroke [12] [13]. Furthermore, antipsychotic drugs such as haloperidol and olanzapine also induce dysphagia [14] [15]. Administration of haloperidol, which is a dopamine D2 receptor antagonist, induces dysphagia clinically and impairs tongue functions in rats [14] [16].

In the present study, we established a dysphagia model in guinea pigs with chronic administration of haloperidol. Furthermore, we investigated swallowing dysfunction using behavioral tests and videofluoroscopy. Finally, we evaluated the effects of ginger (zingibers rhizome), which has a positive effect on swallowing in humans [17]. In addition to ginger, we evaluated kikyoto (containing platycodi radix and glycyrrhizae radix), which have the anti-allergic and anti-inflammatory actions [18] [19], and a mixture of ginger and kikyoto.

2. Materials and Methods

2.1. Animals

Male Hartley guinea pigs were used in the experiments. Guinea pigs were housed at $24°C \pm 2°C$ under a 12:12 hr light:dark cycle (lights on from 8:00 to 20:00), and had *ad libitum* access to food and water. All animal care and treatment procedures were conformed to animal care guidelines of the Animal Experiment Committee of Gifu Pharmaceutical University. All efforts were made to minimize both suffering and the number of animals used.

2.2. Generation of a Haloperidol-Induced Dysphagia Model

Haloperidol was obtained from Wako (Osaka, Japan). It was dissolved in saline solution containing 1% acetic acid. Haloperidol (1 mg/kg, at volume of 1 ml/kg) or vehicle (saline containing 1% acetic acid, at volume of 1 ml/kg) was administered subcutaneously twice a day for 15 days. The behavioral tests were performed on day 8 and 9. On days 13 and 15, swallowing ability was investigated with computed tomography (CT) and videofluoroscopy, respectively.

2.3. Videofluoroscopic Examination of Swallowing

Before the experiment, guinea pigs were fasting for 3.5 hr. The number of swallows was measured with videofluoroscopy after oral administration of various volumes of the contrast medium (140, 280, 420, 560, and 700 μl). The contrast medium contained barium sulfate and glucose in a ratio of 5:2, and was administered into the upper part of the pharynx. After administration, guinea pigs were placed into a box, and swallowing was recorded for 1 min using videofluoroscopic examination. Swallowing was defined as passage of the contrast medium from the pharynx to the stomach.

2.4. Behavioral Test

On days 8 and 9, the number of tongue movements was measured. Swallowing was induced by oral administration of distilled water (400, 500, and 600 μl) into the upper part of the pharynx. Tongue movement was defined as the protrusion of the tongue. Tongue movements were measured for 1 min after the injection of distilled water based on visual inspection.

2.5. Treatments in the Haloperidol-Induced Dysphagia Model

Ginger emulsion and kikyoto were obtained from Taiho Pharmaceutical Co. Ltd. (Tokushima, Japan). They were suspended in 0.5% sodium carboxymethyl cellulose (CMC). Ginger emulsion (30 or 100 μl/kg/day), kikyoto (10 or 30 mg/kg/day), the mixture of ginger emulsion (30 μl/kg/day) and kikyoto (10 mg/kg/day), or vehicle (0.5% CMC) were administered orally at volume of 2 ml/kg for 7 days. On day 8, behavioral tests were performed.

2.6. Statistical Analysis

Data are presented as mean ± standard error of the mean (S.E.M.). Statistical comparisons were performed using the Pearson's test for correlation, and the one-tailed Student's t-test and one- or two-sided Dunnett's tests for other statistics. We used the JSTAT software (Vector, Tokyo, Japan) or SPSS (IBM, Armonk, NY, USA) for the statistical analysis. Probability (p) values of less than 0.05 were considered statistically significant.

3. Results

3.1. Chronic Administration of Haloperidol Impaired Swallowing, as Examined Using Videofluoroscopy

We investigated the swallowing ability of the guinea pigs with videofluoroscopic examination. We evaluated frequency of the deglutition as the outcome measure of the ability of the deglutition as described previously [7].

The ratio of $BaSO_4$ to glucose in the contrast medium was 5:2 (n = 2).

We used a C-arm fluoroscope to perform the videofluoroscopic examination of swallowing (the equipment used is shown in **Figure 1(a)** and **Figure 1(b)**). Firstly, we administered several volumes of contrast medium orally, and measured the number of swallows in untreated guinea pigs. Delivery of the contrast medium from the pharynx to the stomach was observed with videofluoroscopy (**Figure 1(c)**). We defined movement of the contrast medium as "swallowing", and counted the number of swallows for 1 min. The number of swallows correlated with volume of the contrast medium (**Table 1**). Because the number of swallows was the highest after oral administration of 700 μl contrast medium, we used this volume in the following examinations. On day 15 of the haloperidol injection, the number of swallows induced by oral administration of 700 μl contrast medium was measured for 1 min using videofluoroscopy (n = 9). The number of swallows in the haloperidol-treated group was significantly decreased compared with the control group (control: 5.78 ± 0.86, haloperidol-treated: 3.33 ± 1.03) (**Figure 1(d)**). Sample movies of the swallows are available for the control (Supplementary Video (A)) and haloperidol-treated animals (Supplementary Video (B)).

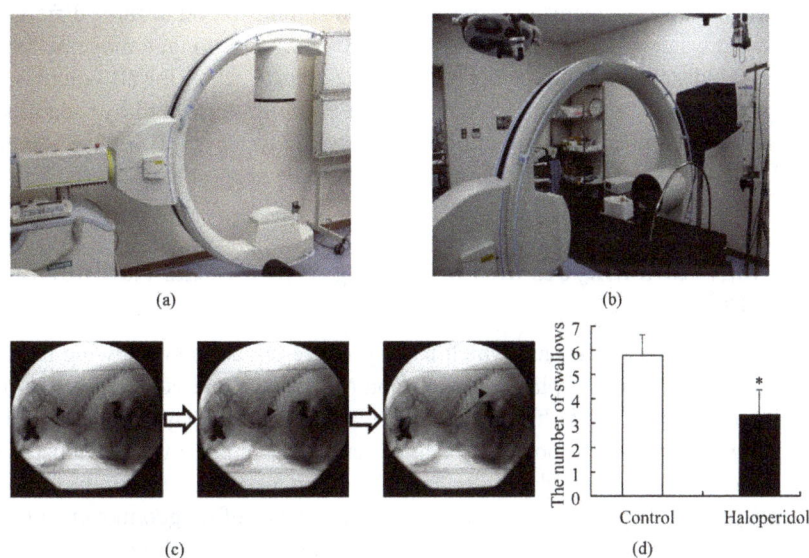

(a)   (b)

(c)   (d)

Figure 1. Videofluoroscopic examination of swallowing in haloperidol-treated guinea pigs. (a) The C-arm X-ray fluoroscopic machine used for the videofluoroscopic examination of swallowing; (b) Experimental setup for the videofluoroscopic examination of swallowing; (c) Representative photographs of swallowing recorded with videofluoroscopy. These photographs show the process of swallowing from left to right. Arrowheads indicate the contrast medium in the digestive system; (d) The number of swallows after the oral administration of 700 μl contrast medium into the upper part of the pharynx in the control and haloperidol-treated animals. Values are expressed as mean ± S.E.M. (n = 9); *p < 0.05, haloperidol-treated group vs. control group (one-tailed Student's t-test).

Table 1. The number of swallows induced by oral administration of the contrast medium measured with videofluoscopy.

Contract medium (µl)	140	280	420	560	700
The number of swallowing	3	4	4.5	6	7.5

3.2. Volume of Cntrast Medium in the Stomach and Intestinum Tenue Measured with CT

Similarly, we investigated swallowing ability using CT (the equipment used for the experiment is shown in **Figure S1(a)** and **Figure S1(b)**). On day 13 of the haloperidol injections, we measured the volume of orally administered contrast medium in the stomach and small intestine (n = 9). There was no difference between the control and haloperidol-treated groups (**Figure S1(c)**).

3.3. Administration of Distilled Water into the Upper Part of the Pharynx Induced a Swallowing Reflex

In previous studies, swallowing ability was investigated by the oral administration of distilled water to guinea pigs [20] [21]. Here, we investigated whether distilled water induced a swallowing reflex. We administered 500 µl distilled water into the upper part of the pharynx of guinea pigs with a feeding needle. The protrusive action of the tongue was observed, and defined as "tongue movement" (**Figure 2(a)**). The number of tongue movements was measured for 1 min after the oral administration of distilled water (n = 4). The number of tongue movements in the group administered distilled water was significantly increased compared to the sham group (without administration) (**Figure 2(b)**). Tongue movements were not detected in the sham group. These results suggest that oral administration of distilled water induced tongue movements.

3.4. Chronic Administration of Haloperidol Decreased the Number of Tongue Movements

We investigated the number of tongue movements in the haloperidol-induced dysphagia model (n = 9). On day 8 and 9, the number of tongue movements induced by the oral administration of three different volumes (400, 500, and 600 µl) of distilled water was measured for 1 min. The number of tongue movements was significantly decreased in the haloperidol-treated group compared with the control group for all volumes (**Figure 3(a)**). Additionally, we observed a correlation between the number of swallows measured by videofluoroscopy and tongue movements induced by the oral administration of 600 µl distilled water (r = 0.4692, p < 0.05) (**Figure 3(b)**), but not 400 or 500 µl distilled water (Data not shown). These results suggest that chronic haloperidol treatment affects the movement of the tongue.

3.5. Effects of Ginger and Kikyoto on Swallowing Action in the Haloperidol-Induced Dysphagia Model

Finally, we evaluated the effect of ginger, which has a positive effect on swallowing in humans [17], on swallowing in the haloperidol-induced dysphagia model [control (vehicle and vehicle treated group), n = 9; haloperidol and vehicle treated group, n = 8; haloperidol and ginger (30 µl/kg/day) treated group, n = 10; haloperidol and ginger (100 µl/kg/day) treated group, n = 9]. Ginger emulsion (ginger) was administrated orally to the haloperidol treated animals for 7 days. On day 8, the number of tongue movements induced by the oral administration of 600 µl distilled water was measured for 1 min. The number of tongue movements was significantly decreased in the haloperidol-treated group compared with the control group. Ginger (100 µl/kg/day), significantly ameliorated the reduced number of tongue movements induced by haloperidol (**Figure 4(a)**). In addition to the evaluation of the effect of ginger, the effect of kikyoto, or the mixture of ginger and kikyoto on swallowing was evaluated in the haloperidol-induced dysphagia model by the similar method [control (vehicle and vehicle treated group, n = 12; haloperidol and vehicle treated group, n = 12; haloperidol and kikyoto (10 m/kg/day) treated group, n = 9; haloperidol and kikyoto (30 m/kg/day) treated group, n = 9; haloperidol and the mixture treated group, n = 8. Kikyoto (30 mg/kg/day), and the mixture of ginger (30 µl/kg/day) and kikyoto (10 mg/kg/day) significantly ameliorated the reduced number of tongue movements induced by haloperidol (**Figure 4(b)**). These results indicate that ginger and kikyoto may improve swallowing in the haloperidol-induced dysphagia model.

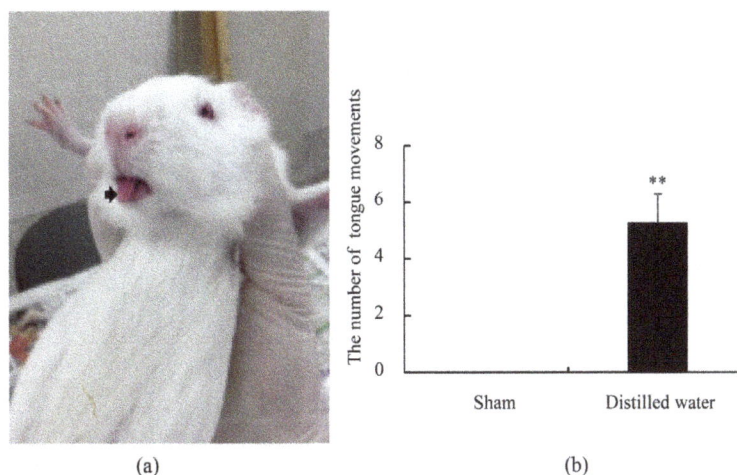

(a)   (b)

Figure 2. The tongue movement induced by distilled water. (a) Picture of the tongue movement. The arrow indicates the evaluated tongue movement; (b) The number of tongue movements in the sham group (no administration of distilled water) and in the animals administered with 500 μl distilled water. Values are expressed as mean ± S.E.M. (n = 4); **p < 0.01, distilled water administered group vs. sham group (two-tailed Student's t-test).

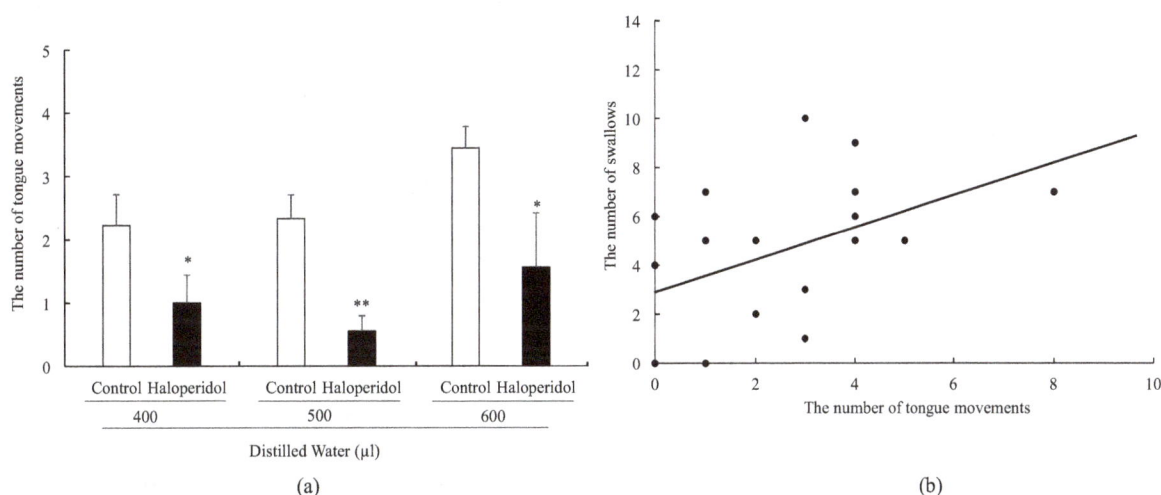

(a)   (b)

Figure 3. Change in the number of tongue movements in the haloperidol-treated guinea pigs. (a) The number of tongue movements induced by the oral administration of 3 different volumes (400, 500, and 600 μl) of distilled water into the upper part of the pharynx in the control and haloperidol-treated groups. Values are expressed as mean ± S.E.M. (n = 9), *p < 0.05 and **p < 0.01, haloperidol-treated group vs. control group (one-tailed Student's t-test); (b) The correlation between the number of tongue movements induced by the oral administration of 600 μl distilled water and the number of swallows measured with videofluoroscopy (Pearson's test).

4. Discussion

One of the main purposes of this study was to establish a dysphagia model using guinea pigs. Videofluoroscopy and behavioral tests were used to evaluate the swallowing ability of guinea pigs.

Videofluoroscopy is an effective clinical method to investigate the process of swallowing [22] [23]. Additionally, advice based on the results of videofluoroscopic examination of swallowing can help to avoid aspiration pneumonia [24]. To date, no studies have evaluated swallowing ability with videofluoroscopy in guinea pigs. In the present study, we showed that it is possible to evaluate the swallowing ability with videofluoroscopy using guinea pigs. It was observed that the number of swallows decreased in the haloperidol-treated guinea pigs. This suggests that chronic administration of haloperidol induces dysphagia in guinea pigs. However, there was no

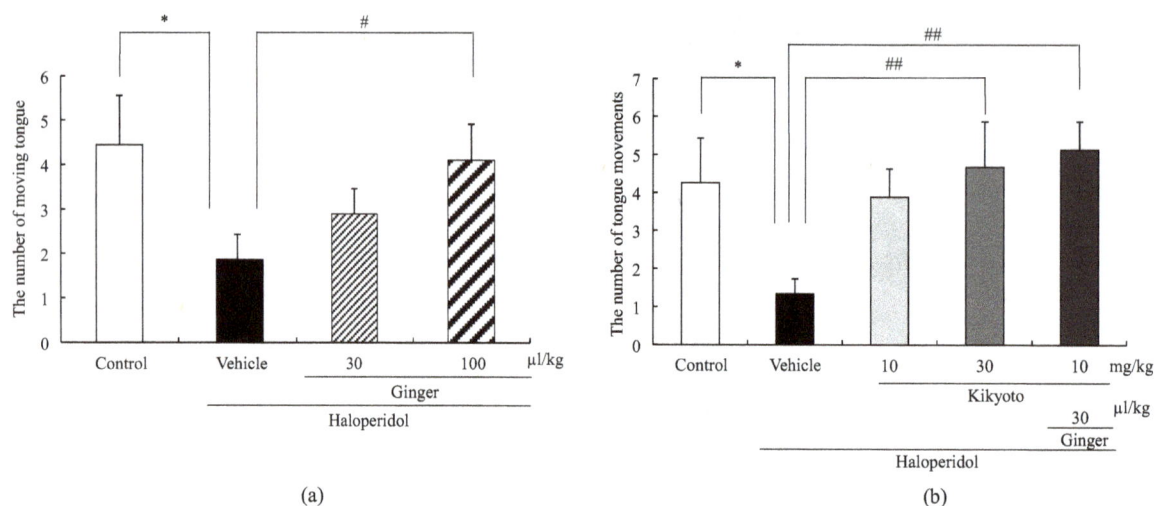

(a)   (b)

Figure 4. Effect of ginger and kikyoto on the haloperidol-induced dysphagia in guinea pigs. (a) The number of tongue movements induced by oral administration of 600 µl distilled water into the upper part of the pharynx of guinea pigs. Values are expressed as mean ± S.E.M.; control (vehicle and vehicle treated group), n = 9; haloperidol and vehicle treated group, n = 8; haloperidol and ginger (30 µl/kg) treated group, n = 10; haloperidol and ginger (100 µl/kg) treated group, n = 9; *p < 0.05, haloperidol and vehicle treated group vs. the control group (one-tailed Student's t-test); $^\#$p < 0.05, haloperidol and ginger (100 µl/kg) treated group vs. haloperidol and vehicle treated group (one-sided Dunnett's test); (b) The number of tongue movements induced by oral administration of 600 µl distilled water into the upper part of the pharynx of guinea pigs. Values are expressed as mean ± S.E.M.; control (vehicle and vehicle treated group), n = 12; haloperidol and vehicle treated group, n = 12; haloperidol and kikyoto (10 mg/kg) treated group, n = 9; haloperidol and kikyoto (30 mg/kg) treated group, n = 9; haloperidol and the mixture treated group, n = 8; *p < 0.05, haloperidol and vehicle treated group vs. control group (one-tailed Student's t-test); $^{\#\#}$p < 0.01, haloperidol and kikyoto (30 mg/kg) or the mixture treated groups vs. haloperidol and vehicle treated group (two-sided Dunnett's test).

difference in the volume of contrast medium in the stomach and small intestine of guinea pigs in the control and haloperidol-treated groups according to CT analysis. It is possible that the contrast medium was mixed with the fluids in the intestine and stomach; thus, amplifying the signal.

Additionally, we evaluated swallowing induced by the administration of distilled water into the upper part of the pharynx using a feeding needle. This behavioral test was evaluated based on visual observations; therefore, this method was easier to perform compared with the videofluoroscopic examination of swallowing. The tongue executes protrusive and retrusive actions during swallowing, and it has been reported that force of the protrusive action is reduced in old rats [25]. Therefore, we focused on the protrusive action of the tongue, and measured this behavior. The number of tongue movements in the haloperidol-treated group was significantly decreased compared with the control group. Additionally, we observed a correlation between the number of swallows measured by videofluoroscopy and the number of tongue movements (for 600 µl). These results suggest that the number of tongue movements might be representative of swallowing ability.

Another purpose of the study was to evaluate the effects of ginger and kikyoto on the haloperidol-induced dysphagia in guinea pigs. Ginger contains numerous pungent phenolic compounds such as 6-gingerol, 6-shagol, 6-paradol, and zingerone [26]. Similar to capsaicin, 6-gingerols are vanilloid receptor 1 agonists [27]. Vanilloid receptor 1 regulates swallowing, and administration of capsaicin improves dysphagia in elderly people and rats with dysphagia induced by middle cerebral artery occlusion [7] [28] [29]. Additionally, it has been reported that gingerol promotes swallowing in young adult women [17]. In the present study, chronic administration of ginger emulsion (100 µl/kg/day) ameliorated the decrease in the number of tongue movements. Kikyoto is a crude drug containing platycodi radix and glycyrrhizae radix extracts. The active ingredient of platycodi radix is saponin and inulin. Glycyrrhizae radix contains glycyrrhizin and other compounds. Kikyoto is reported to have various effects, such as anti-allergic and anti-inflammatory actions; however, no reports implicate its effect in dysphagia [18] [19]. In our animal model, chronic administration of kikyoto (30 mg/kg/day) increased the number of tongue movements, suggesting that kikyoto might improve dysphagia. Further examinations are necessary to reveal its mechanism of action in dysphagia. Finally, the mixture of ginger and kikyoto improved swallowing dysfunction at doses that were not efficient individually. This finding indicates that ginger and kikyoto might have different mechanisms of action and thus their effects are additive.

5. Conclusion

In conclusion, chronic administration of haloperidol induced dysphagia in guinea pigs, and ginger and kikyoto were effective for alleviating swallowing dysfunction in this model. Therefore, our model might be useful to clarify the pathogenesis of dysphagia and to test compounds that might improve swallowing.

Acknowledgements

We thank Mr. Eiji Naito, and Miss. Kanae Oyake (Department of Veterinary Medicine, Faculty of Applied Biological Sciences, Gifu University, Gifu, Japan) for technical support.

Disclosure Statement

Prof. Hideaki Hara has received a research grant from Taiho Pharmaceutical Co. Ltd. (Tokushima, Japan). The other authors declare that have no conflict of interest.

References

[1] Martin, B.J., Corlew, M.M., Wood, H., Olson, D., Golopol, L.A., Wingo, M. and Kirmani, N. (1994) The Association of Swallowing Dysfunction and Aspiration Pneumonia. *Dysphagia*, **9**, 1-6. http://dx.doi.org/10.1007/BF00262751

[2] Taniguchi, M.H. and Moyer, R.S. (1994) Assessment of Risk Factors for Pneumonia in Dysphagic Children: Significance of Videofluoroscopic Swallowing Evaluation. *Developmental Medicine & Child Neurology*, **36**, 495-502. http://dx.doi.org/10.1111/j.1469-8749.1994.tb11879.x

[3] Harkness, G.A., Bentley, D.W. and Roghmann, K.J. (1990) Risk Factors for Nosocomial Pneumonia in the Elderly. *American Journal of Medicine*, **89**, 457-463. http://dx.doi.org/10.1016/0002-9343(90)90376-O

[4] Ohkubo, T., Chapman, N., Neal, B., Woodward, M., Omae, T. and Chalmers, J. (2004) Effects of an Angiotensin Converting Enzyme Inhibitor-Based Regimen on Pneumonia Risk. *American Journal of Respiratory and Critical Care Medicine*, **169**, 1041-1045. http://dx.doi.org/10.1164/rccm.200309-1219OC

[5] Shinohara, Y. (2006) Antiplatelet Cilostazol Is Effective in the Prevention of Pneumonia in Ischemic Stroke Patients in the Chronic Stage. *Cerebrovascular Diseases*, **22**, 57-60. http://dx.doi.org/10.1159/000092922

[6] Nakagawa, T., Wada, H., Sekizawa, K., Arai, H. and Sasaki, H. (1999) Amantadine and Pneumonia. *Lancet*, **353**, 1157. http://dx.doi.org/10.1016/S0140-6736(98)05805-X

[7] Sugiyama, N., Nishiyama, E., Nishikawa, Y., Sasamura, T., Nakade, S., Okawa, K., Nagasawa, T. and Yuki, A. (2014) A Novel Animal Model of Dysphagia Following Stroke. *Dysphagia*, **29**, 61-67. http://dx.doi.org/10.1007/s00455-013-9481-x

[8] Daniels, S.K., Brailey, K., Priestly, D.H., Herrington, L.R., Weisberg, L.A. and Foundas, A.L. (1998) Aspiration Inpatients with Acute Stroke. *Archives of Physical Medicine and Rehabilitation*, **79**, 14-19. http://dx.doi.org/10.1016/S0003-9993(98)90200-3

[9] Smithard, D.G., O'Neill, P.A., Park, C., England, R., Renwick, D.S., Wyatt, R., Morris, J. and Martin, D.F. (1998) Canbedside Assessment Reliably Exclude Aspiration Following Acute Stroke? *Age Ageing*, **27**, 99-106. http://dx.doi.org/10.1093/ageing/27.2.99

[10] Ali, G.N., Wallace, K.L., Schwartz, R., DeCarle, D.J., Zagami, A.S. and Cook, I.J. (1996) Mechanisms of Oralpharyngeal Dysphagia in Patients with Parkinson's Disease. *Gastroenterology*, **110**, 383-392. http://dx.doi.org/10.1053/gast.1996.v110.pm8566584

[11] Ertekin, C., Aydogdu, I., Yuceyar, N., Kiylioglu, N., Tarlaci, S. and Uludag, B. (2000) Pathophysiological Mechanisms of Oropharyngeal Dysphagia in Amyotrophic Lateral Sclerosis. *Brain*, **123**, 125-140. http://dx.doi.org/10.1093/brain/123.1.125

[12] Palmer, J.B., Drennan, J.C. and Baba, M. (2000) Evaluation and Treatment of Swallowing Impairments. *American Family Physician*, **61**, 2453-2462.

[13] Smithard, D.G., O'Neill, P.A., England, R.E., Park, C.L., Wyatt, R., Martin, D.F. and Morris, J. (1997) The Natural History of Dysphagia Following a Stroke. *Dysphagia*, **12**, 188-193. http://dx.doi.org/10.1007/PL00009535

[14] Nagamine, T. (2008) Serum Substance P Levels in Patients with Chronic Schizophrenia Treated with Typical or Atypical Antipsychotics. *Neuropsychiatric Disease and Treatment*, **4**, 289-294. http://dx.doi.org/10.2147/NDT.S2367

[15] Sagar, R., Varghese, S.T. and Balhara, Y.P. (2005) Olanzapine-Induced Double Incontinence. *Indian Journal of Medical Sciences*, **59**, 163-164. http://dx.doi.org/10.4103/0019-5359.16123

[16] Ciucci, M.R. and Connor, N.P. (2009) Dopaminergic Influence on Rat Tongue Function and Limb Movement Initiation. *Experimental Brain Research*, **194**, 587-596. http://dx.doi.org/10.1007/s00221-009-1736-2

[17] Krival, K. and Bates, C. (2012) Effects of Club Soda and Ginger Brew on Lingua-Palatal Pressures in Healthy Swallowing. *Dysphagia*, **27**, 228-239. http://dx.doi.org/10.1007/s00455-011-9358-9

[18] Oh, Y.C., Kang, O.H., Choi, J.G., Lee, Y.S., Brice, O.O., Jung, H.J., Hong, S.H., Lee, Y.M., Shin, D.W., Kim, Y.S. and Kwon, D.Y. (2011) Anti-Allergic Activity of a Platycodon Root Ethanol Extract. *International Journal of Molecular Sciences*, **11**, 2746-2758. http://dx.doi.org/10.3390/ijms11072746

[19] Parihar, M., Chouhan, A., Harsoliya, M.S., Pathan, J.K., Banerjee, S., Khan, N. and Patel, V.M. (2011) A Review—Cough & Treatments. *International Journal of Natural Products Research*, **1**, 9-18.

[20] Jin, Y., Sekizawa, K., Fukushima, T., Morikawa, M., Nakazawa, H. and Sasaki, H. (1994) Capsaicin Desensitization Inhibits Swallowing Reflex in Guinea Pigs. *American Journal of Respiratory and Critical Care Medicine*, **149**, 261-263. http://dx.doi.org/10.1164/ajrccm.149.1.7509247

[21] Jia, Y.X., Sekizawa, K., Ohrui, T., Nakayama, K. and Sasaki, H. (1998) Dopamine D1 Receptor Antagonist Inhibits Swallowing Reflex in Guinea Pigs. *American Journal of Physiology*, **274**, R76-R80.

[22] Holas, M.A., De Pippo, K.L. and Reding, M.J. (1994) Aspiration and Relative Risk of Medical Complications Following Stroke. *Archives of Neurology*, **51**, 1051-1053. http://dx.doi.org/10.1001/archneur.1994.00540220099020

[23] Teasell, R.W., McRae, M., Marchuk, Y. and Finestone, H.M. (1996) Pneumonia Associated with Aspiration Following Stroke. *Archives of Physical Medicine and Rehabilitation*, **77**, 707-709. http://dx.doi.org/10.1016/S0003-9993(96)90012-X

[24] Cappabianca, S., Reginelli, A., Monaco, L., Del Vecchio, L., Di Martino, N. and Grassi, R. (2008) Combined Video Fluoroscopy and Manometry in the Diagnosis of Oropharyngeal Dysphagia: Examination Technique and Preliminary Experience. *La Radiologia Medica*, **113**, 923-940. http://dx.doi.org/10.1007/s11547-008-0290-5

[25] Nagai, H., Russell, J.A., Jackson, M.A. and Connor, N.P. (2008) Effect of Aging on Tongue Protrusion Forces in Rats. *Dysphagia*, **23**, 116-121. http://dx.doi.org/10.1007/s00455-007-9103-6

[26] Surh, Y.J., Lee, E. and Lee, J.M. (1998) Chemoprotective Properties of Some Pungent Ingredients Present in Redpepper and Ginger. *Mutation Research*, **402**, 259-267. http://dx.doi.org/10.1016/S0027-5107(97)00305-9

[27] Dedov, V.N., Tran, V.H., Duke, C.C., Connor, M., Christie, M.J., Mandadi, S. and Roufogalis, B.D. (2002) Gingerols: A Novel Class of Vanilloid Receptor (VR1) Agonists. *British Journal of Pharmacology*, **137**, 793-798. http://dx.doi.org/10.1038/sj.bjp.0704925

[28] Ebihara, T., Takahashi, H., Ebihara, S., Okazaki, T., Sasaki, T., Watando, A., Nemoto, M. and Sasaki, H. (2005) Capsaicin Troche for Swallowing Dysfunction in Older People. *Journal of the American Geriatrics Society*, **53**, 824-828. http://dx.doi.org/10.1111/j.1532-5415.2005.53261.x

[29] Watando, A., Ebihara, S., Ebihara, T., Okazaki, T., Takahashi, H., Asada, M. and Sasaki, H. (2004) Effect of Temperature on Swallowing Reflex in Elderly Patients with Aspiration Pneumonia. *Journal of the American Geriatrics Society*, **52**, 2143-2144. http://dx.doi.org/10.1111/j.1532-5415.2004.52579_3.x

Supplementary Material and Methods
Computed Tomography (CT)

On day 13, CT was performed. Before the experiment, guinea pigs were fasting for 12 hr. The contrast medium used for the experiment consisted of 500 µl of barium sulfate and 200 µl of glucose. Guinea pigs were placed in the box afteroral administration of the contrast medium. CT images were exposed at 1, 3, 5, 9, and 15 min after the administration. The volume of orally administered contrast medium in the stomach and small intestine was measured with OsiriX (OsiriX Foundation, Geneva, Switzerland).

Supplementary Video
Sample Movies of Videofluoroscopic Examination of Swallowing

(A) A sample movie of control group.
https://drive.google.com/file/d/0B0bQSsm7L31aNTRuRDZ1WTNTT1k/view?usp=sharing
(B) A sample movie of haloperidol-treated group.
https://drive.google.com/file/d/0B0bQSsm7L31ab2RLbXBLdmI1Zm8/view?usp=sharing

The number of swallows in haloperidol-treated group was significantly decreased with compared with control group.

Supplementary Figure

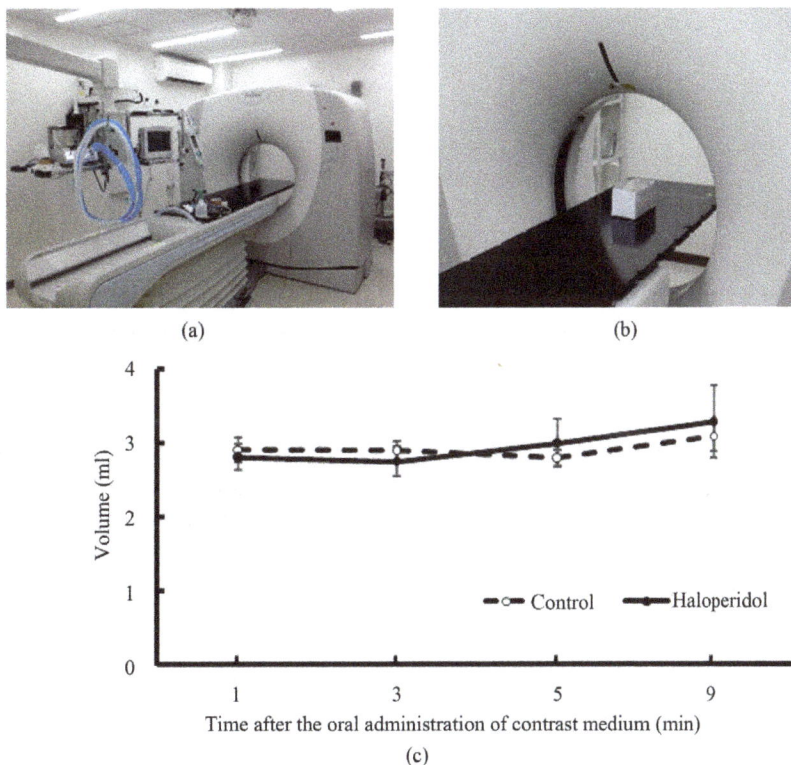

Figure S1. CT in haloperidol-treated guinea pigs. (a) CT machine used for computed tomography (CT); (b) Experimental setup for CT; (c) The volume of orally administered contrast medium in stomach and small intestine. Values are expressed as the mean ± S.E.M. (n = 9).

26

Pharmacokinetics and Tissue Residues of Tylosin in Broiler Chickens

Ahmed M. Soliman[1]*, Mahmoud Sedek[2]

[1]Department of Pharmacology, Faculty of Veterinary Medicine, Cairo University, Giza, Egypt
[2]Department of Poultry and Fish Diseases, Faculty of Veterinary Medicine, Damanhour University, Damanhour, Egypt
Email: *galalpharma@hotmail.com, galalpharma@cu.edu.eg

Abstract

The pharmacokinetics and tissue residue of tylosin in broiler chickens were studied after I.V. and oral administrations in a dose of 50 mg tylosin/kg.b.wt. Tylosin was obeyed a two-compartment open model following I.V. administration at a dose of 50 mg/kg.b.wt. The disposition kinetics of tylosin following I.V. administration revealed that tylosin was highly distributed with $V_{d(area)}$ of 6 L/kg and eliminated with half-life $(t_{1/2\beta})$ equal to 7.29 hours. The disposition kinetics of tylosin following oral administration revealed that the maximum blood concentration (C_{max}) was 3.40 μg/ml attained at (t_{max}) of 1.08 hour. Tylosin was eliminated with half-life $(t_{1/2\beta})$ equal to 5.78 hours. The mean systemic bioavailability of tylosin after oral administration was 90.29%. Following repeated oral administration of 50 mg tylosin base/kg.b.wt once daily for 5 consecutive days, the blood (μg/ml) and tissue (μg/g) residues of tylosin showed that liver, kidney and lung contained the highest tylosin residues and completely disappeared from those tissues at 6 days after the last oral dose. Chickens should not be slaughtered for human consumption within the treatment and 6 days after the last oral administrations of tylosin.

Keywords

Pharmacokinetics, Tylosin, Broiler Chickens, Bioavailability, Tissue Residue

1. Introduction

Antibiotics, normally administrated via food or drinking water, are used by veterinarians for therapy, prophylaxis and growth promotion in broilers and laying hens. As a result there is concern that residues of this drug may be retained in meat or eggs from treated hens. It is therefore essential to obtain data for the target tissues for

---

*Corresponding author.

this drug in chickens [1] [2]. The macrolide antibiotics are a group of structurally similar compounds, most of which are derived from various species of *Streptomyces* soil-borne bacteria [3]. Tylosin is a macrolide antibiotic registered exclusively for veterinary use and was first described by [4]. Tylosin is active against Gram-positive bacteria, anaerobic bacteria and mycoplasmas [5]. It is indicated primarily for the treatment of chronic respiratory disease complex caused by *Mycoplasma gallisepticum* and synoviae in chickens and infectious sinusitis in turkeys [2] [6] [7]. Tylosin, erythromycin and tilmicosin have found the most clinical applications of the macrolide class in veterinary medicine. New derivatives such as azithromycin are increasing in popularity. Other macrolides such as oleandomycin and carbomycin have been used as feed additives for growth promotion in food animals [7]. The antibacterial action of tylosin is due to inhibition of protein synthesis by binding to the 50S, ribosomal subunit of organisms [8] [9]. Although most authors have listed macrolides as bacteriostatic at therapeutic concentrations [10], they can be slowly bactericidal action with time dependent effects [11].

Despite the extensive use of tylosin in poultry industry, limited information is currently available about pharmacokinetic disposition of tylosin in broiler [2]. Accordingly, the main purpose of this study is to investigate and provide an overview of the pharmacokinetics, blood and tissue residues of tylosin in Tylan Soluble® to determine the withdrawal time in healthy broiler chickens.

2. Materials and Methods

2.1. Drugs

Tylan Soluble® (Elanco, UK) is a water soluble powder dispensed as tylosin tartrate 100 g.

2.2. Experimental Design

Ten single comb white leghorn healthy broiler chickens (2 months of age) weighing 2000 - 2250 gm were chosen from Tanta Poultry Farm, Egypt. They were kept individually in cages, within a ventilated, heated room (20°C) and 14 hours of day light. They received a standard commercial ration free from any antibiotics for 30 days before starting the experiment (to withdraw any antibiotic residues) and water *ad libitum*. All procedures involving animals were reviewed and approved by the Institutional Animal Care and Use Committee (IACUC) of Cairo University.

2.3. Pharmacokinetics Study

Ten chickens were used to study the pharmacokinetics of tylosin following intravenous and oral administrations. Chickens were injected intravenously in the left wing vein with 50 mg tylosin base/kg.b.wt (from tylosin tartarate, Sigma Aldrich® according to the product instruction). Chicken were left for 15 days to ensure complete excretion of the tylosin from their bodies and were administered orally (intracrop) with Tylan Soluble® in a dose of 50 mg tylosin base/kg.b.wt.

2.4. Tissue Residues Study

Fifteen clinically normal Hubbard chickens of 2 - 3 months, weighing 1800 - 2200 g were chosen randomly from Tanta Poultry Farm, Egypt. Chicken were fed on a balanced ration free from antibiotic for 2 weeks to withdraw any antibiotic residues.

Tissue residue of tylosin in Tylan Soluble® was determined following repeated oral administrations of 50 mg tylosin base/kg.b.wt once daily for 5 consecutive days. After the end of the fifth day of repeated oral administration, three chickens were slaughtered at 24, 48, 72, 96 and 120 hours for both drugs, respectively.

2.5. Blood and Tissue Samples

One ml of blood was collected from right wing vein after a single intravenous or oral administrations at intervals of 5, 15, 30 minutes, 1, 2, 4, 6, 8, 12 and 24 hours. Blood samples were collected in dry centrifuge tubes. Serum was separated by centrifugation (2000 r.p.m/10 minutes) and stored at −20°C until tylosin assay.

After the end of the fifth day of repeated oral administrations of Tylan Soluble®, three chickens were slaughtered at 24, 48, 72, 96 and 120 hours, from each slaughtered chicken, blood, lung, liver, kidney and muscles were taken for drug assay. Samples were frozen and stored at −20°C until tylosin assay.

2.6. Analytical Procedure

The analytical procedure was described by Arret *et al.*, 1971 [12] and modified by Tsai and Konda, 2001 [13], a cylinder plate diffusion assay technique which used with a single layer of agar medium II (Difco). About 1 ml of the spore suspension of *Bordetella bronchiseptica* (ATCC 4617) obtained from the Department of Microbiology, Faculty of Veterinary Medicine, Cairo University, Egypt. The organism was added to 100 ml agar II (at 55°C - 60°C). The mixture was shacked thoroughly till complete mixing of the test organism with the agar. Petri dishes (120 × 20 mm) with flat ad even bottoms were placed on a levels glass plate, and about 25 ml of inoculated medium was added to each dish by using a sterile cylinder (25 ml capacity) to form a thin layer of uniform thickness. After complete solidification six wells were made on the surface of inoculated agar using stainless steel cylinder with sharp edges (10 ± 0.1 mm length, 8 ± 0.1 mm outside diameter, and 6 ± 0.1 mm inside diameter) careful vertical punching creates ells that were clean and symmetric. A paper grid system under the plate facilitates the even spacing of the wells that allows for triplicate determination of standards and samples.

Three plates were used for each sample; three wells on each plate were filled with the reference concentration (5 μg of tylosin per milliliter free serum or phosphate buffer). The other three wells were filled with the sample (serum or tissues). The plates were incubated at 37°C for 16 - 18 hours. The diameter of each inhibition zone was measured. The average diameter of the inhibition zone of the samples was corrected by using the zone diameter of the reference concentration, the concentration corresponding to the corrected values of the zone diameter was obtained.

2.7. Pharmacokinetic and Statistical Analysis

The pharmacokinetic parameters of tylosin were calculated by using a non-compartmental software program (WinNonlin® software, version 5.2, Pharsight Corporation, NC, USA). The area under the serum concentration-time curve (AUC) was calculated using the trapezoidal rule with extrapolation to infinity. The maximum concentration (C_{max}) and the corresponding peak time (t_{max}) were determined by the inspection of the individual drug serum concentration-time profiles. The slope of the terminal phase of the time-concentration curve was determined by linear regression and converted to an elimination half-life ($t_{1/2\beta}$) by multiplying the reciprocal by 0.693.

2.8. Bioavailability

The rate of absorption after oral administration was determined by comparing the area under the serum concentration-time curve (AUC) oral with that obtained following intravenous injection (AUC) i.v. in the same chicken.

$$\text{Bioavailability} = \frac{(AUC)_{oral} \times D_{i.v}}{(AUC)_{i.v} \times D_{oral}} \times 100$$

where: D_{iv} = Dose of intravenous injection;

D_{oral} = Dose of oral administration.

Data were expressed as X ± SE and were statistically analyzed using analysis of variance. Mean comparisons were performed using Tukey's test. The differences were considered significant when p < 0.05. These calculations were performed using Prism 5.0 (GraphPad).

3. Results

The mean serum concentration-time curve of tylosin in Tylan Soluble® following I.V. and oral administration is plotted and presented graphically in **Figure 1**. The pharmacokinetic parameters of tylosin in Tylan Soluble® following I.V. and oral administration of tylosin 50 mg/kg.b.wt in broiler chickens were calculated and showed in **Table 1, Table 2**. The disposition kinetics of tylosin following I.V. administration revealed that tylosin was highly distributed with $V_{d(area)}$ of 6 L/kg and eliminated with half-life ($t_{1/2\beta}$) equal to 7.29 hours. The disposition kinetics of tylosin in Tylan Soluble® following oral administration of 50 mg/kg.b.wt tylosin base/kg.b.wt revealed that the maximum blood concentration [C_{max}] was 3.40 μg/ml and attained at [t_{max}] of 1.08 hours. Tylosin in Tylan Soluble® was eliminated with half-life [$t_{1/2\beta}$] equal to 5.78 hours. The mean systemic bioav-ailability of tylosin following oral administration in broiler chickens was 90.29%. The oral bioavailability of Tylan Soluble®

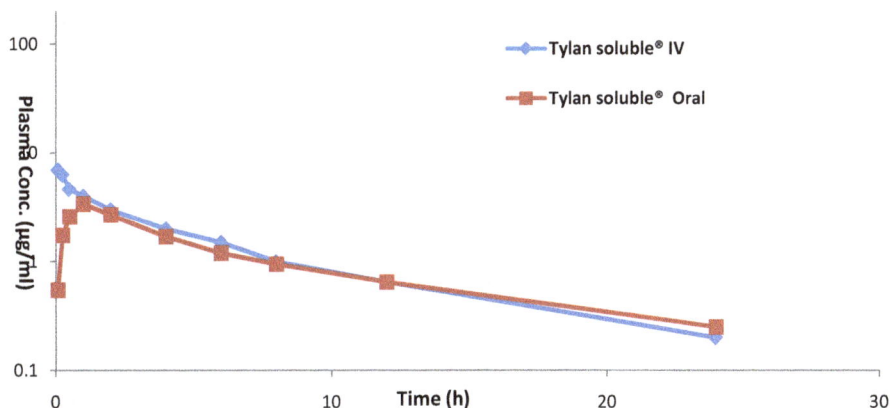

Figure 1. Semilogarthimic plot showing the serum concentrations-time profile of tylosin in Tylan Soluble® following intravenous and oral administration in broiler chickens (n = 10).

Table 1. Pharmacokinetic parameters of tylosin in Tylan Soluble® following I.V. administration of 50 mg tylosin base/kg.b.wt in broiler chickens (n = 10), mean ± S.E.

Parameters	Unit	Tylan Soluble®
C^0	µg/ml	4.50 ± 0.25
$t_{1/2\alpha}$	h	0.385 ± 0.08
V_c	L/kg	2.60 ± 0.15
$V_{d(area)}$	L/kg	6.00 ± 0.65
V_{dss}	L/kg	5.30 ± 0.40
K_{12}	h^{-1}	0.77 ± 0.05
K_{21}	h^{-1}	0.82 ± 0.05
$t_{1/2\beta}$	h	7.29 ± 0.75
Cl_B	L/kg/h	0.005 ± 0.008
$AUC_{0-\infty}$	µg·h/ml	20.60 ± 2.05

C^0 = Drug concentration in serum at zero time immediately after a single intravenous injection; $AUC_{0-\infty}$ = area under the concentration-time curve from zero up to ∞ with extrapolation of the terminal phase; $t_{1/2\beta}$ = half-life of the elimination; V_c = volume of the central compartment; Vd_{area} = Volume calculated by the area method; V_{dss} = apparent volume of distribution at steady-state; Cl_B = clearance from the body. K_{12} = First order transfer rate constant for drug distribution from central to peripheral compartment ; K_{21} =First order transfer rate constant for drug distribution from peripheral to central compartment.

Table 2. Pharmacokinetic parameters of tylosin in Tylan Soluble® following oral administration of 50 mg tylosin base/kg.b.wt in broiler chickens (n = 10), Mean ± S.E.

Parameters	Unit	Tylan Soluble®
k_{ab}	h^{-1}	3.60 ± 0.65
$t_{1/2ab}$	h	0.19 ± 0.08
$t_{1/2\beta}$	h	5.78 ± 0.50
$t_{max.}$	h	1.08 ± 0.20
$C_{max.}$	µg/ml	3.40 ± 0.25
Cl_B	L/kg/h	0.002 ± 0.005
AUC	µg·h/ml	18.60 ± 1.50
Bioavailability	%	90.29 ± 2.10

C_{max} = maximal concentration; t_{max} = when the maximal serum concentration is reached; AUC_{0-t} = area under serum concentration-time curve; $t_{1/2\beta}$ = Elimination half-life; K_{ab} = first-order absorption rate constant; $t_{1/2ab}$ = The absorption half-life (h).

Table 3. Blood levels (µg/ml) and tissue concentrations (µg/g) of tylosin in Tylan Soluble® following repeated oral administrations of 50 mg tylosin base/kg.b.wt once daily for five consecutive days in broiler chickens (n = 3), Mean ± S.E.

Blood and tissues	Time after the last dose (hours)					
	24	48	72	96	120	144
Blood	3.85 ± 0.16	1.40 ± 0.09	0.35 ± 0.01	N.D	N.D	N.D
Lung	39.0 ± 3.37	21.0 ± 1.78	8.35 ± 0.75	1.0 ± 0.05	N.D	N.D
Liver	42.0 ± 4.11	26.0 ± 3.18	13.0 ± 1.11	4.0 ± 0.50	1.0 ± 0.04	N.D
Kidney	55.0 ± 5.93	33.0 ± 4.48	16.0 ± 2.59	7.0 ± 0.46	2.0 ± 0.06	N.D
Muscles	15.0 ± 1.13	6.0 ± 1.25	2.0 ± 0.45	0.50 ± 0.03	N.D	N.D

N.D = Not detected. After the end of the fifth day of repeated oral administrations, three chickens were slaughtered at 24, 48, 72, 96, 120 and 144 hours.

indicated a good absorption from GIT which indicated that this formulation is advised to be given orally in case of acute systemic bacterial infections.

Blood and tissue residues of tylosin in Tylan Soluble® in slaughtered chickens following repeated oral administrations of 50 mg/kg.b.wt tylosin base/kg.b.wt once daily for 5 consecutive days are recorded in **Table 3**. The represented data revealed a good spread distribution of tylosin in Tylan Soluble® in lung, liver, kidney and muscles.

4. Discussion

Antibiotics are widely used as veterinary drugs or as feed additives to promote growth. Some studies had induced pharmacokinetic data in poultry [14]-[19]. Tylosin was obeyed a two compartments open model following I.V. administration at a dose of 50 mg/kg.b.wt. This result is consistent with [20]. Tylosin in Tylan Soluble® was highly distributed with great extent to all tissues V_c, $V_{d\ area}$ and V_{dss}; (exceeded one liter/kg). This correlated with the rapid transfer of tylosin from central compartment to the peripheral one (k_{12}) than its passage from peripheral to the central compartment (k_{21}) [21] [22]; a factor revealed that tylosin is the drug of choice for attacking the systemic infections caused by sensitive organisms.

Tylosin in Tylan Soluble® following IV administration obeyed a two compartments-open model. This indicated that tylosin distributed in the body of chicken in two compartments; a central one which represent blood and highly perfused organs (kidney-liver-spleen-heart) and a 2nd peripheral compartment which represented by skin and connective tissues [2] [23].

The disposition kinetics of tylosin in Tylan Soluble® following oral administration of 50 mg tylosin/kg.b.wt revealed that the maximum blood concentration [$C_{max.}$] were 3.40 µg/ml and attained at [t_{max}] of 1.08 hours and was eliminated with half-lives ($t_{1/2\beta}$) equal to 5.78 hours. These results are consistent with those recorded in cows [24] and some avian species [25]-[27]. The higher volume of distribution of tylosin was also recorded in chickens [2] [22].

The mean systemic bioavailability of tylosin in Tylan Soluble® following oral administration was 90.29%. [2] and [28] stated that tylosin had good absorption from the GIT and no enteric coating is required to maintain the stability of the compound in the stomach. It is widely distributed to basically the same tissues as described for tylosin, metabolized by the liver and excreted via the bile and feces.

Blood and tissue residues of tylosin in Tylan Soluble® in slaughtered chickens following repeated oral administrations of 50 mg tylosin/kg.b.wt once daily for 5 consecutive days revealed a wide spread distribution of tylosin in Tylan Soluble® in lung, liver, kidney, muscles. Liver, kidney and lung contained the highest drug residues, while the lowest concentration showed in blood. Tylan Soluble® was completely cleared from blood and all tissues at 5 days (120 hours) after the last dose. These data were consistent with those reported by [17].

[29] concluded and recommended that microbiological ADI of 6 µg/kg.b.wt (360 µg per 60 kg person) was established for tylosin.

Tylosin residues in Tylan Soluble® was the MRLs approved by [30]. These results are consistent with those investigated in broiler chickens [2] [22] [26].

5. Conclusion

The oral bioavailability of tylosin in Tylan Soluble® indicated a good absorption from GIT. This indicated that Tylan Soluble® is advised to be given orally in case of acute bacterial attacks in blood and other organs. In addition, chickens should not be slaughtered for human consumption within the treatment and 6 days after the last oral administration of tylosin in Tylan Soluble®.

Acknowledgements

The authors would like to express their sincere gratitude to Dr. Ahmed Samir (Department of Microbiology, Faculty of Veterinary Medicine, Cairo University) for his great effort in preparation of microbial suspension and helping in the bio-assay technique in this project.

Conflict of Interests

The author declares that there is no conflict of interests regarding the publication of this paper.

References

[1]   Furusawa, N. (1999) Spiramycin, Oxytetracycline and Sulphamono-Methoxine Contents of Eggs and Egg-Forming Tissues of Laying Hens. *Journal of Veterinary Medicine Series A*, **46**, 599-603. http://dx.doi.org/10.1046/j.1439-0442.1999.00247.x

[2]   Kowalski, C., Rolinski, Z., Zan, R. and Wawron, W. (2002) Pharmacokinetics of Tylosin in Broiler Chickens. *Polish Journal of Veterinary Science*, **5**, 127-130.

[3]   Scott, P.R., McGowan, M., Sargison, N.D., Penny, C.D. and Lowman, B.G. (1996) Use of Tilmicosin in a Severe Outbreak of Respiratory Disease in Weaned Beef Calves. *Australian Veterinary Journal*, **73**, 62-64. http://dx.doi.org/10.1111/j.1751-0813.1996.tb09967.x

[4]   Stark, W.M., Daily, W.A. and McGuire, J.M. (1961) A Fermentation Study of the Biosynthesis of Tylosin in Synthetic Media. *Scientific Report of the Istituto Superiore di Sanita*, **1**, 340-354.

[5]   Giguere, S. (2006) Lincosamindes, Macrolides, and Pleuromutilins. In: *Antimicrobial Therapy in Veterinary Medicine*, 4th Edition, Wiley Blackwell, Ames, 179-190.

[6]   Montesissa, C., DeLiguoro, M., Santi, A., Capolongo, F. and Biancotto, G. (1999) Tylosin Depletion in Edible Tissues of Turkeys. *Food Additives and Contaminants*, **16**, 405-410. http://dx.doi.org/10.1080/026520399283795

[7]   Kong, K., Yuan, Z., Fan, S., Wang, D., Qin, I.T., Zhou, S., Yang, E. and Cai, J. (1999) HPLC Analysis of Erythromycin Residues in Broiler Tissues. *Chinese Journal of Veterinary Science*, **19**, 489-491.

[8]   Musser, J., Mechor, G.D., Grohn, Y.T., Dubovi, E.J. and Shin, S. (1996) Comparison of Tilmicosin with Long-Acting Oxytetracyline for Treatment of Respiratory Tract Disease in Calves. *Journal of the American Veterinary Medical Association*, **208**, 102-106.

[9]   Gaynor, M. and Mankin, A.S. (2005) Macrolide Antibiotics: Binding Site, Mechanism of Action, Resistance. *Frontiers in Medicinal Chemistry*, **2**, 21-35. http://dx.doi.org/10.2174/1567204052931113

[10] Wilson, R.C. (1984) Macrolides in Veterinary Medicine. In: Omura, S., Ed., *Macrolide Antibiotics. Chemistry, Biology, and Practice*, Academic Press, Inc., 301-347.

[11] Carbon, C. (1998) Pharmcodynamics of Macrolides, Azalides, and Streptogramins: Effect on Extracellular Pathogens. *Clinical Infectious Disease*, **27**, 28-32. http://cid.oxfordjournals.org/content/27/1/28.full.pdf http://dx.doi.org/10.1086/514619

[12] Arret, B., Johnson, D.P. and Kirshbaum, A. (1971) Outline of Details for Microbiological Assay of Antibiotics. 2nd Revision. *Journal of Pharmaceutical Sciences*, **60**, 1689-1694. http://dx.doi.org/10.1002/jps.2600601122

[13] Tsai, G.E. and Kondo, F. (2001) Improved Agar Diffusion Method for Detecting Residual Antimicrobial Agents. *Journal of Food Protection*, **64**, 361-366.

[14] Yoshida, M., Kubota, D., Yonezawa, S., Nakamura, H., Azechi, H. and Terakado, N. (1971) Transfer of Dietary Spiramycin into the Eggs and Its Residue in the Liver of Laying Hen. *Japan Poultry Science*, **8**, 103-110. https://www.jstage.jst.go.jp/article/jpsa1964/8/2/8_2_103/_pdf http://dx.doi.org/10.2141/jpsa.8.103

[15] Yoshida, M., Kubota, D., Yonezawa, S., Nakamura, H., Yamaoka, R. and Yoshimura, H. (1973) Transfer of Dietary Erythromycin into the Eggs and Its Residue in the Liver of Laying Hen. *Japan Poultry Science*, **10**, 29-36. http://dx.doi.org/10.2141/jpsa.10.29

[16] Roudaut, B., Moretain, J.P. and Biosseau, J. (1987) Excretion of Oxytetracycline in Egg after Medication of Laying Hens. *Food Additives and Contaminants*, **4**, 297-307. http://dx.doi.org/10.2141/jpsa.10.29

[17] Roudaut, B. and Moretain, J.P. (1990) Residues of Macrolide Antibiotics in Eggs Following Medication of Laying Hens. *British Poultry Science*, **31**, 661-675. http://dx.doi.org/10.1080/00071669008417297

[18] Yashimura, M., Osawa, D., Rasa, F.C.S., Hermawati, D., Werdiningsihi, S., Isriyanthi, N.M.R. and Sugimoto, T. (1991) Residues of Doxycycline and Oxytetracycline in Eggs after Medication via Drinking Water to Laying Hens. *Food Additives and Contaminants*, **8**, 65-69. http://dx.doi.org/10.1080/02652039109373956

[19] Omija, B., Mittema, E.S. and Maitho, T.E. (1994) Oxytetracycline Residue Levels in Chicken Eggs after Oral Administration of Medicated Drinking Water to Laying Hens. *Food Additives and Contaminants*, **11**, 641-647. http://dx.doi.org/10.1080/02652039409374265

[20] Ji, L.-W., Dong, L.-L., Ji, H., Feng, X.-W., Li, D., Ding, R.-L. and Jiang, S.-X. (2014) Comparative Pharmacokinetics and Bioavailability of Tylosin Tartrate and Tylosin Phosphate after a Single Oral and i.v. Administration in Chickens. *Journal of Veterinary Pharmacology and Therapeutics*, **37**, 312-315. http://dx.doi.org/10.1111/jvp.12092

[21] Burrows, G.E., Barto, P.B., Martin, B. and Tripp, M.L. (1983) Comparative Pharmacokinetics of Antibiotics in Newborn Calves: Chloramphenical, Lincomycin and Tylosin. *American Journal of Veterinary Research*, **44**, 1053-1057.

[22] Atef, M., El-Gendi, A.Y.I., Amer, A.M. and Kamel, G.M. (2009) Pharmacokinetic Assessment of Tylosin Concomitantly Administered with Two Anticoccidials; Diclazuril and Halofuginone in Broiler Chickens. *Advances in Environmental Biology*, **3**, 210-218. http://www.insipub.com/aensi/aeb/2009/210-218.pdf

[23] Atef, M., Youssef, S.A., Atta, A.H. and El-Maaz, A.A. (1991) Disposition of Tylosin in Goats. *British Veterinary Journal*, **147**, 207-215. http://dx.doi.org/10.1016/0007-1935(91)90045-O

[24] Gingerich, D., Baggot, J. and Kowalski, J. (1977) Erythromycin Antimicrobial Activity and Pharmacokinetics in Cows. *Canadian Veterinary Journal*, **18**, 96-100.

[25] Locke, D., Bush, M. and Carpenter, J.W. (1982) Pharmacokinetics and Tissue Concentrations of Tylosin in Selected Avian Species. *American Journal of Veterinary Research*, **43**, 1807-1810.

[26] Cezary, K. and Malgorzata, P. (2006) Evaluation of Bioequivalence of Two Tylosin Formulations after Oral Administration in Broiler Chickens. *ANNALES*, **3**, 25-29.

[27] Abu-Basha, E.A., Al-Shunnaq, A.F. and Gehring, R. (2012) Comparative Pharmacokinetics and Bioavailability of Two Tylosin Formulations in Chickens after Oral Administration. *Journal of the Hellenic Veterinary Medical Society*, **63**, 159-165.

[28] Ziv, G. and Sulman, F.G. (1973) Passage of Polymyxins from Serum into Milk in Ewes. *American Journal of Veterinary Research*, **34**, 317-322.

[29] European Agency for the Evaluation of European Medicines Agency (EMEA) (2002) Committee for Veterinary Medicinal Products (Tylosin) Extension to Eggs; Summary Report (4). The European Agency for the Evaluation of Medicinal Products; London.

[30] European Agency for the Evaluation of European Medicines Agency (EMEA) (2000) Committee for Veterinary Medicinal Products (Tylosin) Extension to Eggs; Summary Report (4). The European Agency for the Evaluation of Medicinal Products; London. http://www.ema.europa.eu/docs/en_GB/document_library/Maximum_Residue_Limits_-_Report/2009/11/WC500015767.pdf

27

Evaluation of the Use of Ketamine for Acute Pain in the Emergency Department at a Tertiary Academic Medical Center

Nahal Beik[1*], Katelyn Sylvester[1], Megan Rocchio[1], Michael B. Stone[2]

[1]Department of Pharmacy, Brigham and Women's Hospital, Boston, USA
[2]Department of Emergency Medicine, Brigham and Women's Hospital, Boston, USA
Email: *nbeik@partners.org

Abstract

Introduction: At subdissociative doses of 0.1 - 0.5 mg/kg, ketamine provides effective analgesia when used alone or as an adjunct to opioid analgesics without causing cardiovascular or respiratory compromise. Ketamine is a beneficial analgesic agent in the emergency department (ED), particularly in patients with opioid-resistant pain or polytrauma patients who are hemodynamically unstable. Purpose: The purpose of this study was to evaluate current practice and describe clinical outcomes associated with the use of low-dose ketamine for acute pain in the ED. Methods: Adult patients receiving ketamine were retrospectively evaluated between March 1, 2012 and March 31, 2013. Patients were included if they were ordered for ketamine in the ED to treat acute pain. Outcomes included dose administered, cumulative doses, concurrent opioid administration, and any efficacy or adverse events documented after the administration of ketamine. Continuous variables are reported as mean (standard deviation [SD]) or median (interquartile range [IQR]). Results: A total of 46 patients were evaluated for inclusion. Of the 25 patients included, 38 doses of ketamine were documented. The mean age was 41 years old with 64% of the patients being female. The average initial ketamine dose was 0.12 ± 0.06 mg/kg and 8 (32%) patients received multiple doses of ketamine (1.5 ± 0.8 doses per patient). Ketamine was added to opioid therapy in 23 (92%) patients. Pain scores decreased post administration of ketamine from 10 (9 - 10) to 5 (4 - 7). Adequate pain relief was documented in 11 (44%) patients (felt comfortable going home); partial pain relief was noted in 5 (20%) patients; 3 (12%) patients reported no pain relief; 3 (12%) patients were able to have a procedure done, and efficacy was not documented in 3 (12%) patients. Anxiety and agitation were documented in 2 (8%) patients. No adverse outcomes were documented in 84% of patients. Conclusion: Administration of low-dose ketamine for acute pain in the ED demonstrated improvement in patients' pain scores with minimal documented adverse outcomes.

---

*Corresponding author.

Keywords

Ketamine, Acute Pain, Emergency Department

1. Introduction

Pain remains one of the most common chief complaints for adults presenting to emergency departments (ED) nationwide. Chest pain, abdominal pain, back pain, headache and injuries are cited as the top five reasons for ED presentation based on national ED survey data from 2006 and 2011 [1] [2]. These same data report that approximately half of all patients presenting to the ED describe their pain as moderate (25%) or severe (20.4%) [1]. Depending on the nature and severity of pain, the standard of care for initial treatment of pain in the ED involves using non-specific analgesics such as a non-steroidal anti-inflammatory agent or an opioid [3].

For some patients, complex past medical histories and concomitant disease states render standard approaches inadequate to treat their pain. In such cases, an alternative analgesic agent such as ketamine should be considered. Ketamine has been shown to be a beneficial analgesic agent in the ED, particularly in patients with opioid-resistant pain (sickle-cell crisis, chronic pain such as cancer and palliative care) or trauma patients who are hemodynamically unstable [3] [4]. The use of ketamine in the ED has been viewed as favorable by both patients and ED physicians [5].

Ketamine is a potent noncompetitive N-methyl-D-aspartate (NMDA) antagonist, best known for its anesthetic properties. At standard doses, it produces profound and rapid anesthesia and analgesia with minimal to no respiratory or hemodynamic compromise and has a predictable duration of action with a relatively short elimination half-life [6] [7]. At subdissociative doses of 0.1 - 0.5 mg/kg, ketamine provides effective analgesic properties, when used alone or as an adjunct to opioid analgesics, with less pronounced psychoactive effects [5] [8]. Additionally, ketamine has a wide margin of safety minimizing the concern for accidental overdose [6]. For these reasons, low-dose ketamine has gained favor as an option for pain management in the ED as reflected by the increased volume of research published in emergency medicine literature over recent years.

At our institution, intravenous (IV) ketamine use is restricted by indication and service, and may be ordered and administered by ED attending physicians for analgesia associated with uncontrolled, incident pain [9]. The purpose of this study was to evaluate current practices and prescribing patterns of ketamine in our ED and to describe clinical outcomes associated with the use of low-dose ketamine for acute pain in the ED.

2. Methods

This was a single-center, retrospective, descriptive analysis of clinical practice of adult patients admitted to our ED who received ketamine for acute pain. Our institutional review board reviewed and approved the study protocol prior to data collection.

Patients were identified between March 1, 2012 and March 31, 2013 via a report generated from the ED Order Entry system. To be included in the analysis, patients had to be >18 years of age and received at least one dose of ketamine for acute pain. Patients were excluded if they received ketamine in the ED for a non-pain indication or if ketamine was ordered but not administered.

Investigators collected data retrospectively, and demographic data collected included age, gender, ethnicity, comorbidities, ketamine indication, home opioid use, and baseline vitals. Outcomes assessed included doses administered, total cumulative doses, concurrent opioid administration, additional therapies used for the treatment of acute pain, and any documented efficacy and safety endpoints in patient charts. Efficacy endpoints were defined as documentation of decreased pain scores and patient reported pain relief after ketamine administration. We assessed safety endpoints by reviewing notes in the patient chart for documentation of patient reported events directly related to ketamine administration as well as medication records for the use of benzodiazepines post ketamine administration as a surrogate for serious behavioral disturbance.

3. Results

During the study timeframe, 46 patients were evaluated for inclusion. Twenty-one patients were excluded: ketamine was ordered and discontinued (7 patients); ketamine was used during rapid sequence intubation (8 patients); ketamine was used for deep procedural sedation (6 patients). A total of 25 patients (54.3%) were included in the final analysis. Demographic information is outlined in **Table 1**. The majority of our patients was opioid tolerant (80%) and presented to the ED with a chief complaint of pain (92%). The top three pain presentations were traumatic pain related to motor vehicle crash or fall (30.4%), abdominal pain (21.7%) and oncology pain (17.4%). Ketamine was prescribed by 10 different emergency medicine attendings.

The mean initial ketamine dose was 0.12 ± 0.06 mg/kg and 8 patients (32%) received multiple doses of ketamine (1.5 ± 0.8 doses per patient). Dosing regimens are outlined in **Table 2**. Ketamine was used as the initial therapy in 5 patients (20%). Ketamine was used concomitantly with opioids in 23 patients (92%).

Table 1. Patient demographics.

Variable	Patients (n = 25)
Age, years*	41 ± 11
Gender—male**	9 (36.0)
Weight, kg*	76.2 ± 20
Ethnicity**	
White	19 (82.6)
Hispanic	3 (13.0)
African American	1 (4.3)
Comorbidities**	
Hypertension	9 (36.0)
End-stage renal disease	1 (4.0)
Congestive heart failure	1 (4.0)
Diabetes	3 (12.0)
Malignancy	7 (28.0)
Tobacco use	9 (36.0)
Alcohol/illicit drug use	11 (44.0)
Indication**	
Pain	23 (92.0)
Traumatic pain	7 (30.4)
Abdominal pain	5 (21.7)
Oncology pain	4 (17.4)
Incision and drainage/abscess	3 (13.0)
Lower extremity pain	2 (8.7)
Back pain	1 (4.3)
Neuropathic pain	1 (4.3)
Sickle cell crisis	1 (4.0)
Back spasms	1 (4.0)
Home opioid use**	20 (80.0)
Baseline vitals*	
Blood pressure, mmHg	135.8/78 ± 20.5/19.8
Heart rate, beats per minute	95.4 ± 16.8
Temperature, F	97.8 ± 1.1
Respiratory rate, breaths per minute	18.5 ± 2.6
Oxygen saturation, %	97.5 ± 1.9
Admitted	15 (60.0)
Attending physicians prescribing	10

*Mean ± SD; **n (%).

Table 2. Ketamine therapy.

Variable	Patients (n = 25)
Ketamine doses administered	38
Initial ketamine dose, mg/kg*	0.12 ± 0.06
Multiple doses administered—patients**	8 (32.0)
Mean doses per patient, mg*	1.5 ± 0.8
Total ketamine administered, mg	520.6
Cumulative dose per patient, mg*	13.2 ± 5.2
Ketamine as initial therapy**	5 (20)
Concomitant therapies**	
Opioids	23 (92)
Benzodiazapines^	7 (28)
Prior to ketamine	5 (71.4)
Simultaneous administration	1 (14.3)
Post ketamine	1 (14.3)
Other^⋈	2 (8)
Pain scores	
Pre ketamine‡	10 (9 - 10)
Post ketamine‡	5 (4 - 7)

*Mean ± SD; **n (%); ‡ Median (IQR); ⋈ Diphenhydramine, tizanidine administered; ^1 patient received post ketamine.

In terms of efficacy, 11 patients (44%) reported adequate pain relief and 5 patients (20%) reported partial pain relief, and 3 patients (12%) reported no pain relief. Efficacy was not documented in 3 patients (12%), and the remaining 3 patients (12%) reported tolerable relief (**Figure 1**).

Subsequent reports of anxiety and agitation were documented on 2 patients (8%) and 1 patient received a benzodiazepine post ketamine administration. There was no documentation of adverse outcomes in 84% of patients (**Figure 2**). Of the 5 patient self-reported adverse events documented, there was 1 instance of feeling weird, 1 instance of feeling anxious, and 1 patient was still in pain. Although there was no documentation of unstable vital signs, there were 2 documented cases of stable vital signs. Of the 25 patients treated with ketamine for pain, 10 patients were discharged from the ED to home (40%).

4. Discussion

The mainstay of treatment for severe acute pain in the ED is IV opioids, and although opioids can provide effective and rapid pain relief, doses needed to achieve adequate pain relief may result in over sedation and respiratory depression [10]. Ketamine is a recognized anesthetic and short-acting analgesic that has been in use for over 30 years [11]. It has a remarkable safety profile and is one of the world's most commonly used agents for procedural sedation and general anesthesia [11]. Since ketamine is an NMDA receptor antagonist, it is a logical choice for controlling pain as well as inducing anesthesia [6] [7]. At subdissociative doses of 0.1 - 0.5 mg/kg, ketamine provides effective analgesic properties with little to no dissociative effects [5] [8]. Studies evaluating the benefit of low-dose ketamine for acute pain have produced favorable results for this indication, however, optimal dosing, specific patient populations, and additional efficacy and safety outcomes (e.g. single bolus vs. repeat dosing, need for rescue analgesia) have not been evaluated [4] [5] [8] [10]-[13].

Low-dose ketamine therapy was studied by Beaudoin, *et al.* [10], evaluating 60 adult patients with acute pain who presented to the ED. Patients were randomized to receive low-dose ketamine as an adjunct to morphine versus standard care with morphine alone. The dosing for ketamine was either 0.15 mg/kg or 0.3 mg/kg. The investigators of the study found that low-dose ketamine is a viable analgesic adjunct to morphine for the treatment of moderate to severe acute pain based on patient-reported pain scores, and that the dosing of 0.3 mg/kg is possibly more effective than 0.15 mg/kg, but may be associated with minor adverse events, such as dysphoria and dizziness.

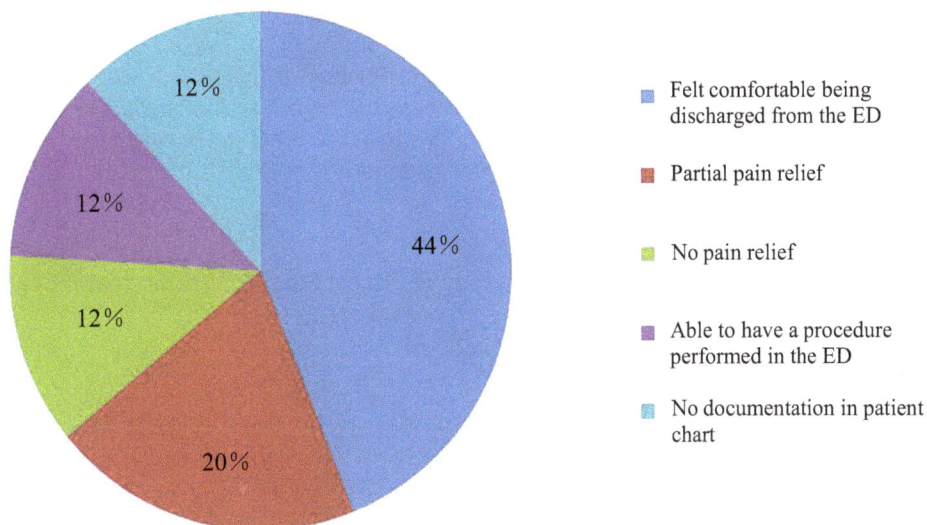

Figure 1. Efficacy data.

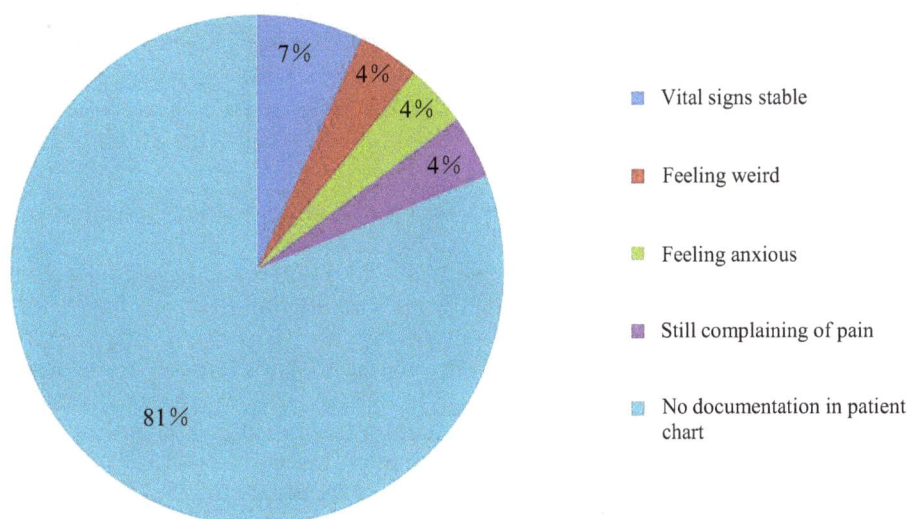

Figure 2. Safety data.

Our study is similar to the study by Beaudoin, *et al.* in that an improvement in patients' pain scores with minimal adverse events was noted. Our analysis contributes to the literature by further discussing the practice of low-dose ketamine administration at a tertiary academic medical center and describes the prescribing practices at this institution. In our experience, ketamine is not used as a first line agent and is typically used after opioid therapy has been ineffective. The patient population that received ketamine included those who were opioid tolerant. Despite the limited number of patients who received ketamine as a first line therapy, this population may benefit from receiving ketamine as a first line treatment option or earlier in their treatment plan. Our analysis differs from the Beaudoin, *et al.* since the mean ketamine dose used in our analysis was lower than the ketamine dose used in the Beaudoin, *et al.* study, which reflects the current practice of our prescribers and may optimize pain control with a lower incidence of adverse effects. Further studies are needed to determine the ideal dose of ketamine.

We acknowledge several limitations in our study; this was a single center, descriptive, retrospective study and has the associated limitations of this design. The retrospective nature of this study may have caused some data to be missed due to inconsistent documentation that was retrospectively reviewed. The sample size is small, and there was inconsistent documentation between the ED Order Entry system and paper medical record documentation and lack of documented safety outcomes.

5. Conclusion

Ketamine, administered at low doses, resulted in an improvement of patients' pain scores while maintaining vital signs. When taking into account the minimal amount of documented adverse outcomes in this patient cohort, ketamine has shown to be a safe and effective option for acute pain relief in the emergency department either as first line therapy or as rescue therapy after opioid administration.

Disclosures

This research was presented in part at the 2014 Society of Critical Care Medicine's Annual Congress in Phoenix, AZ.

References

[1] Pitts, S.R., Niska, R.W., Xu, J. and Burt, C.W. (2008) National Hospital Ambulatory Medical Care Survey: 2006 Emergency Department Summary. *National Health Statistics Reports*, **2**, 1-39.

[2] Weiss, A.J., Wier, L.M., Stocks, C. and Blanchard, J. (2011) Overview of Emergency Department Visits in the United States. HCUP Statistical Brief #174. Agency for Healthcare Research and Quality, Rockville. http://www.hcup-us.ahrq.gov/reports/statbriefs/sb174-Emergency-Department-Visits-Overview.pdf

[3] Thomas, S.H. (2013) Management of Pain in the Emergency Department. *ISRN Emergency Medicine*, **2013**, Article ID: 583132. http://dx.doi.org/10.1155/2013/583132

[4] Herring, A.A., Ahern, T.L., Stone, M.S. and Frazee, B.W. (2013) Emerging Applications of Low-Dose Ketamine for Pain in the ED. *American Journal of Emergency Medicine*, **31**, 416-419. http://dx.doi.org/10.1016/j.ajem.2012.08.031

[5] Richards, J.R. and Rockford, R.E. (2013) Low-Dose Ketamine Analgesia: Patient and Physician Experience in the ED. *American Journal of Emergency Medicine*, **31**, 390-394. http://dx.doi.org/10.1016/j.ajem.2012.07.027

[6] (2013) Ketamine Package Insert. Hospira, Inc.

[7] Haas, D.A. and Harper, D.G. (1992) Ketamine: A Review of Its Pharmacologic Properties and Use in Ambulatory Anesthesia. *Anesthesia Progress*, **39**, 61-68.

[8] Ahern, T.L., Herring, A.A., Stone, M.S. and Frazee, B.W. (2013) Effective Analgesia with Low-Dose Ketamine and Reduced Dose Hydromorphone in ED Patients with Severe Pain. *American Journal of Emergency Medicine*, **31**, 847-851. http://dx.doi.org/10.1016/j.ajem.2013.02.008

[9] (2005) Ketamine Drug Administration Guideline. Brigham and Women's Hospital. Approved by the Pharmacy and Therapeutics Committee.

[10] Beaudoin, F.L., Lin, C., Guan, S. and Merchant, R.C. (2014) Low-Dose Ketamine Improves Pain Relief in Patients Receiving Intravenous Opioids for Acute Pain in the Emergency Department: Results of a Randomized, Double-Blind, Clinical Trial. *Academic Emergency Medicine*, **21**, 1194-1202. http://dx.doi.org/10.1111/acem.12510

[11] Schmid, R.L., Sandler, A.N. and Katz, J. (1999) Use and Efficacy of Low-Dose Ketamine in the Management of Acute Postoperative Pain: A Review of Current Techniques and Outcomes. *Pain*, **82**, 111-125. http://dx.doi.org/10.1016/S0304-3959(99)00044-5

[12] Ahern, T.L., Herring, A.A., Anderson, E.S., Madia, V.A., Fahimi, J. and Frazee, B.W. (2015) The First 500: Initial Experience with Widespread Use of Low-Dose Ketamine for Acute Pain Management in the ED. *American Journal of Emergency Medicine*, **33**, 197-201. http://dx.doi.org/10.1016/j.ajem.2014.11.010

[13] Sin, B.S., Ternas, T. and Motov, S.M. (2015) The Use of Subdissociative-Dose Ketamine for Acute Pain in the Emergency Department. *Academic Emergency Medicine*, **22**, 251-257. http://dx.doi.org/10.1111/acem.12604

Abbreviations

ED: Emergency Department.
SD: Standard Deviation.
IQR: Interquartile Range.

28

Sphaeranthus indicus: Traditional Wisdom to Modern Medicine—An Orally Active, Potent Cytokine Inhibitor for the Management of Inflammatory Disorders

Jacqueline Trivedi, Firuza Kharas, Sapna Parikh, Roda Dalal, Aurelio Lobo, Lyle Fonseca, Mahesh Jadhav, Shruta Dadarkar, Asha Almeida, Ankita Srivastava, Ashish Suthar[*]

Department of Herbal Development, Piramal Life Sciences India Limited, Mumbai, India
Email: [*]ashish.suthar@piramal.com

Abstract

Tumor necrosis factor (TNF-α) is a key regulator of the inflammatory and tissue destructive pathways in rheumatoid arthritis (RA). The clinical success of anti-TNF-α and anti-IL-17 biologics has validated the concept that cytokine blockade is beneficial in RA. However, as these drugs are parenterally administered, our efforts are directed at identifying a novel orally active TNF-α inhibitor with a therapeutic profile similar to that of biologics. Since plants are natural immunomodulators, we explored the immunomodulatory potential of *Sphaeranthus indicus* extract. In our studies, the extract dose-dependently inhibited the release of cytokines in stimulated human peripheral blood mononuclear cells (hPBMCs), and their spontaneous release in synovial cells derived from patients suffering from RA. TNF-α and IFN-γ induced release of p40 subunit of IL-12/IL-23, and p19 subunit of IL-23 in differentiated THP-1 cells is potently blocked. The expression of endothelial cell adhesion molecules in TNF-α-stimulated HUVECs was also potently inhibited. The oral treatment significantly and dose-dependently reduced LPS-induced TNF-α and IL-1β production in mice. Disease regression was seen in collagen-induced arthritis in DBA/1J mice, which was validated along with radiological and histopathological evaluation. Therefore, the extract of *Sphaeranthus indicus* could be used in the management of inflammatory conditions.

Keywords

Sphira, Rheumatoid Arthritis, Psoriasis, Cytokine Inhibition

---

[*]Corresponding author.

1. Introduction

Immune mediated inflammatory disease is a group of unrelated inflammatory conditions that share common inflammatory pathways. This definition encompasses disorders as diverse as rheumatoid arthritis (RA), inflammatory bowel disease (IBD), psoriatic arthritis (PsA), type 1 diabetes, multiple sclerosis, vasculitis, ankylosing spondylitis (AS), and juvenile chronic arthritis (JCA). Treatment of these conditions incurs substantial costs to patients and society at large. Numerous cytokines have been identified in such diseased tissues across a range of immune mediated inflammatory diseases. Since then, cytokine mediated strategy is one of the most successful remedial efforts that have resulted in regression of IMIDs. One such example is RA.

In the case of RA, laboratory and preclinical animal model studies in the late 1980s and early 1990s identified tumor necrosis factor-α (TNF-α) as a key pathogenic molecule [1]. Data from numerous clinical trials, initially with the anti-TNF agents infliximab and etanercept [2] and later with adalimumab [3], have confirmed the validity of TNF-α as a therapeutic target in RA. The success of clinical trials in RA has prompted investigation of the therapeutic efficacy of anti-TNF-α agents in several other immune-mediated inflammatory diseases in which its pathogenicity has been implicated.

In a psoriatic skin plaque, there is a predominance of interferon-γ, IL-2, IL-12, IL-17 and IL-23 [4]. TNF-α is expressed in the epidermis and dermis and potentially contributes to the accumulation of inflammatory cells in these tissues by inducing expression of intercellular adhesion molecule-1 (ICAM-1) on endothelial cells and keratinocytes [5]. The validity of TNF-α as a therapeutic target in psoriasis has been confirmed in double-blind, placebo-controlled randomized trials using the anti-TNF agents etanercept (25 mg or 50 mg twice weekly) and infliximab (5 mg/kg) [6] [7], where patients have experienced a rapid and high degree of clinical benefit. Recent data on IL-17 and IL-23 have indicated that these cytokines also play a significant role in inducing and maintaining the inflammatory nexus in skin lesions of psoriatic patients. Clinical data emerging with antibodies directed towards each of these cytokines have shown marked disease regression and better efficacy than with anti-TNF-α antibodies [8] [9]. Hence, modern approaches towards therapeutic enhancement of inflammatory diseases include targeting both cytokines, and combinatorial approaches involving TNF-α and IL-17.

Plant sterols and sterolins are natural immunomodulators found in some raw fruits and vegetables and in the alga, spirulina. *S. indicus* is a well-known Indian herb known as Gorakhmundi, Mundi or Munditika, which is also known to have immuno-modulatory as well as anti-inflammatory activities. According to Ayurvedic literature, *S. indicus* is useful in bronchitis, tuberculosis, elephantiasis, anemia, inflammatory conditions of pelvis in women, asthma and glandular swelling in the neck [10] [11]. In our approach to explore the anti-inflammatory potential of this plant, we have initiated studies to evaluate the holistic extracts prepared from fruiting and flowering bodies and their active constituents for anti-TNF activity by using various pharmacological models *in vitro* and *in vivo*.

2. Materials and Methods

2.1. Extraction and Preparation of Sphira (NPS31807)

The extraction and preparation of *S. indicus* was performed as described previously [12]. Various extracts were evaluated for their anti-TNF activity. The methanolic extract was found to be the most potent (data not shown). This extract was further evaluated for its anti-inflammatory potential, and will henceforth be referred to as Sphira (NPS31807).

2.2. *In Vitro* Screening of Sphira for Its Anti-Inflammatory Potential

The anti-inflammatory potential of Sphira was evaluated using various *in vitro* screening models of inflammation. Blood was collected from healthy donors after obtaining Independent Ethics Committee approval and written informed consent. Briefly, peripheral blood was collected in potassium EDTA vacutainer tubes (BD Biosciences). hPBMC were isolated by density gradient centrifugation using Histopaque-1077 solution (Sigma Aldrich; St. Louis, MO). Isolated hPBMC were re-suspended in Rosewell Park Memorial Institute (RPMI) 1640 culture medium (Sigma Aldrich) containing 10% heat inactivated fetal bovine serum (FBS; JRH), 100 U/ml penicillin (Sigma Chemical Co.; St. Louis, MO) and 100 μg/ml streptomycin (Sigma Chemical Co.). The hPBMCs were uniformly plated in 96-well tissue culture plates at a seeding density of 1×10^6 cells/ml. Cells were then treated to different concentrations of Sphira (0.03 - 100 μg/ml) dissolved in DMSO (the final concentration of

DMSO maintained at 0.5%), or 0.5% DMSO (control), and incubated for 30 minutes. Incubation in all the *in vitro* screening assays was in a humidified atmosphere at 37°C, 5% CO_2.

Cytokine release assay: This assay measures LPS-induced cytokine release from hPBMCs, specifically to evaluate TNF-α inhibition. The procedure followed was similar to that described previously [13]. After being exposed to the test compounds, 1 µg/ml LPS (*Escherichia coli* 0127:B8, Sigma Chemical Co., St. Louis, MO) was added per well to stimulate cytokine production. The cells were further incubated for 5 h, following which supernatants were collected, stored at −70°C and assayed later for TNF-α, IL-1β, IL-6 and IL-8 by ELISA (OptiEIA ELISA sets, BD Biosciences, Pharmingen). In all experiments, a parallel plate was run to ascertain the toxicity of test extracts. The toxicity was determined using the MTS (3-(4,5-dimethylthiazol-2-yl)-5-(3-carboxymethoxyphenyl)-2-(4-sulfonyl)-2H-tetrazolium) reagent.

IL-17 release assay: After treatment with test compounds, the cells were stimulated with 25 ng/ml of PMA (phorbol 12-myristate 13-acetate; SIGMA) and 1 µM ionomycin. The plates were further incubated for 48 h, after which the supernatant from the cells were collected and ELISA was performed to detect the levels of IL-17.

2.3. Evaluation of Sphira in Synovial Cells from RA Patients

The ability of Sphira to inhibit the spontaneous release of cytokines from freshly isolated human synovial tissue cells was determined in a manner similar to that described by Brennan *et al.* [14]. After informed consent and Independent Ethics Committee approval, synovial tissue was obtained from RA patients undergoing knee replacement surgery. The tissue was minced and digested in RPMI medium containing 100 U/ml penicillin-G, 100 µg/ml streptomycin, 50 ng/ml amphotericin B (GIBCO), 1.33 mg/ml collagenase Type I (Worthington Biochemical Corporation, New Jersey), 0.5 µg/ml DNase Type I (Sigma Aldrich) and 8.33 U/ml heparin (Biological E. Limited, India) for 3 h at 37°C, 5% CO_2. Isolated cells were uniformly plated in 96-well tissue culture plates at a seeding density of 1×10^6 cells/ml and exposed to various concentrations of Sphira (0.03 - 100 µg/ml) dissolved in DMSO. The plates were incubated for 16 h. Subsequently, the supernatants were harvested and stored at −70°C. The amounts of TNF-α, IL-1β, IL-6 and IL-8 in the supernatants were assayed using OptiEIA ELISA sets (BD BioSciences Pharmingen). The protocol followed was as per manufacturer's instructions.

2.4. *In Vitro* Screening of Sphira for Its Anti-Psoriatic Potential

The anti-psoriatic potential of Sphira was evaluated in an *in vitro* screening model targeting p40, a subunit shared by human interleukin-12 and human Interleukin-23 (IL-12/IL-23 p40). Differentiated THP-1 cells were treated with varying concentrations of Sphir aranging from 0.1 to 100 µg/ml, and later on with a combination of TNF-α and IFN-γ. The levels of IL-12/IL-23p40, IL-23p19 and IL-12p70 were estimated by ELISA [15].

2.5. NFκB Transcription Assay

CEM-κB (a kind gift from Dr. Shigeki Miyamoto, University of Wisconsin, Madison, WI) is a CEM cell line transfected with κB binding element linked to green florescence protein (GFP) promoter. CEM-κB was maintained in RPMI-1640 supplemented with 10% FBS and 0.1% G418 (Sigma Aldrich). The experiment was done as described previously [16]. Briefly, the cells were seeded at a density of 50,000 cells/ml, in a 6-well plate. The cells were treated with 0.1, 0.5, 1, 3, 10 and 30 µg/ml of Sphira dissolved in DMSO, 0.5% DMSO (vehicle control) or BAY 11-7082, an IKKα inhibitor (positive control), and incubated for 30 minutes. The cells were then stimulated with 0.5 ng/ml TNF-α and incubated for 16 h. After 16 h, the shift in NFκB expression was measured using BD FACS Calibur. The GFP fluorescence measured is directly proportional to NFκB expression.

2.6. Evaluation of Sphira for Its Potential to Affect Cell Adhesion Molecules

The surface expression of endothelial cell adhesion molecules was quantified using cell ELISA, as described previously [17]. Briefly, confluent HUVECs (Cascade biologics) in 96-well fibronectin-coated plates were pretreated with various concentrations of Sphira for 30 minutes, before being stimulated with 1 ng/mL TNF-α for the indicated time. The expressions of ICAM-1 and VCAM-1 were evaluated after TNF-α stimulation for 4 h, and expression of E-selectin was evaluated after 6 h of stimulation. The cells were fixed with 1% paraformaldehyde and blocked using bovine serum albumin (2% in DPBS). The cells were then washed and incubated with monoclonal mouse anti-human ICAM-1, VCAM-1, E-selectin or the isotype control mouse IgG1 for 2 - 4 h at

4°C. Subsequently, cells were washed and incubated with a horseradish peroxidase-conjugated goat anti-mouse IgG for 90 minutes. Binding of the secondary antibody was determined by incubating with 3, 3, 5, 5' tetramethylbenzidine (TMB) substrate and then terminating the reaction by 2N sulphuric acid. Surface expression of adhesion molecules was quantified by measuring absorbance at 490 nm in an automated microtitre plate reader.

Monocytic cells and endothelial cell adhesion assay: The human monocytic leukemia cell line, THP-1 was used as a model for monocytic cells. Leukocyte adhesion assays were performed under static conditions as previously described by Kim HK [18], with minor modifications. Briefly, THP-1 cells were labeled with BCECF-AM in serum-free RPMI 1640 media for 30 minutes at RT in the dark, then washed with DPBS to remove surplus dye and suspended in M200 medium. Confluent HUVEC monolayers were pretreated with various concentrations of Sphira for 30 minutes, prior to 4 h exposure to 1 ng/mL TNF-α. Labeled THP-1 (6×10^5 cells/ml) were seeded onto control or treated HUVECs, and incubated for 10 minutes at RT in the dark. The unbound cells were removed by gentle washing with medium and the images were obtained at 485 nm excitation and 538 nm emission using a NIKON Eclipse 80i fluorescence microscope. For adhesion quantification, THP-1 cells bound to HUVECs were lysed with 0.1% Triton-X-100 in 0.1 M Tris buffer, pH 8.8, and fluorescence intensity was measured by a spectrofluorometer with emission at 520 nm and excitation at 485 nm. Adherent cells were quantified using standard curves of BCECF and expressed as % adhesion of added cells. Furthermore, a duplicate set of flasks were kept aside and counterstained with hematoxylin to simultaneously evaluate the morphology of HUVECs and monocytic cells.

2.7. Anti-Inflammatory Effect of the Oral Formulation of Sphira in Balb/c Mice

To evaluate the anti-inflammatory effect of Sphira, the "Inhibition of Lipopolysaccharide (LPS)-induced TNF-α release in BALB/c mice" model was used. All animal experiments were approved by Institutional Animal Ethics Committee of Piramal Life Sciences Limited. The procedure followed is as described in Moreira, AL [19]. Balb/c mice (procured from The Jackson Laboratory, U.S.A.) of either sex weighing between 18 - 22 g (n = 10) were orally administered Sphira at a dose of 30, 100 and 300 mg/kg. All suspensions were freshly prepared in 0.5% CMC. One hour later, LPS (1 and 2 mg/kg, i.p. for TNF-α and IL-1β release, respectively) (*Escherichia coli*, serotype 0127:B8, Sigma Chemical Co., St. Louis, MO) dissolved in sterile pyrogen-free saline was administered intra-peritoneally to the control group, standard treatment group (Rolipram, 30 mg/kg, p.o.) and test groups (Sphira), except the negative control group which received only normal saline. Post LPS-challenge (1.5 h for TNF-α and 4 h for IL-1β), blood samples were collected from anesthetized mice, with heparin as an anti-coagulant (25 IU per sample), centrifuged at 10,000 rpm for 10 min, and the resultant plasma samples were analyzed for levels of cytokines by ELISA, as described by the manufacturer (OptiEIA ELISA sets, BD BioSciences Pharmingen). Percent inhibition of TNF-α and IL-1β release was calculated by comparing the levels of the treatment groups with those of the control group.

2.8. Anti-Arthritic Activity of Sphira in Collagen-Induced Arthritis Model

The anti-arthritic potential of Sphira was evaluated using collagen-induced arthritis mouse model in a manner similar to that described previously [20]. Male DBA/1J mice (procured from The Jackson Laboratory, U.S.A.), aged 8 - 10 weeks were immunized with an emulsion equivalent to 200 µg of type II collagen in Freund's Complete Adjuvant, injected intra-dermally at the base of the tail. A booster shot with the same emulsion was given 21 days later. Sphira was tested in the therapeutic regime, from day 23 following primary immunization. Mice were examined once daily for signs of RA, using the articular index and paw thickness as parameters. Articular index scoring was performed employing the following criteria:

Scoring for forelimbs: Scale 0-3, where, 0: No redness or swelling; 1: Redness, but no swelling; 2: Redness and swelling of the paw; 3: Redness and severe swelling of the paw. *Scoring for hind limbs*: Scale 0-4, where, 0: No redness or swelling; 1: Redness and mild swelling of paw; 2: Redness and moderate swelling of paw and/or swelling of at least one of the digits; 3: Redness and moderate/severe swelling of paw, swelling of ankle joint and/or swelling of one or more digits; 4: Redness and severe swelling of paw, digits and ankle joint, with joint stiffness and altered angle of digits.

Mice with a minimum hind paw score of 2 were inducted into the study. Mice were randomized into the various study groups and orally administered the vehicle (0.5% CMC, 1 ml/kg), test compound (Sphira, 600 mg/kg, twice daily) or standard compound (Enbrel, 3 mg/kg, s.c., once daily). Each group had a minimum of 8 - 10 mice. The dosing of the compounds was done for 13 days. Parameters such as body weight, articular index, paw thickness (in mm, using a tension-free caliper) and any significant observation regarding the condition of the animal were observed and recorded daily. On the last day, 1 h after the compound treatment, the animals were sacrificed, blood withdrawn, and plasma collected for drug level analysis. Also, the limbs of all the animals were preserved for histopathological evaluations.

Histological analysis: Mice were humanely euthanized and the hind paws were harvested from each animal, fixed in 10% neutral buffered formalin, decalcified in 10% EDTA and embedded in paraffin. Section were stained with either hematoxylin and eosin or safranin O and evaluated microscopically. Histopathological changes were scored as follows: mild (score = 1), moderate (score = 2) or severe (score = 3) for the parameters of cellular infiltration, bone erosions and cartilage damage, graded separately. Cartilage depletion was indicated visually by diminished safranin O staining of proteoglycan matrix. The mean total score was compared to that of vehicle treated group. In case of histological scoring, Kruskal-Wallis analysis was followed by Dunn's multiple comparison tests to evaluate the statistical difference between two groups. Values of $P < 0.05$ were considered significant.

2.9. Statistical Analysis

All statistical analysis were performed by Student's t-test, where $^{*}P < 0.05$, $^{**}P < 0.01$, $^{***}P < 0.001$, were considered statistically significant.

3. Results

3.1. Sphira Inhibits the Release of Cytokines in LPS-Induced hPBMC

The anti-inflammatory potential of methanolic extract of *S. indicus* was confirmed *in vitro*. Sphira was studied in 12 donors at eight different concentrations (0.3 - 100 µg/ml) in LPS-induced TNF-α, IL-1β, IL-6 and IL-8 release in hPBMCs. It was observed that it dose-dependently inhibits the release of LPS-induced TNF-α (IC_{50} 4.31 ± 0.78 µg/ml), IL-1β (IC_{50} 1.96 ± 0.56 µg/ml), IL-6 (IC_{50} 10.17 ± 10.47 µg/ml) and IL-8 (IC_{50} 28.33 ± 2.97 µg/ml) in hPBMCs. It was also found to be non-toxic at the doses tested (**Figure 1(A)**). Thus, our data clearly demonstrated that the extract could significantly modulate inflammatory cytokine secretion from monocyte-macrophage lineage in the advent of LPS mediated stimulatory signals.

3.2. Sphira Inhibits IL-17 Production in hPBMCs Stimulated with PMA-Ionomycin

To study the effect of the extract on T-cell mediated cytokines such as IL-17, hPBMC were treated with different doses of Sphira, and the supernatant evaluated for secreted IL-17 levels in presence of PMA-ionmycin stimulus. The effect of the extract on the viability of these cells was also measured simultaneously. It is well demonstrated that Sphira blocked IL-17 (IC_{50} 2.1 ± 0.67 µg/ml) and TNF-α (IC_{50} 1.8 ± 0.9 µg/ml) production by PMA-ionomycin stimulated hPBMCs. The extract did not have any toxic manifestations on normal resting cells, but effectively blocked proliferation of stimulated cells (**Figure 1(C)**).

3.3. Sphira Inhibits the Release of Cytokines in Synovial Cells Isolated from RA Patients

Sphira was evaluated at eight different concentrations in synovial cells obtained from RA patients undergoing knee replacement surgery [14]. This study was performed in 10 donors. The extract inhibited the spontaneous release of TNF-α (IC_{50} 13.10 ± 3.19 µg/ml), IL-1 β (IC_{50} 5.33 ± 1.76 µg/ml), and IL-6 (IC_{50} 16.33 ± 2.91 µg/ml) in a dose-dependent manner, in synovial cells. It was found to be toxic at the highest concentration (100 µg/ml) (**Figure 1(B)**).

3.4. Sphira Inhibits the Release of IL-12/IL-23 p40 and IL-23 p19 from TNF-α and IFN-γ Stimulated THP-1 Cells

Anti-IL-12/23 antibodies have successfully been targeted to the common IL-12p40 subunit; both cytokines are implicated in inflammatory diseases. Ustekinumab and ABT-874, inhibitors of IL-12p40, have shown efficacy in psoriasis [21] [22]. Our studies show that Sphira potently inhibits the release of IL-12/IL-23 p40 (IC_{50} 1.0 ±

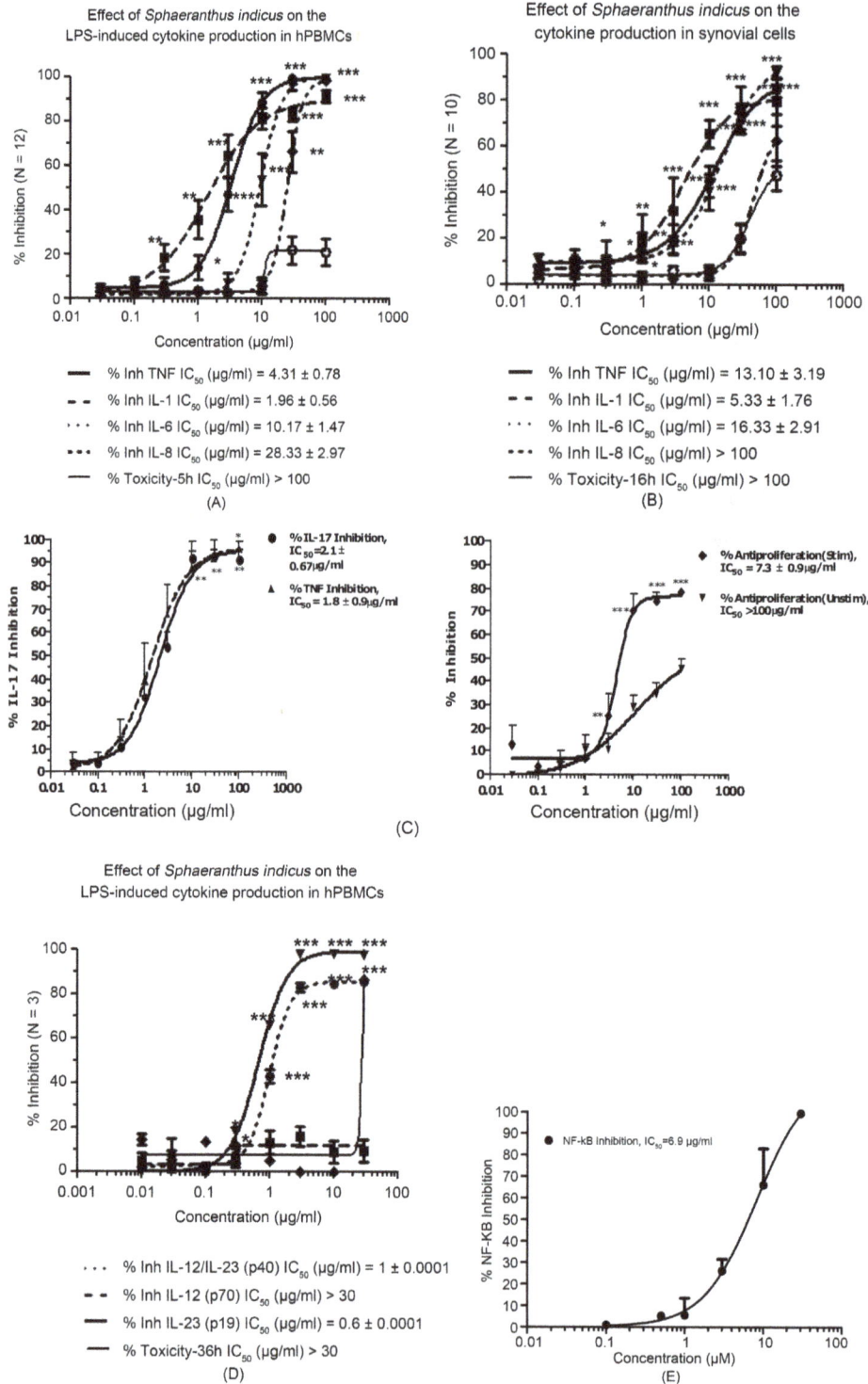

Figure 1. Sphira potently inhibits pro-inflammatory cytokine release. (A) Pretreatment with Sphira induced a concentration dependent reduction in levels of TNF-α, IL-1β, IL-6 and IL-8 in LPS stimulated hPBMCs; (B) Sphira inhibits the spontaneous release of cytokines from synovial cells isolated from RA patients; (C) Pretreatment with Sphira induced a concentration dependent reduction in levels of IL-17 in PMA + ionomycin stimulated hPBMCs; (D) Sphira inhibits the release of IL-12/IL-23 p40 and IL-23 p19 from TNF-α and IFN-γ stimulated THP-1 cells; (E) Sphira inhibits TNF-α induced NFκB activation in CEM cell line transfected NFκB promoter. The graph represents the percent inhibition (mean ± SD). Statistical significance was associated with *P < 0.05, **P < 0.01, ***P < 0.001.

0.0001 µg/ml) and IL-23 p19 (IC$_{50}$ 0.6 ± 0.0001 µg/ml), with no toxicity up to the highest concentration tested (**Figure 1(D)**).

3.5. Sphira Inhibits TNF-α Induced NFκB Activation in CEM Cell Line Transfected NFκB Promoter

NF-κB is an important transcription factor required for T-cell proliferation and other immunological functions. Sphira dose dependently inhibited NFκB activation (IC$_{50}$ 6.9 µg/ml) in TNF-α stimulated CEM-κB cells (**Figure 1(E)**).

3.6. Sphira Decreases the Cell Surface Expression of ICAM-1, VCAM-1 and E-Selectin in TNF-α-Stimulated HUVECs

As cell adhesion molecules play an important role during inflammation, we analyzed the effect of different concentrations of Sphira on TNF-α-induced cell surface expression of these molecules. In accordance with previous studies, ICAM-1 and E-selectin were expressed at low levels in unstimulated HUVECs, but their expression increased after TNF-α stimulation (data not shown). As shown in **Figure 2(A)**, Sphira, at the highest concentration of 10 µg/mL, significantly inhibited the expression of TNF-α-induced ICAM-1 (61% ± 14%), VCAM-1 (69% ± 8%) and E-selectin (90% ± 7%) respectively. The IC$_{50}$ values of ICAM-1, VCAM-1 and E-selectin expression

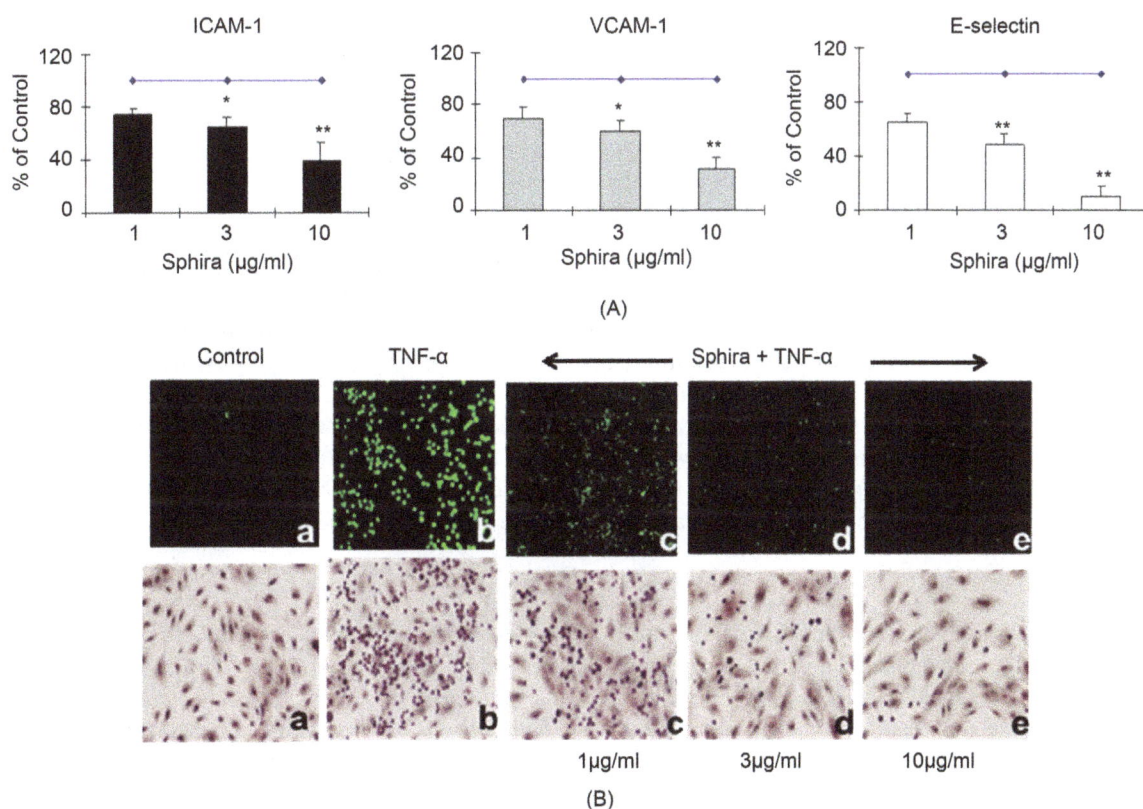

(A)

(B)

Figure 2. Sphira potently inhibits the expression of cell adhesion molecules. (A) The expression of ICAM-1, VCAM-1 and E-selectin in TNF-α-stimulated HUVECs determined by cell ELISA. HUVECs were pretreated with Sphira (1, 3 and 10 µg/mL) for 30 min, followed by TNF-α stimulation (1 ng/mL) for 4 h (ICAM-1, E-selectin) and 6 h (VCAM-1). Data are expressed as the mean ± SEM of 6 experiments (VCAM-1) and 4 experiments (ICAM-1 and E-selectin) in triplicates. *P < 0.05 and **P < 0.01, as compared with TNF-α -stimulated HUVECs; (B) Upper panel: Representative fluorescence photomicrographs showing effects of Sphira on TNF-α induced adhesion of BCECF-labeled human monocytic cells to HUVECs (40×). Lower panel: Bright-field images showing the population of intact endothelial cells and bound monocytic cells counterstained with hematoxylin (100×). (a) Untreated control HUVEC; (b) HUVECs stimulated by TNF-α; (c)-(e) HUVECs treated with 1, 3 and 10 µg/ml Sphira, followed by TNF-α stimulation (1 ng/ml).

were 7.6, 3.7 and 2.9 µg/ml, respectively. Taken together, these findings indicate that Sphira specifically inhibits the cytokine-induced expression of ECAMs in a dose-dependent manner.

3.7. Sphira Inhibits the Binding of THP-1 Cells to TNF-α-Stimulated HUVECs

The functional significance of inhibition of cell adhesion molecules was evaluated by analyzing the adhesion of monocytic cells to endothelial cells in the presence of Sphira (**Figure 2(B)**). Unstimulated confluent HUVEC monolayers exhibited minimal binding to THP-1 (**Figure 2(B)**, Panel a). However, there was a marked increase in the THP-1 cell adherence to HUVECs treated with TNF-α (**Figure 2(B)**, Panel b). Pretreatment of confluent HUVECs with Sphira (1, 3 and 10 µg/mL) drastically inhibited THP-1 adhesion to HUVECs in a dose-dependent manner (**Figure 2(B)**, Panels c-e), with maximum inhibition at 10 µg/mL ($P < 0.01$; n = 5). By counterstaining with hematoxylin, the bright-field images (100×) show that the morphology of HUVECs was maintained, and monocytic cells were shown to be intact in each individual condition (**Figure 2(B)**, lower panel). These results demonstrate that Sphira is effective in blocking adhesion of THP-1 to endothelial cells by inhibiting the TNF-α-induced expression of ICAM-1, VCAM-1 and E-selectin.

3.8. Sphira Extract Inhibits the Release of Cytokines in the *in Vivo* LPS Model of Inflammation

The anti-inflammatory effect of oral formulations of Sphira was evaluated in the *in vivo* LPS model of inflammation [23]. Percent inhibition of TNF-α and IL-1β release was calculated by comparing the cytokine levels in the Sphira-treated groups with those of the control group. Dose-dependent inhibition of cytokine release was noted (**Figure 3(A)**).

3.9. Sphira Extract Arrests Collagen-Induced Arthritis When Administered Orally in the Therapeutic Regimen

The extract was evaluated in a chronic model of arthritis, *i.e.* the well-established mouse collagen-induced arthritis (CIA) model. As reported earlier [24], the CIA in DBA/1J mice was manifested with significant increases in paw thickness and articular index, and these clinical signs of arthritic disease were significantly reduced in mice receiving Sphira 600 mg/kg, orally, twice daily (**Figure 3(B)**). Histological analyses of paw tissues of diseased mice treated with placebo revealed severe destruction in the joints characterized by synovitis, pannus formation, articular cartilage erosion and pronounced infiltration of inflammatory cells invading bony cortex at multiple foci (**Figure 3(C)**). In contrast, the hind paws of treated mice (either with 600 mg/kg Sphira orally, or Enbrel) showed maintenance of joint architecture with diminished pannus formation and reduced infiltration of inflammatory cells (**Figure 3(C)**). The degree of macroscopic protection provided by Sphira 600 mg/kg, p.o., was statistically similar to the protection demonstrated by Enbrel treated with placebo control (**Figure 3(C)**).

4. Discussion

All drugs which modify immune response are generally categorized as immunomodulators. Since plants are known to be immunomodulators, we investigated the methanolic extract of *S. indicus* (Sphira) for its immunomodulatory potential. Our data clearly demonstrates that Sphira robustly treats CIA by selectively inhibiting a spectrum of signal transduction pathways central to the pathogenesis of RA. Sphira abrogates multiple cytokines from human peripheral blood mononuclear cells as well as human RA synovial cells. Abrogation of these cytokines is mediated by mitigating NF-κB activation, which is a transcription factor central to all inflammatory signaling cascades. Sphira potently inhibits diverse cellular responses that play critical roles in driving synovitis, pannus formation, and joint destruction in RA, and hence exerts a multitude of responses which are successful in protecting against inflammation.

In the synovial cells of patients with RA, activation of the NF-κB pathway results in the transactivation of a multitude of responsive genes that contribute to the inflammatory phenotype, including TNF-α from macrophages, matrix metalloproteinases from synovial fibroblasts and chemokines that recruit immune cells to the inflamed pannus [25]. Using CEM cell line transfected NFκB promoter, we demonstrated that Sphira inhibits TNF-α-induced NFκB activation.

The destruction of synovial tissue in RA is mediated by cytokines and matrix metalloproteinases produced by

(A)

(B)

(C)

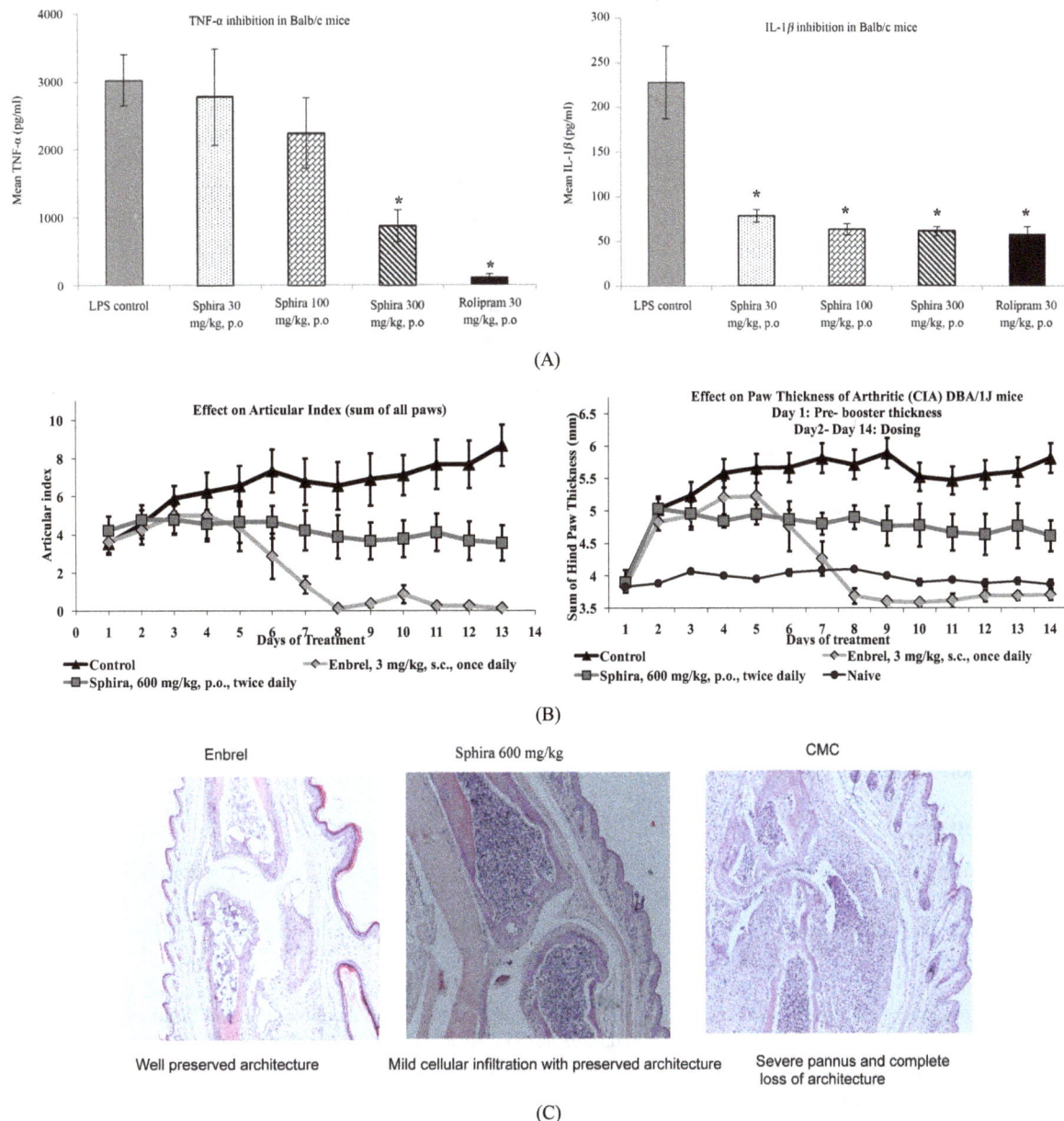

Figure 3. Effect of Sphira in *in vivo* models of inflammation. (A) Sphira inhibits the release of cytokines in the *in vivo* LPS model of inflammation: Sphira was orally administered 1 hr before LPS challenge. Plasma levels of TNF-α and IL-1β were evaluated by ELISA. Data represents mean ± SEM (n = 10). Statistical evaluation was performed by Student's t-test. Statistical difference was observed between control and treated mice, where *P < 0.05; (B) Sphira treats CIA: Following the development of clinical arthritis (average visual arthritis score of 4), DBA/1J mice with CIA were randomized and treated with placebo (n = 10), 600 mg/kg Sphira (n = 10), or 3 mg/kg enbrel (n = 10). The disease was monitored using a visual arthritis scoring system and paw thickness measurements. Values from the presented results are the mean ± SEM for this representative experiment. *P < 0.05, **P < 0.01, ***P < 0.001 compared with placebo-treated mice; (C) Histological effects of Sphira in CIA: The vehicle control shows extensive pannus formation. Enbrel treated mice show well-preserved joint architecture. Sphira treated mice (600 mg/kg, p.o., twice daily) show mild cellular infiltration and a preserved architecture, comparable to Enbrel.

macrophages and fibroblasts, and seems to be controlled by lymphocytes. Activation, circulation, and migration of mononuclear cells to inflammatory sites are regulated by adhesion molecules such as ICAM-1, VCAM-1, or E-selectin [26]. Therefore, cell adhesion molecules (CAMs) and endothelial growth factors have an important role in the infiltration of rheumatoid synovium with mononuclear cells and seem to play a part in the initiation and progression of the disease. In our study, we have shown that Sphira inhibited the expression of cell adhesion molecules, thus implying its protective role in RA.

Evidence shows that IL-17 is present at sites of inflammatory arthritis and that, in synergistic interactions, it amplifies the inflammation induced by other cytokines, primarily TNF-α. In several animal models of arthritis, inhibition of IL-17 limits inflammation and joint erosion. Initial observations from phase I trials show that signs and symptoms of RA are significantly suppressed following treatment with anti-IL-17 antibodies, without notable adverse effects [27]. Our studies showed that Sphira inhibits IL-17 production in hPBMCs stimulated with PMA-ionomycin. Sphira also inhibits IL-6, TGF-β and IL-1β induced IL-17 production and accumulation in CD4+ T-cells (data not shown). mRNA expression studies done showed that Sphira inhibits Th17 differentiation markers in normal CD4 cells like IL-17A, IL-21 and IL-22 (data not shown).

In vivo studies in mice using the CIA model showed that treatment with Sphira reduced arthritic clinical score and paw swelling significantly. Histopathologic analysis was performed on hind paws harvested from mice receiving Sphira. The evaluation, by an investigator blinded to treatment group, demonstrated that Sphira resulted in statistically significant reductions in synovitis, pannus, and erosion scores in established CIA treatment.

In addition to potentially providing benefit in RA, it is anticipated that Sphira could also provide efficacy in other autoimmune diseases like psoriasis, as exhibited by our experiments which show a reduction in expression of IL-12/IL-23. Previous studies done at our research center has shown that Sphira inhibits the inflammatory, migratory and proliferative activity in keratinocytes and immune cells [12].

5. Conclusion

In conclusion, we have shown that Sphira potently treats CIA and inhibits multiple signal transduction pathways that drive pathogenic cellular responses in RA. Our results provide further rationale for prospective clinical trials to determine whether Sphira provides efficacy in RA and other autoimmune diseases.

Conflict of Interest

The authors declare no commercial or financial conflict of interest.

References

[1]   Feldmann, M. (2008) Many Cytokines Are Very Useful Therapeutic Targets in Disease. *The Journal of Clinical Investigation*, **118**, 3533-3536. http://dx.doi.org/10.1172/JCI37346

[2]   Taylor, P.C. (2001) Anti-TNF Therapy for Rheumatoid Arthritis and Other Inflammatory Diseases. *Molecular Biotechnology*, **19**, 153-168. http://dx.doi.org/10.1385/mb:19:2:153

[3]   Weinblatt, M.E., Keystone, E.C., Furst, D.E., Moreland, L.W., Weisman, M.H., Birbara, C.A. and Teoh, L.A. (2003) Adalimumab, a Fully Human Anti-Tumor Necrosis Factor α Monoclonal Antibody, for the Treatment of Rheumatoid Arthritis in Patients Taking Concomitant Methotrexate: The ARMADA Trial. *Arthritis & Rheumatism*, **48**, 35-45. http://dx.doi.org/10.1002/art.10697

[4]   Uyemura, K., Yamamura, M., Fivenson, D.F., Modlin, R.L. and Nickoloff, B.J. (1993) The Cytokine Network in Lesional and Lesion-Free Psoriatic Skin Is Characterized by a T-Helper Type 1 Cell-Mediated Response. *Journal of Investigative Dermatology*, **101**, 701-705. http://dx.doi.org/10.1111/1523-1747.ep12371679

[5]   Ettehadi, P., Greaves, M., Wallach, D., Aderka, D. and Camp, R. (1994) Elevated Tumour Necrosis Factor-Alpha (TNF-α) Biological Activity in Psoriatic Skin Lesions. *Clinical & Experimental Immunology*, **96**, 146-151. http://dx.doi.org/10.1111/j.1365-2249.1994.tb06244.x

[6]   Mease, P.J., Goffe, B.S., Metz, J., Vander Stoep, A., Finck, B. and Burge, D.J. (2000) Etanercept in the Treatment of Psoriatic Arthritis and Psoriasis: A Randomised Trial. *The Lancet*, **356**, 385-390. http://dx.doi.org/10.1016/S0140-6736(00)02530-7

[7]   Reich, K., Nestle, F.O., Papp, K., Ortonne, J.-P., Evans, R., Guzzo, C., Li, S., Dooley, L.T. and Griffiths, C.E. (2005) Infliximab Induction and Maintenance Therapy for Moderate-to-Severe Psoriasis: A Phase III, Multicentre, Double-Blind Trial. *The Lancet*, **366**, 1367-1374. http://dx.doi.org/10.1016/S0140-6736(05)67566-6

[8]   Leonardi, C., Matheson, R., Zachariae, C., Cameron, G., Li, L., Edson-Heredia, E., Braun, D. and Banerjee, S. (2012) Anti-Interleukin-17 Monoclonal Antibody Ixekizumab in Chronic Plaque Psoriasis. *New England Journal of Medicine*, **366**, 1190-1199. http://dx.doi.org/10.1056/NEJMoa1109997

[9]   Yeilding, N., Szapary, P., Brodmerkel, C., Benson, J., Plotnick, M., Zhou, H., Goyal, K., *et al.* (2011) Development of the IL-12/23 Antagonist Ustekinumab in Psoriasis: Past, Present, and Future Perspectives. *Annals of the New York*

Academy of Sciences, **1222**, 30-39. http://dx.doi.org/10.1111/j.1749-6632.2011.05963.x

[10] Rohit, R., Mahendra, S., Richa, S., Kavitha, M. and Vikram, S.S. (2014) A Clinical Study on the effect of *Punarnavadi churna*, *Singhanada guggulu* in the management of *Amavata* (Rheumatoid Arthritis). *International Journal of Ayurveda and Pharma Research*, **2**, 46-54.

[11] Ramachandran, S. (2013) Review on *S. indicus* Linn. (Koṭṭaikkarantai). *Pharmacognosy Reviews*, **7**, 157-169. http://dx.doi.org/10.4103/0973-7847.120517

[12] Chakrabarti, D., Suthar, A.S., Jayaraman, G., Muthuvelan, B., Sharma, S. and Padigaru, M. (2012) NPS31807, a Standardized Extract from *Sphaeranthus indicus*, Inhibits Inflammatory, Migratory and Proliferative Activity in Keratinocytes and Immune Cells. *Pharmacology & Pharmacy*, **3**, 178-194. http://dx.doi.org/10.4236/pp.2012.32025

[13] Jansky, L., Reymanova, P. and Kopecky, J. (2003) Dynamics of Cytokine Production in Human Peripheral Blood Mononuclear Cells Stimulated by LPS, or Infected by Borrelia. *Physiological Research*, **52**, 593-598.

[14] Brennan, F.M., Chantry, D., Jackson, A., Maini, R. and Feldmann, M. (1989) Inhibitory Effect of TNF Alpha Antibodies on Synovial Cell Interleukin-1 Production in Rheumatoid Arthritis. *Lancet*, **334**, 244-247. http://dx.doi.org/10.1016/S0140-6736(89)90430-3

[15] Kamata, M., Tada, Y., Tatsuta, A., Kawashima, T., Shibata, S., Mitsui, H., Asano, Y., Sugaya, M., Kadono, T., Kanda, N., Watanabe, S. and Sato, S. (2013) Ciclosporin A Inhibits Production of Interleukin-12/23p40 and Interleukin-23 by the Human Monocyte Cell Line, THP-1. *Clinical and Experimental Dermatology*, **38**, 545-548. http://dx.doi.org/10.1111/ced.12110

[16] Balachandran, S., Gadekar, P.K., Parkale, S., Yadav, V.N., Kamath, D., Ramaswamy, S., Sharma, S., Vishwakarma, R.A. and Dagia, N.M. (2011) Synthesis and Biological Activity of Novel MIF Antagonists. *Bioorganic & Medicinal Chemistry Letters*, **21**, 1508-1511. http://dx.doi.org/10.1016/j.bmcl.2010.12.127

[17] Béchard, D., Scherpereel, A., Hammad, H., Gentina, T., Tsicopoulos, A., Aumercier, M., Pestel, J., *et al.* (2001) Human Endothelial-Cell Specific Molecule-1 Binds Directly to the Integrin CD11a/CD18 (LFA-1) and Blocks Binding to Intercellular Adhesion Molecule-1. *The Journal of Immunology*, **167**, 3099-3106. http://dx.doi.org/10.4049/jimmunol.167.6.3099

[18] Kim, K., Choi, Y., Lee, N., Park, K., Kim, G., Park, J., Kim, B., Lim, Y., *et al.* (2011) 5-Hydroxymethylfurfural from Black Garlic Extract Prevents TNFα-Induced Monocytic Cell Adhesion to HUVECs by Suppression of Vascular Cell Adhesion Molecule-1 Expression, Reactive Oxygen Species Generation and NF-κB Activation. *Phytotherapy Research*, **25**, 965-974. http://dx.doi.org/10.1002/ptr.3351

[19] Moreira, L., Wang, J., Sarno, N. and Kaplan, G. (1997) Thalidomide Protects Mice against LPS-Induced Shock. *Brazilian Journal of Medical and Biological Research*, **10**, 1199-1207. http://dx.doi.org/10.1590/s0100-879x1997001000010

[20] Terato, K., Karen, H., Michael, C., John, S., Alexander, T. and Andrew, K. (1985) Collagen-Induced Arthritis in Mice. Localization of an Arthritogenic Determinant to a Fragment of the Type II Collagen Molecule. *The Journal of Experimental Medicine*, **162**, 637-646. http://dx.doi.org/10.1084/jem.162.2.637

[21] Papp, A., Langley, G., Lebwohl, M., Krueger, G., Szapary, P. and Yeilding, N. (2008) Efficacy and Safety of Ustekinumab, a Human Interleukin-12/23 Monoclonal Antibody, in Patients with Psoriasis: 52-Week Results from a Randomised, Double-Blind, Placebo-Controlled Trial (PHOENIX 2). *Lancet*, **371**, 1675-1684. http://dx.doi.org/10.1016/S0140-6736(08)60726-6

[22] Ding, C., Xu, J. and Li, J. (2008) ABT-874, a Fully Human Monoclonal Anti-IL-12/IL-23 Antibody for the Potential Treatment of Autoimmune Diseases. *Current Opinion in Investigational Drugs*, **9**, 515-522.

[23] Fukuda, T., Sumichika, H., Murata, M., Hanano, T., Adachi, K. and Hisadome, M. (2000) A Novel Dual Regulator of Tumour Necrosis Factor-α and Interleukin-10 Protects Mice from Endotoxin-Induced Shock. *European Journal of Pharmacology*, **391**, 317-320. http://dx.doi.org/10.1016/S0014-2999(00)00096-0

[24] Wooley, H., Luthra, S., Krco, J., Stuart, M. and David, S. (1984) Type II Collagen—Induced Arthritis in Mice. *Arthritis & Rheumatism*, **27**, 1010-1017. http://dx.doi.org/10.1002/art.1780270907

[25] Simmonds, R.E. and Foxwell, B.M. (2008) Signalling, Inflammation and Arthritis: NF-κB and Its Relevance to Arthritis and Inflammation. *Rheumatology*, **5**, 584-590. http://dx.doi.org/10.1093/rheumatology/kem298

[26] Klimiuk, P., Sierakowski, S., Latosiewicz, R., Cylwik, J., Cylwik, B., Skowronski, J. and Chwiecko, J. (2002) Soluble Adhesion Molecules (ICAM-1, VCAM-1, and E-Selectin) and Vascular Endothelial Growth Factor (VEGF) in Patients with Distinct Variants of Rheumatoid Synovitis. *Annals of the Rheumatic Diseases*, **9**, 804-809. http://dx.doi.org/10.1136/ard.61.9.804

[27] Van den Berg, B. and Miossec, P. (2009) IL-17 as a Future Therapeutic Target for Rheumatoid Arthritis. *Nature Reviews Rheumatology*, **10**, 549-553. http://dx.doi.org/10.1038/nrrheum.2009.179

29

Gentamicin Renal Excretion in Rats: Probing Strategies to Mitigate Drug-Induced Nephrotoxicity

Aruna Dontabhaktuni[1], David R. Taft[1], Mayankbhai Patel[1,2]*

[1]Long Island University, Brooklyn, USA
[2]Current Address: Takeda Pharmaceuticals International Co., Cambridge, USA
Email: *mayankbhai.patel@takeda.com

Abstract

The renal excretion of gentamicin, an aminoglycoside antibiotic, was studied in the isolated perfused rat kidney (IPRK) model. Dose-linearity experiments were carried out at four doses (400, 800, 1600, 3200 µg), targeting initial perfusate levels of 5, 10, 20 and 40 µg/ml. Additionally, gentamicin was co-perfused with sodium bicarbonate (0.25 mM) and/or cimetidine (2 mM) to evaluate the effect of urinary alkalization and secretory inhibition on gentamicin excretion and kidney accumulation. Gentamicin displayed net reabsorption in the IPRK, consistent with extensive luminal uptake. Kinetic analysis indicated that luminal transport of gentamicin (kidney → urine) is the rate-determining step for gentamicin urinary excretion. Clearance and cumulative excretion decreased with increased gentamicin dose. Gentamicin kidney accumulation, estimated by mass balance, ranged from ~20% - 30%. Urinary alkalization significantly increased gentamicin excretion, with no effect on kidney accumulation. Conversely, cimetidine co-administration did not affect gentamicin clearance in the IPRK, but kidney accumulation was significantly reduced. When both sodium bicarbonate and cimetidine were administered together, gentamicin kidney accumulation decreased ~80% with corresponding increases in clearance and excretion ratio (XR) compared to gentamicin alone. A main strategy to reduce the incidence of nephrotoxicity with gentamicin therapy (up to ~25%) involves reducing kidney accumulation of the compound. The results of this research suggest that the combination of urinary alkalization and inhibition of basolateral secretion (blood → kidney) may be a viable approach to mitigate aminoglycoside toxicity, and warrants further investigation.

Keywords

Gentamicine, Isolated Perfused Kidney Component, Nephrotoxicity, pH Effect, Cimetidine

---

*Corresponding author.

1. Introduction

Aminoglycosides have been used for many decades to treat serious infections [1]. Gentamicin is the most commonly prescribed aminoglycoside, in part due to its low resistance levels and low cost [1]. Gentamicin is active against most strains of gram negative and some gram positive bacteria, with relatively low incidences of tolerance [2]. The therapeutic use of gentamicin has generally been restricted to life threatening infections, as the compound is nephrotoxic at therapeutic doses [3] [4]. The incidence of aminoglycoside nephrotoxicity in patients is approximately 25% [5]. However, because of the emergence of multi-drug resistance of bacteria to less toxic antimicrobial medications, clinicians are forced to consider aminoglycoside therapy for nosocomial infections in hospitalized patients and enterococcal endocarditis [6]. Thus, gentamicin is frequently used as a first or second choice drug in the clinic [4]. Given its continued use in drug therapy, considerable research has been aimed at developing approaches to reduce aminoglycoside toxicity in patients.

Despite significant research in this field, the molecular mechanism associated with gentamicin nephrotoxicity is not completely understood. Gentamicin is a hydrophilic cationic compound that does not readily penetrate cell membranes [7]. *In vivo*, approximately 90% of a gentamicin dose is recovered in the urine [8]. However, the drug selectively accumulates in the proximal tubule at concentrations much higher than those measured in plasma, and with a longer half-life in the tubular cell [1]. Once inside the kidney cell, gentamicin concentrates in lysosomes, endosomes and within the Golgi complex [9]. As drug concentrations rise, gentamicin empties into the cytosol, where it induces apoptosis and necrosis and inhibits various kidney membrane transporters leading to altered tubular reabsorption and reduced cellular viability [5].

The mechanisms of gentamicin uptake and accumulation in the kidney have been the subject of numerous published reports [1] [7] [10]-[17]. Elucidation of these pathways can provide insight into the mechanism of aminoglycoside nephrotoxicity. A study comparing renal accumulation in filtering and non-filtering kidneys demonstrated that gentamicin uptake proceeded via reabsorption across the luminal membrane of the proximal tubular cell [18]. Subsequently, it was established that aminoglycoside uptake involves absorptive endocytosis mediated by megalin [10], although other reports suggest that other transport pathways may be involved that do not require endocytosis [7] [17]. Thus, it appears that gentamicin uptake and accumulation may involve multiple processes.

Two general strategies have been proposed to protect against aminoglycoside nephrotoxicity [4] [9]. The first strategy involves reducing drug accumulation in the kidney. Administering gentamicin as a single daily dose has been suggested to be less nephrotoxic, due to saturation of luminal uptake resulting in reduced concentrations in the kidney [1] [5] [9] [19]. Alternatively, inhibitions of megalin-mediated endocytosis or other transport pathways through direct competition or other approaches have also been tested [10] [20]. A second strategy aims to reduce toxicity through co-administration of renoprotective compounds, including antioxidants [21]-[23].

The objective of this investigation was to explore alternative methods to reduce gentamicin uptake into the proximal tubule cell, the critical step leading to aminoglycoside nephrotoxicity. Experiments were performed using the isolated perfused rat kidney (IPRK) model. The IPRK can be used to study numerous aspects of renal drug disposition. Applications of the model include elucidating renal excretion mechanisms, screening for potential drug-drug interactions, and assessing renal drug metabolism [24]. Thus, it is a useful preclinical tool for the current investigation.

The specific aims of the research were: 1) to assess the dose-linearity of gentamicin excretion over a range of clinically-relevant concentrations; and 2) to probe potential strategies for reducing the kidney accumulation of gentamicin, including urinary alkalization and transporter-inhibition. Urinary alkalization was induced through administration of sodium bicarbonate ($NaHCO_3$), and the effect of increased urine pH on gentamicin excretion was determined. Transport inhibition studies were carried out using cimetidine, a known inhibitor of organic cation transport in the kidney [25].

2. Material and Methods

2.1. Chemicals

Fraction V bovine serum albumin (molecular weight range 69,000 to 78,000 D), dextran (clinical grade, molecular weight range 60,000 to 90,000 D), inulin (from chicory root), amino acids, potassium chloride, sodium chloride, sodium bicarbonate, magnesium sulfate, calcium chloride, glucose, sodium bicarbonate ($NaHCO_3$), cimetidine and gentamicin (sulfate salt) were purchased from Sigma-Aldrich (St. Louis, MO). Sodium hydroxide and pH calibration standards were obtained from VWR Scientific Products (West Chester, PA). Solvents used for HPLC were obtained from J & H Berge Co. (Plainfield, NJ). Amicon Centrifree YM-30 (molecular weight cut off 30 K) centrifugal filter devices were obtained from Millipore Corporation (Billerica, MA).

2.2. Animals

Male Sprague Dawley rats (250 - 350 g) were used for perfusion experiments. The rats were purchased from Harlan Laboratories (Indianapolis, IN). All rats were caged in stainless steel cages and fed standard chow and water *ad libitum*. The Institutional Animal Care and Usage Committee (IACUC) of Long Island University approved the experimental protocol for this investigation.

2.3. Isolated Perfused Rat Kidney Preparation

IPRK experiments were carried out as described previously [24] [26]. The surgical procedure involved cannulation of the right kidney via the superior mesenteric artery, using a technique that maintained a continuous flow of perfusate to the kidney, thereby decreasing the possibility of ischemia during the isolation of the kidney [26]. The perfusate consisted of Krebs-Henseleit buffer (pH 7.4) containing BSA (4%), dextran (1.67%), glucose (0.1%), inulin (GFR marker, 0.06%) and amino acids.

Anesthesia was induced with an intraperitoneal injection of sodium pentobarbital (40 mg/kg). A midline incision was made and the renal segment of the aorta exposed. A ligature was passed under the right renal artery close to the aorta, and distal and proximal ligatures placed around the superior mesenteric artery. The right ureter was catheterized with polyethylene (PE-10) tubing in order to facilitate urine collection. A cannula was then threaded through the mesenteric artery, across the aorta, and into the right renal artery in situ. The ligatures were tied, securing the cannula in place. The right kidney was then excised from the animal, trimmed of adhering tissue and transferred to the *in vitro* recirculating perfusion apparatus.

2.4. Treatment Groups

Control perfusions were conducted to test system suitability and viability of the study model, and to assess effects of treatments on kidney function. The renal excretion of gentamicin was determined over a range of doses targeting initial perfusate concentrations between 5 and 40 µg/ml. A total of four doses were studied (5, 10, 20 and 40 µg/ml). Three additional study groups were carried out to determine the effect of urinary alkalization and/or transport inhibition on gentamicin excretion: 1) Gentamicin (10 µg/ml) co-administered with NaHCO$_3$ (0.25 mM); 2) Gentamicin (10 µg/ml) co-administered with cimetidine (2 mM) (OCT inhibitor); and 3) Gentamicin co-administered with NaCO$_3$ (0.25 mM) and cimetidine (2 mM). A total of five perfusion experiments were conducted for each study group.

2.5. Experimental Design

Each IPRK experiment was conducted over a 2-hour period. Once the kidney was placed in the perfusion apparatus, a stabilization period (10 minutes) preceded any pharmacokinetic experimentation. For the dose linearity experiments, a bolus dose of vehicle (KHS buffer, dose linearity perfusions), NaHCO$_3$ or cimetidine (or both) was administered following the stabilization period. After a ten minute distribution phase, gentamicin was then added to the perfusion reservoir as a bolus dose. The time was denoted as time zero for pharmacokinetic calculations.

A perfusate sample was collected 5 minutes post-dose and every 10 minutes thereafter for a total of 100 minutes. Urine was collected in 10-minute intervals throughout the experiment. After each collection interval, urine volume was determined gravimetrically and pH was measured. Perfusate and urine samples were analyzed for electrolytes (sodium, chloride) and glucose using a Beckman Synchron CX-3 Clinical Chemistry Analyzer (Beckman-Coulter, Brea CA). Inulin (GFR marker) was measured using colorimetric method [27]. Urine and perfusate samples were stored at −20°C prior to the analysis of gentamicin.

During the course of the experiment, the perfusion pressure was maintained at 100 ± 10 mm Hg by adjusting the perfusate flow rate as needed. The volume of the recirculating perfusate (80 mL) was maintained constant by addition of the replenishing solution that was prepared with a 1:1 dilution of the perfusate and deionized water. At the end of the experiment, the kidney was removed, blotted dry, and weighed. Kidney function and viability was assessed by the following parameters: GFR, reabsorption of electrolytes and glucose, urine flow rate, and urine pH.

2.6. Perfusate Binding of Gentamicin

Perfusate binding of gentamicin was measured by ultrafiltration. Four concentrations of gentamicin were studied: 1, 5, 10, and 40 μg/ml. Perfusate samples were incubated at 37°C under constant stirring for 60 min to ensure binding equilibrium. After incubation, an aliquot of sample was collected for the determination of total drug perfusate concentration. A second aliquot (1 ml) was added to an Amicon Centrifree Micropartition System (Millipore Corporation, Bedford, MA) and the device was centrifuged at 1500 × g for 15 min. After centrifugation, the resulting ultrafiltrate was stored at −20°C for subsequent determination of free drug concentration. Preliminary studies determined that the drug binding to the device was negligible. All studies were performed in triplicate. The fraction of gentamicin unbound in perfusate (f_u) was calculated as the ratio of unbound and total concentration.

Further studies were performed to evaluate nonspecific binding to IPRK apparatus for all gentamicin doses used in current investigation. These studies were performed using KHS buffer and gentamicin was added as a bolus dose. Samples were collected 5 min post-dose and every 10 min thereafter over 2 hour.

2.7. HPLC Analysis

Structurally, gentamicin does not possess ultraviolet light absorbing properties, and therefore the compound cannot be analyzed directly by UV or fluorescence detection. Consequently, HPLC methods for gentamicin typically include pre-column or post-column derivatization. There are a number of published methods for gentamicin involving various derivatizing agents [28]-[33], which were used by other investigators. In the present investigation new HPLC method was developed and validated [34]. The method utilized in this investigation involves pre-column derivatization of gentamicin with O-phthalaldehyde (OPA) and 2-mercaptoethanol (MPE). In contrast to published gentamicin HPLC assays, 1) this assay requires a low sample volume; 2) involves simple and less time-consuming derivatization process, 3) the derivative produced is more stable (up to 4 hours) at room temperature and 4) the sensitivity of assay is higher, thus it can be used to measure gentamicin concentrations at therapeutic doses.

Gentamicin was quantified using an HPLC method with fluorescence detection. Test samples (perfusate, urine, ultrafiltrate) were treated with 1% $ZnSO_4$ (1:1 ratio) to precipitate proteins. Derivatizing agents were spiked directly into the resulting sample extract. Analyte separation was accomplished using a Hypersil ODS C18 column (150 mm × 4.6 mm, 5 um particle size). The mobile phase consisted of 0.02 M sodium heptanesulfonic acid in methanol-glacial acetic acid-water (70:5:25) (pH 3.4). Analysis was conducted at ambient temperature at a constant flow rate of 2.0 mL/min using isocratic elution. Gentamicin was detected at an excitation maximum of 360 nm and emission maximum of 430 nm.

A standard addition method [35] was used to increase the sensitivity of the assay in perfusate. The method involved the addition of known quantities of gentamicin to multiple aliquots of a perfusate sample. The standard samples were analyzed, and the concentration of gentamicin in the sample was determined from a plot of detector response (peak height) versus gentamicin concentration.

2.8. Data Analysis

For each urine collection period, the renal clearance of inulin (GFR) was calculated using the following equation:

$$GFR = UFR \times \frac{U_{inulin}}{P_{inulin}} \qquad (1)$$

where UFR represents the urine flow rate, U_{inulin} is the concentration of inulin in urine, and P_{inulin} is the perfusate concentration of inulin sampled at the midpoint of the urine collection interval.

The following equation was used to calculate clearance (Cl) of gentamicin in the IPRK:

$$Cl = \frac{X_u}{AUC} \qquad (2)$$

X_u refers to the cumulative urinary excretion of gentamicin and AUC is the area under the curve over the duration of the perfusion experiment (100 minutes). AUC was estimated using the trapezoidal rule.

Renal excretion ratio (XR) is a parameter used to determine net mechanisms of renal excretion. XR was calculated as follows:

$$XR = \frac{Cl}{f_u \times GFR} \qquad (3)$$

Kidney accumulation of gentamicin was estimated using mass balance analysis; that is, as the difference between the administered dose and the total amount of drug remaining in the perfusate and recovered in the urine at the end of the perfusion experiment.

2.9. Statistical Analysis

Estimates of IPRK viability parameters for control and drug treatment groups were compared using analysis of variance (ANOVA). Post-hoc analysis (Dunnett's Test) was utilized to identify study groups that differed from control perfusions in terms of viability criteria. Consequently, alterations in kidney functions induced by drug administration or NaHCO₃ were determined. Likewise, mean values for gentamicin pharmacokinetic parameters were compared using ANOVA. Post-hoc analysis (Tukey HSD) was once again used to identify differences among the various treatment groups in an effort to identify differences in gentamicin excretion as a function of dose or co-administration of NaHCO₃ and/or cimetidine.

3. Results

3.1. Quantification of Gentamicin

In current investigation, pre-column derivatization with 2-mercaptoethanol (MPE) with OPA was used to improve assay sensitivity. The derivative was found to be stable in the mobile phase for up to 4 hours at room temperature. The variability of the method with regard to reproducibility, accuracy, and precision was within acceptable limits (**Table S1, Table S2**). Nearly complete recovery of the drug from the matrix was obtained. Limit of detection (LOQ) of the HPLC assay method was high (10 μg/ml). In order to measure gentamicin perfusate concentration in the clinically relevant range, a standard addition method was employed. The method involved the addition of known quantities of gentamicin to multiple aliquots of a plasma sample. The standard samples were analyzed, and the concentration of gentamicin in the sample was determined from a plot of detector response (peak height) versus gentamicin concentration. This approach lowered the LOQ of the method in perfusate to 1 μg/ml. Gentamicin was stable in all matrices for 24 hr at room temperature and up to 1 month at −20°C.

3.2. Gentamicin Perfusate Binding

Gentamicin binding in IPRK perfusate was constant over the range of concentrations tested (5 - 40 μg/ml). Binding was estimated as 12% ± 0.9% (f_u = 0.88). In a separate experiment, gentamicin was not found to undergo non-specific binding of gentamicin to the IPRK apparatus.

3.3. Dose Linearity Assessment

A summary of the parameters used to assess IPRK suitability is presented in **Table 1**. Control (drug-naive) studies were performed to establish the viability of the preparation and to assess the effect of varying doses of gentamicin on kidney function. The data presented in the table are consistent with published values [24] [26] [36] [37]. There were no significant differences in parameter estimates among any of the treatment groups compared to control (p-value > 0.05), indicating that that kidney function was well preserved in the presence of varying doses of gentamicin over the duration of the IPRK experiments.

Estimates for gentamicin renal excretion parameters are provided in **Table 2**. To correct for inter-kidney variability, GFR and clearance estimates were normalized for kidney weight. Although the drug appeared to exhibit dose-linearity with respect to AUC, the data indicate a non-linear renal excretion profile with increasing dose. Gentamicin excretion ratio (XR) was less than one across all groups, consisted with net reabsorption by the

Table 1. IPRK viability parameters: dose proportionality experiments.

Viability parameter[a]	Control (drug-naïve)	Gentamicin concentration			
		5 µg/ml	10 µg/ml	20 µg/ml	40 µg/ml
Perfusion flow rate (ml/min)	22.7 (2.5)	23 (5.7)	29 (1.1)	28 (1.2)	24 (3.1)
Urine flow rate (ml/min)	0.06 (0.03)	0.10 (0.03)	0.11 (0.02)	0.10 (0.04)	0.08 (0.04)
Urine pH	7.2 (0.04)	7.3 (0.14)	7.1 (0.17)	7.1 (0.16)	7.3 (0.16)
GFR[b] (ml/min/g)	0.49 (0.15)	0.57 (0.15)	0.52 (0.12)	0.46 (0.15)	0.45 (0.15)
$FR_{Glucose}$[c]	0.96 (0.02)	0.96 (0.01)	0.97 (0.01)	0.95 (0.02)	0.96 (0.02)
FR_{Sodium}[d]	0.94 (0.03)	0.92 (0.04)	0.88 (0.03)	0.90 (0.05)	0.92 (0.07)
$FR_{Chloride}$[e]	0.92 (0.04)	0.89 (0.04)	0.85 (0.03)	0.88 (0.06)	0.90 (0.04)

[a]Data reported as mean (standard deviation) representing five perfusion (n = 5) per treatment group. Ten excretion periods were analyzed for each perfusion experiment; [b]Glomerular filtration rate, normalizes per kidney weight; [c]Fractional reabsorption of glucose; [d]Fractional reabsorption of sodium; [e]Fractional reabsorption of chloride.

Table 2. Gentamicin renal excretion parameters in IPRK: dose proportionality experiments.

Parameter	Gentamicin concentration			
	5 µg/ml	10 µg/ml	20 µg/ml	40 µg/ml
GFR[a] (ml/min/g)	0.57 (0.15)	0.52 (0.12)	0.46 (0.15)	0.45 (0.15)
Clearance (ml/min/g)[b]	0.14 (0.02)**	0.18 (0.03)**	0.08 (0.02)	0.09 (0.02)
Excretion ratio[c]	0.31 (0.05)	0.47 (0.11)**	0.26 (0.11)	0.26 (0.07)
Cumulative excretion (% Dose)	22.1 (1.75)**	26.2 (3.76)**	14.2 (3.21)	15.6 (1.81)
Kidney accumulation (% Dose)[e]	19.7 (4.92)	29.1 (3.32)*	26.5 (5.78)*	20.9 (5.18)
Dose normalized AUC_{0-t} (min-µg/ml)[e]	1.0 (0.08)	0.94 (0.04)	1.1 (0.09)***	1.0 (0.02)

[a]Glomerular filtration rate, normalized for kidney weight; [b]Calculated as the ratio of cumulative urinary excretion and AUC for duration of IPRK experiment (data are corrected for kidney weight); [c]Calculated are ratio of clearance (clearance/(f_u × GFR)); [d]Estimated from mass balance analysis at end of experiment (dose-cumulative excretion-amount remaining in perfusate); [e]Area under the curve was estimated using trapezoidal rule. Estimates were divided by gentamicin dose; *Indicates values that are significantly different from all other treatment groups; **Indicates values that are significantly different from 20 µg/ml and 40 µg/ml treatment groups; ***Indicates values that are significantly different from 10 µg/ml treatment group.

kidney. Likewise, clearance and cumulative excretion decreased with increased gentamicin dose. Gentamicin kidney accumulation, estimated by mass balance, ranged from ~20% - 30% among the treatment groups.

3.4. Interaction Studies

A second set of perfused experiments was carried out to assess whether the excretion profile and kidney accumulation of gentamicin could be altered through changes in pH or transport inhibition. Accordingly, gentamicin was co-perfused with $NaHCO_3$ (to ↑ urine pH) and/or cimetidine (inhibitor of basolateral transport). As presented in the **Table 3**, there were no significant differences in perfusion flow rate, urine flow rate, GFR and $FR_{Chloride}$ among all study groups. Urine pH was significantly higher in $NaHCO_3$-treated perfusions, which is relevant to the study design of those experiments. Although differences in glucose and sodium reabsorption were noted treatments, parameter estimates within acceptable ranges [24].

A plot of gentamicin perfusate concentrations vs. time is presented in **Figure 1**. The graph shows the cimetidine co-administration decreased the gentamicin elimination from the IPRK, whereas perfusate levels decreased more rapidly in the presence of $NaHCO_3$. As noted in **Figure 2**, gentamicin urinary excretion was increased in the presence of $NaHCO_3$.

Renal excretion parameters for these interaction experiments are summarized in **Table 4**. The data illustrate that $NaHCO_3$ co-perfusion increased gentamicin elimination in the IPRK, as clearance, cumulative excretion and XR were all significantly increased compared to experiments with gentamicin alone. Whereas gentamicin clearance was apparently not impacted by cimetidine administration, kidney accumulation was significantly reduced.

Table 3. IPRK viability parameters: interaction experiments.

Viability parameter	Treatment groups					
	Control drug naïve	NaHCO$_3$	Gentamicin 10 µg/ml	Gentamicin + NaHCO$_3$	Gentamicin + Cimetidine	Gentamicin + Cimetidine + NaHCO$_3$
Perfusion flow rate (ml/min)	22.7 (2.50)	24.8 (3.74)	29.0 (1.10)	23.5 (4.87)	23.7 (7.21)	28.9 (4.97)
Urine flow rate (ml/min)	0.06 (0.03)	0.12 (0.05)	0.11 (0.02)	0.12 (0.01)	0.08 (0.02)	0.11 (0.01)
Urine pH	7.2 (0.04)	8.1 (0.58)*	7.1 (0.17)	8.1 (0.05)*	7.0 (0.08)	8.2 (0.04)*
GFR^a (ml/min/g)	0.49 (0.15)	0.51 (0.09)	0.52 (0.12)	0.48 (0.04)	0.43 (0.03)	0.32 (0.01)
FR$_{Glucose}$^{b}	0.96 (0.02)	0.94 (0.01)	0.97 (0.01)	0.93 (0.01)	0.95 (0.01)	0.88 (0.01)**
FR$_{Sodium}$^{c}	0.94 (0.03)	0.86 (0.03)*	0.88 (0.03)	0.85 (0.02)*	0.94 (0.03)	0.84 (0.01)*
FR$_{Chloride}$^{d}	0.92 (0.04)	0.86 (0.06)	0.85 (0.03)	0.87 (0.03)	0.91 (0.01)	0.85 (0.01)

^{a}GFR normalized per kidney weight; ^{b}Fraction reabsorption of glucose; ^{c}Fraction reabsorption of sodium; ^{d}Fraction reabsorption of chloride; *Indicates values that are significantly different from control, gentamicin and gentamicin + cimetidine treatment groups; **Indicates values that are significantly different from all other treatment groups.

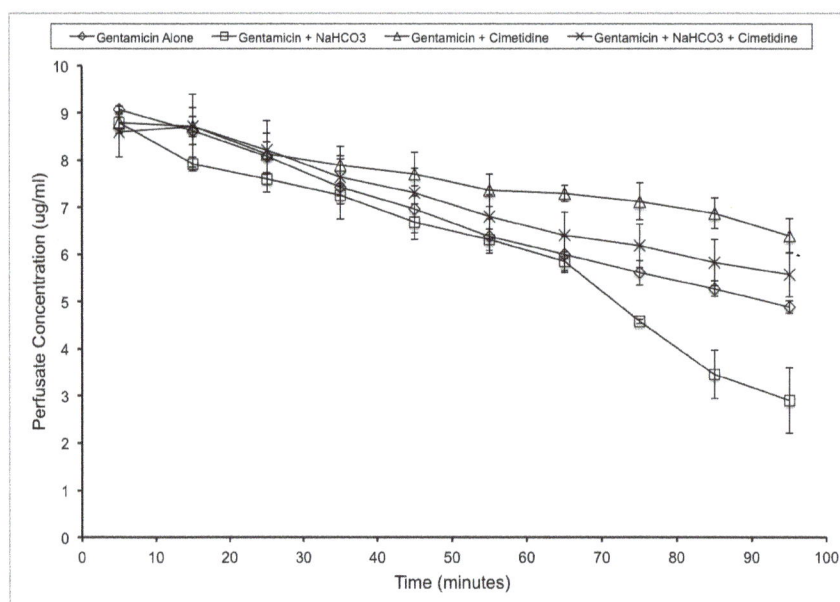

Figure 1. Plot of gentamicin perfusate concentration vs. time in the IPRK: Effect of co-administration of NaHCO$_3$ and/or cimetidine.

When both NaHCO$_3$ and cimetidine were administered together, gentamicin kidney accumulation decreased ~80%, with corresponding increases in clearance and XR compared to gentamicin alone.

4. Discussion

Despite their toxicity profile, the clinical use of aminoglycosides has increased in recent years following the emergence of multidrug resistant pathogens [38]. Since the incidence of aminoglycoside nephrotoxicity is ~25%, various strategies have been proposed to circumvent this toxicity either by reducing drug accumulation in the kidney or by co-administering renoprotective compounds [1] [4].

It is well established that aminoglycosides are substrates for megalin, a multiligand endocytotic receptor in the luminal membrane of the kidney, and this is thought to be a major pathway for accumulation of aminoglycosides on the kidney [7] [39]. Accordingly, this pathway is a proposed target to prevent aminoglycoside toxicity, and research has showed that gentamicin binding can be inhibited by megalin ligands and small peptides [10]. However, concern has been raised about the clinical consequences of interfering with megalin-mediated

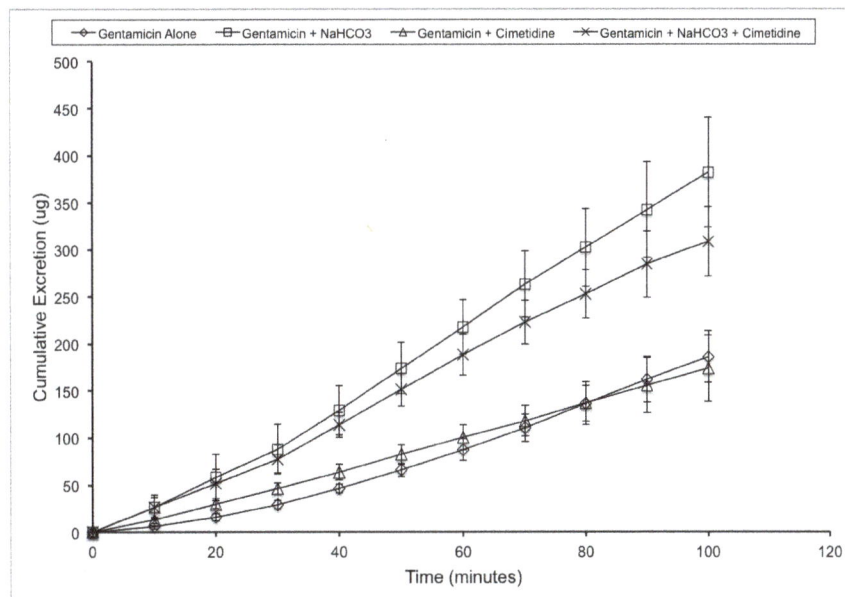

Figure 2. Plot of gentamicin cumulative urinary excretion vs. time in the IPRK: Effect of co-administration of NaHCO$_3$ and/or cimetidine.

Table 4. Gentamicin renal excretion parameters in IPRK: interaction experiments.

Parameter	Gentamicin 10 µg/ml	Interactant (concentration)		
		NaHCO$_3$ (0.25 mM)	Cimetidine (2 mM)	Cimetidine (2 mM) + NaHCO$_3$ (0.25mM)
GFR[a] (ml/min/g)	0.52 (0.12)	0.48 (0.04)	0.43 (0.03)	0.32 (0.01)
Clearance (ml/min/g)[b]	0.18 (0.03)	0.40 (0.09)[*,***]	0.16 (0.03)[**]	0.25 (0.04)[*]
Excretion ratio[c]	0.47 (0.11)	0.94 (0.22)[*]	0.41 (0.05)[**,***]	0.89 (0.16)[*]
Cumulative excretion (% Dose)	26.2 (3.76)	47.7 (7.24)[*]	21.7 (4.43)[**,***]	36.0 (5.55)
Kidney accumulation[d] (% Dose)	29.10 (3.32)	25.50 (7.34)[***]	14.30 (1.22)[*,**]	6.16 (0.74)[*]
AUC$_{0-t}$[e] (min*µg/ml)	708 (32.0)	636 (16.1)	780 (27.1)[**]	695 (72.2)

[a]Glomerular filtration rate, normalized for kidney weight; [b]Calculated as the ratio of cumulative urinary excretion and AUC for duration of IPRK experiment (data are corrected for kidney weight); [c]Calculated are ratio of clearance (Clearance/(f$_u$ × GFR)); [d]Estimated from mass balance analysis at end of experiment (dose-cumulative excretion-amount remaining in perfusate); [e]Area under the curve was estimated using trapezoidal rule; [*]Indicates values that are significantly different from gentamicin alone; [**]Indicates values that are significantly different from NaHCO$_3$ treatment group; [***]Indicates values that are significantly different from Cimetidine + NaHCO$_3$ treatment group.

endocytosis [4]. Additionally, several preclinical studies have demonstrated reduced aminoglycoside nephrotoxicity through co-administration of antioxidants [21]-[23], so this is an avenue for further exploration.

In the present study, gentamicin excretion was evaluated in the IPRK model, a versatile *ex vivo* technique that can be used to study numerous aspects of renal drug disposition. Some of the earliest evidence that luminal uptake was responsible for the renal tubular uptake of gentamicin came from IPRK experiments in filtering and non-filtering kidneys [18]. The present work extended application of the IPRK to assess dose-linearity of gentamicin excretion and to probe ways to reduce kidney accumulation.

Dose linearity experiments were carried at four doses (400, 800, 1600 and 3200 µg) targeting initial concentrations from 5 - 40 µg/ml. These concentrations encompass the clinical range of expected peak levels of gentamicin following a conventional dosing regimen (1 - 2 mg/kg every 8 hours, targeting peak serum concentrations of 5 - 10 µg/ml) or a "once daily" dosing regimen (5 - 7.5 mg/kg every 24 hours, targeting peak serum concentrations as high as 30 - 40 µg/ml) [40] [41].

Estimates of gentamicin clearance in the IPRK have been reported by Bekersky *et al.* (0.25 - 0.30 ml/min, reference 25) and Collier *et al.* (0.32 ml/min, reference 18). These findings are based on studies performed at an initial drug concentration of 10 μg/ml. The results of the present investigation are consistent with these values. The mean gentamicin clearance (not kidney weight corrected, 10 μg/ml dosing group) was 0.29 ± 0.033 ml/min.

Approximately 50% - 60% of the administered gentamicin dose was eliminated from the perfusate over the duration of the IPRK experiment (100 minutes). Comparing the temporal profiles of urinary excretion rate with perfusate concentrations (**Figure 3**), there is a distributional delay in the renal excretion of gentamicin; that is, the luminal transport of gentamicin (kidney $\Rightarrow$ urine) appears to be the rate-determining step for drug excretion. However, this observation is consistent with slow removal of drug from the proximal tubule [7], and would therefore lead to renal accumulation with successive dosing.

Gentamicin displayed nonlinear excretion in the IPRK, with significant decreases in clearance and cumulative excretion with increasing dose (**Table 2**). However, kidney accumulation (% dose) did not decrease with dose. Although "once a day" dosing is thought to decrease kidney accumulation through saturation of aminoglycoside reabsorption [1] [5] [9], the nonlinear behavior seen in the present study does not support this hypothesis. Aminoglycoside uptake into the kidney involves pathways other than absorptive endocytosis [7], and it appears that one of these pathways is responsible for the nonlinearity in gentamicin excretion in the IPRK.

One of the goals of this investigation was to test potential strategies to decrease the kidney accumulation of gentamicin: urinary alkalization and co-administration of cimetidine. Administration of $NaHCO_3$ (0.25 mM) to the IPRK caused a significant increase in urine pH from ~7.1 to ~8.1, and this effect was constant for the duration of the experiment. Under these conditions, gentamicin excretion was significantly increased, as reflected in differences in clearance (0.40 ml/min/g vs. 0.18 ml/min/g), excretion ratio (0.47 to 0.94) and cumulative excretion (47.7% vs. 26.2%) compared to gentamicin alone.

Gentamicin tubular uptake has been studied extensively in the last decade. Ionized gentamicin binds to the acidic phospholipids on brush-border membrane of the renal tubular cell. Thus, altering the ionized fraction of gentamicin can ameliorate its nephrotoxicity. Gentamicin is weak base with a pKa = 7.4. Thus, increasing urine pH to 8.1 decreased the ionization of gentamicin to ~17%. Since luminal reabsorption of gentamicin is an electrostatic process [42], altering the cationic charge on the molecule adversely impacted epithelial uptake of gentamicin by reduced charged affinity for the luminal membrane. However, increased gentamicin excretion was not associated with decreased kidney accumulation (**Table 4**).

The effect of urinary alkalization on gentamicin kidney uptake and nephrotoxicity has previously been studied in rats. Whereas Chiu *et al*. observed a decrease in gentamicin accumulation in the kidney cortex when urine pH was increased [43], Elliott reported that pre-treatment with $NaHCO_3$ was not associated with reduced gentamicin nephrotoxicity [44]. The results from these IPRK experiments suggest that while gentamicin excretion is increased

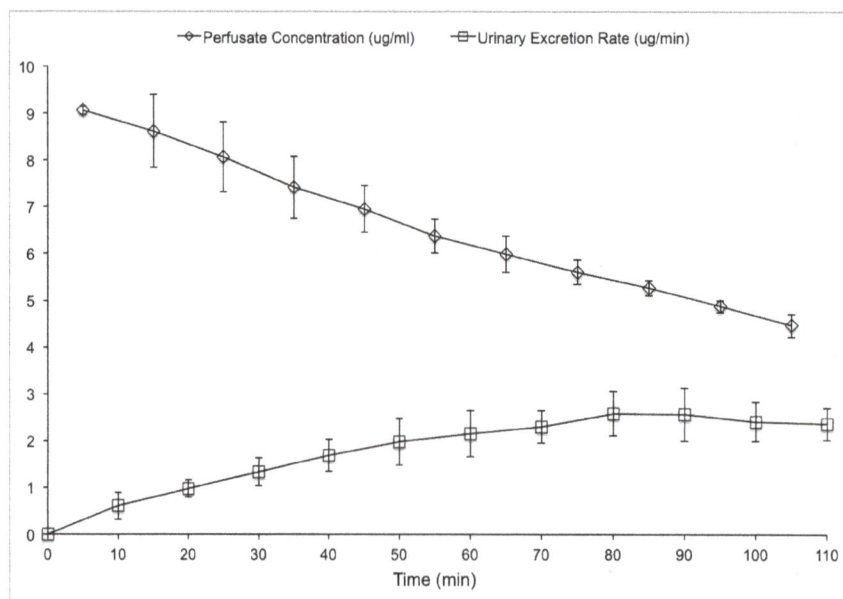

Figure 3. Comparison of the temporal changes in gentamicin perfusate concentration and urinary excretion rate following bolus dosing (800 μg) in the IPRK.

when co-administered with $NaHCO_3$, this strategy would likely not reduce the risk of nephrotoxicity, as kidney accumulation was not altered with this treatment.

IPRK experiments also investigated the effect of co-administration of cimetidine on gentamicin excretion and kidney accumulation. Although luminal transport has been the principle target for reducing aminoglycoside accumulation in the kidney, there is evidence to suggest that gentamicin is secreted across the basolateral membrane [45] [46]. Cimetidine is a known inhibitor of basolateral organic cation transport (OCT2). Although cimetidine had no apparent effect on gentamicin clearance and urinary excretion in the IPRK (**Table 4**), there was a slight increase in AUC (**Figure 1**) and a significant reduction in kidney accumulation (~50%). These results indicate that basolateral transport (blood → kidney) is a promising target for reducing aminoglycoside accumulation. Whereas tubular secretion may contribute significantly to the urinary excretion of aminoglycosides (*i.e.*, inhibition of basolateral transport would not alter renal clearance), the pathway appears to be an important determinant of aminoglycoside toxicity.

In a final set of experiments, the effect of both basolateral transport inhibition and urinary alkalization on gentamicin disposition in the IPRK was explored. Co-administration with both cimetidine and $NaHCO_3$ not only increased renal excretion of gentamicin, but kidney accumulation was also reduced 80% (**Table 4**). Thus, it appears that urinary alkalization combined with basolateral transport inhibition is a potential strategy to limit the renal accumulation of gentamicin and to reduce the risk of drug-induced nephrotoxicity.

5. Conclusion

While further studies are needed to confirm the results of this investigation and to evaluate the synergistic protective effect of $NaHCO_3$ and cimetidine, an advantage of this approach over other proposed strategies is that both compounds are clinically available. A recent clinical study found that oral administration of sodium bicarbonate (4 g every 8 hours) was able to achieve a urine pH above 8 with no apparent adverse effects, although the authors acknowledge that more research is needed to investigate efficacy of longer periods of treatment [46]. Cimetidine is a commercially available medication used to treat gastric ulcers, gastroesophegeal reflux disease, and other conditions. While further studies are needed to confirm that kidney accumulation of gentamicin can be reduced at therapeutic doses of cimetidine, the findings of the present investigation are promising and merit continued exploration.

Funding Information

This research received no specific grant from any funding agency in the public, commercial, or not-for-profit sectors.

References

[1]   Nagai, J. and Takano, M. (2004) Molecular Aspects of Renal Handling of Aminoglycosides and Strategies for Preventing the Nephrotoxicity. *Drug Metabolism and Pharmacokinetics*, **19**, 159-170. http://dx.doi.org/10.2133/dmpk.19.159

[2]   Weinstein, M.J., Luedemann, G.M., Oden, E.M., Wagman, G.H., Rosselet, J.P., Marquez, J.A., Coniglio, C.T., Charney, W., Herzog, H.L. and Black, J. (1963) Gentamicin, a New Antibiotic Complex from Micromonospora. *Journal of Medicinal Chemistry*, **6**, 463-464. http://dx.doi.org/10.1021/jm00340a034

[3]   Ali, B.H. (1995) Gentamicin Nephrotoxicity in Humans and Animals: Some Recent Research. *General Pharmacology*, **26**, 1477-1487. http://dx.doi.org/10.1016/0306-3623(95)00049-6

[4]   Lopez-Novoa, J.M., Quiros, Y., Vicente, L., Morales, A.I. and Lopez-Hernandez, F.J. (2011) New Insights into the Mechanism of Aminoglycoside Nephrotoxicity: An Integrative Point of View. *Kidney International*, **79**, 33-45. http://dx.doi.org/10.1038/ki.2010.337

[5]   Wargo, K.A. and Edwards, J.D. (2014) Aminoglycoside-Induced Nephrotoxicity. *Journal of Pharmacy Practice*, **27**, 573-577. http://dx.doi.org/10.1177/0897190014546836

[6]   Destache, C.J. (2014) Aminoglycoside-Induced Nephrotoxicity—A Focus on Monitoring: A Review of Literature. *Journal of Pharmacy Practice*, **27**, 562-566. http://dx.doi.org/10.1177/0897190014546102

[7]   Nagai, J. and Takano, M. (2014) Entry of Aminoglycosides into Renal Tubular Epithelial Cells via Endocytosis-Dependent and Endocytosis-Independent Pathways. *Biochemical Pharmacology*, **90**, 331-337. http://dx.doi.org/10.1016/j.bcp.2014.05.018

[8]   Triggs, E. and Charles, B. (1999) Pharmacokinetics and Therapeutic Drug Monitoring of Gentamicin in the Elderly.

Clinical Pharmacokinetics, **37**, 331-341. http://dx.doi.org/10.2165/00003088-199937040-00004

[9] Mingeot-Leclercq, M.P. and Tulkens, P.M. (1999) Aminoglycosides: Nephrotoxicity. *Antimicrobial Agents and Chemotherapy*, **43**, 1003-1012.

[10] Nagai, J., Saito, M., Adachi, Y., Yumoto, R. and Takano, M. (2006) Inhibition of Gentamicin Binding to Rat Renal Brush-Border Membrane by Megalin Ligands and Basic Peptides. *Journal of Controlled Release*, **112**, 43-50. http://dx.doi.org/10.1016/j.jconrel.2006.01.003

[11] Feldman, S., Wang, M.Y. and Kaloyanides, G.J. (1982) Aminoglycosides Induce a Phospholipidosis in the Renal Cortex of the Rat: An Early Manifestation of Nephrotoxicity. *Journal of Pharmacology and Experimental Therapeutics*, **220**, 514-520.

[12] Ghosh, P. and Chatterjee, S. (1987) Effects of Gentamicin on Sphingomyelinase Activity in Cultured Human Renal Proximal Tubular Cells. *Journal of Biological Chemistry*, **262**, 12550-12556.

[13] Inui, K., Saito, H., Iwata, T. and Hori, R. (1988) Aminoglycoside-Induced Alterations in Apical Membranes of Kidney Epithelial Cell Line (LLC-PK1). *American Journal of Physiology*, **254**, C251-C257.

[14] Kosek, J.C., Mazze, R.I. and Cousins, M.J. (1974) Nephrotoxicity of Gentamicin. *Laboratory Investigation*, **30**, 48-57.

[15] Moriyama, T., Nakahama, H., Fukuhara, Y., Horio, M., Yanase, M., Orita, Y., Kamada, T., Kanashiro, M. and Miyake, Y. (1989) Decrease in the Fluidity of Brush-Border Membrane Vesicles Induced by Gentamicin. A Spin-Labeling Study. *Biochemical Pharmacology*, **38**, 1169-1174. http://dx.doi.org/10.1016/0006-2952(89)90264-5

[16] Silverblatt, F.J. and Kuehn, C. (1979) Autoradiography of Gentamicin Uptake by the Rat Proximal Tubule Cell. *Kidney International*, **15**, 335-345. http://dx.doi.org/10.1038/ki.1979.45

[17] Karasawa, T., Wang, Q., Fu, Y., Cohen, D.M. and Steyger, P.S. (2008) TRPV4 Enhances the Cellular Uptake of Aminoglycoside Antibiotics. *Journal of Cell Science*, **121**, 2871-2879. http://dx.doi.org/10.1242/jcs.023705

[18] Collier, V.U., Lietman, P.S. and Mitch, W.E. (1979) Evidence for Luminal Uptake of Gentamicin in the Perfused Rat Kidney. *Journal of Pharmacology and Experimental Therapeutics*, **210**, 247-251.

[19] Rybak, M.J., Abate, B.J., Kang, S.L., Ruffing, M.J., Lerner, S.A. and Drusano, G.L. (1999) Prospective Evaluation of the Effect of an Aminoglycoside Dosing Regimen on Rates of Observed Nephrotoxicity and Ototoxicity. *Antimicrobial Agents and Chemotherapy*, **43**, 1549-1555.

[20] Watanabe, A., Nagai, J., Adachi, Y., Katsube, T., Kitahara, Y., Murakami, T. and Takano, M. (2004) Targeted Prevention of Renal Accumulation and Toxicity of Gentamicin by Aminoglycoside Binding Receptor Antagonists. *Journal of Controlled Release*, **95**, 423-433. http://dx.doi.org/10.1016/j.jconrel.2003.12.005

[21] Koyner, J.L., Sher Ali, R. and Murray, P.T. (2008) Antioxidants. Do They Have a Place in the Prevention or Therapy of Acute Kidney Injury? *Nephron Experimental Nephrology*, **109**, e109-e117. http://dx.doi.org/10.1159/000142935

[22] Sardana, A., Kalra, S., Khanna, D. and Balakumar, P. (2015) Nephroprotective Effect of Catechin on Gentamicin-Induced Experimental Nephrotoxicity. *Clinical and Experimental Nephrology*, **19**, 178-184. http://dx.doi.org/10.1007/s10157-014-0980-3

[23] Morsy, M.A., Ibrahim, S.A., Amin, E.F., Kamel, M.Y., Rifaai, R.A. and Hassan, M.K. (2014) Sildenafil Ameliorates Gentamicin-Induced Nephrotoxicity in Rats: Role of iNOS and eNOS. *Journal of Toxicology*, **2014**, Article ID: 489382. http://dx.doi.org/10.1155/2014/489382

[24] Taft, D.R. (2004) The Isolated Perfused Rat Kidney Model: A Useful Tool for Drug Discovery and Development. *Current Drug Discovery Technologies*, **1**, 97-111. http://dx.doi.org/10.2174/1570163043484824

[25] Urakami, Y., Kimura, N., Okuda, M. and Inui, K. (2004) Creatinine Transport by Basolateral Organic Cation Transporter hOCT2 in the Human Kidney. *Pharmaceutical Research*, **21**, 976-981. http://dx.doi.org/10.1023/B:PHAM.0000029286.45788.ad

[26] Bekersky, I. (1983) Use of the Isolated Perfused Kidney as a Tool in Drug Disposition Studies. *Drug Metabolism Reviews*, **14**, 931-960. http://dx.doi.org/10.3109/03602538308991417

[27] Poola, N.R., Bhuiyan, D., Ortiz, S., Savant, I.A., Sidhom, M., Taft, D.R., Kirschenbaum, H. and Kalis, M. (2002) A Novel HPLC Assay for Pentamidine: Comparative Effects of Creatinine and Inulin on GFR Estimation and Pentamidine Renal Excretion in the Isolated Perfused Rat Kidney. *Journal of Pharmacy and Pharmaceutical Sciences*, **5**, 135-145.

[28] Barends, D.M., van der Sandt, J.S. and Hulshoff, A. (1980) Micro Determination of Gentamicin in Serum by High-Performance Liquid Chromatography with Ultraviolet Detection. *Journal of Chromatography B: Biomedical Sciences and Applications*, **182**, 201-210. http://dx.doi.org/10.1016/S0378-4347(00)81624-2

[29] Larsen, N.E., Marinelli, K. and Heilesen, A.M. (1980) Determination of Gentamicin in Serum Using Liquid Column Chromatography. *Journal of Chromatography B: Biomedical Sciences and Applications*, **221**, 182-187. http://dx.doi.org/10.1016/S0378-4347(00)81023-3

[30] Maitra, S.K., Yoshikawa, T.T., Hansen, J.L., Nilsson-Ehle, I., Palin, W.J., Schotz, M.C. and Guze, L.B. (1977) Serum Gentamicin Assay by High-Performance Liquid Chromatography. *Clinical Chemistry*, **23**, 2275-2278.

[31] Walker, S.E. and Coates, P.E. (1981) High-Performance Liquid Chromatographic Methods for Determination of Gentamicin in Biological Fluids. *Journal of Chromatography B: Biomedical Sciences and Applications*, **223**, 131-138. http://dx.doi.org/10.1016/S0378-4347(00)80075-4

[32] White, L.O., Lovering, A. and Reeves, D.S. (1983) Variations in Gentamicin C1, C1a, C2, and C2a Content of Some Preparations of Gentamicin Sulphate Used Clinically as Determined by High-Performance Liquid Chromatography. *Therapeutic Drug Monitoring*, **5**, 123-126. http://dx.doi.org/10.1097/00007691-198303000-00014

[33] Yusuf, A., Al-Rawithi, S., Raines, D., Frayha, H., Toonsi, A., Al-Mohsen, I. and El-Yazigi, A. (1999) Simplified High-Performance Liquid Chromatographic Method for the Determination of Gentamicin Sulfate in a Microsample of Plasma: Comparison with Fluorescence Polarization Immunoassay. *Therapeutic Drug Monitoring*, **21**, 647-652. http://dx.doi.org/10.1097/00007691-199912000-00012

[34] Dontabhaktuni, A., Sidhom, M.B. and Taft, D.R. (2005) An Alternative HPLC Assay for Gentamicin. *AAPS Annual Meeting*, Nashville, 6-10 November 2005.

[35] Bader, M. (1980) A Systematic Approach to Standard Addition Methods in Instrumental Analysis. *Journal of Chemical Education*, **57**, 703. http://dx.doi.org/10.1021/ed057p703

[36] Maack, T. (1980) Physiological Evaluation of the Isolated Perfused Rat Kidney. *American Journal of Physiology*, **238**, F71-F78.

[37] Ajavon, A.D., Bonate, P.L. and Taft, D.R. (2010) Renal Excretion of Clofarabine: Assessment of Dose-Linearity and Role of Renal Transport Systems on Drug Excretion. *European Journal of Pharmaceutical Sciences*, **40**, 209-216. http://dx.doi.org/10.1016/j.ejps.2010.03.014

[38] Poulikakos, P., Tansarli, G.S. and Falagas, M.E. (2014) Combination Antibiotic Treatment versus Monotherapy for Multidrug-Resistant, Extensively Drug-Resistant, and Pandrug-Resistant Acinetobacter Infections: A Systematic Review. *European Journal of Clinical Microbiology & Infectious Diseases*, **33**, 1675-1685. http://dx.doi.org/10.1007/s10096-014-2124-9

[39] Schmitz, C., Hilpert, J., Jacobsen, C., Boensch, C., Christensen, E.I., Luft, F.C. and Willnow, T.E. (2002) Megalin Deficiency Offers Protection from Renal Aminoglycoside Accumulation. *The Journal of Biological Chemistry*, **277**, 618-622. http://dx.doi.org/10.1074/jbc.M109959200

[40] Schentag, J.J., Meagher, A.K. and RW, J. (2006) Aminoglycosides. In: Burton, M.E., Shaw, L., Schentag, J.J. and Evans, E., Eds., *Applied Pharmacokinetics & Pharmacodynamics: Principles of Therapeutic Drug Monitoring*, Lippincott Williams & Wilkins, New York, 306.

[41] Freeman, C.D., Nicolau, D.P., Belliveau, P.P. and Nightingale, C.H. (1997) Once-Daily Dosing of Aminoglycosides: Review and Recommendations for Clinical Practice. *Journal of Antimicrobial Chemotherapy*, **39**, 677-686. http://dx.doi.org/10.1093/jac/39.6.677

[42] Sastrasinh, M., Knauss, T.C., Weinberg, J.M. and Humes, H.D. (1982) Identification of the Aminoglycoside Binding Site in Rat Renal Brush Border Membranes. *Journal of Pharmacology and Experimental Therapeutics*, **222**, 350-358.

[43] Chiu, P.J., Miller, G.H., Long, J.F. and Waitz, J.A. (1979) Renal Uptake and Nephrotoxicity of Gentamicin during Urinary Alkalinization in Rats. *Clinical and Experimental Pharmacology and Physiology*, **6**, 317-326. http://dx.doi.org/10.1111/j.1440-1681.1979.tb01253.x

[44] Elliott, W.C., Parker, R.A., Houghton, D.C., Gilbert, D.N., Porter, G.A., DeFehr, J. and Bennett, W.M. (1980) Effect of Sodium Bicarbonate and Ammonium Chloride Ingestion in Experimental Gentamicin Nephrotoxicity in Rats. *Research Communications in Chemical Pathology and Pharmacology*, **28**, 483-495.

[45] Pastoriza-Munoz, E., Bowman, R.L. and Kaloyanides, G.J. (1979) Renal Tubular Transport of Gentamicin in the Rat. *Kidney International*, **16**, 440-450. http://dx.doi.org/10.1038/ki.1979.149

[46] Cohen, B., Laish, I., Brosh-Nissimov, T., Hoffman, A., Katz, L.H., Braunstein, R., Sagi, R. and Michael, G. (2013) Efficacy of Urine Alkalinization by Oral Administration of Sodium Bicarbonate: A Prospective Open-Label Trial. *The American Journal of Emergency Medicine*, **31**, 1703-1706. http://dx.doi.org/10.1016/j.ajem.2013.08.031

Supplementary

Table S1. Summary of calibration curve of gentamicin HPLC method in IPRK perfusate and KHS buffer.

Matrix	Concentration range (µg/ml)	Correlation[a] (r^2)	Slope[a]	Intercept[a]
Perfusate[b]	1 - 40	0.99 ± 0.01	21.5 ± 1.46	1.20 ± 1.33
KHS buffer	10 - 100	0.99 ± 0.01	3.96 ± 0.12	0.91 ± 3.96

[a]Data presented as mean ± standard deviation of six calibration curves; [b]Data obtained after the application of standard addition method.

Table S2. Precision of gentamicin quantification method by HPLC in IPRK perfusate and KHS buffer.

Matrix	Concentration (µg/ml)	Concentration predicted[a] (µg/ml)	Mean prediction error (%)	CV%
Perfusate[b]	1	1.17 ± 0.10	17.50	9.31
	2	2.18 ± 0.22	9.23	10.00
	3	3.04 ± 0.09	1.37	3.03
	5	4.56 ± 0.29	−8.77	6.50
	10	9.64 ± 0.66	−3.57	6.84
	20	20.6 ± 1.00	2.94	4.88
	40	40.6 ± 0.94	1.43	2.32
KHS buffer	10	10.6 ± 1.15	6.59	10.80
	15	15.5 ± 0.35	3.45	2.27
	20	20.8 ± 1.04	3.74	4.99
	40	39.2 ± 1.35	−2.04	3.45
	60	59.3 ± 1.88	−1.12	3.17
	80	79.3 ± 2.09	−0.82	2.63
	100	103 ± 2.74	3.15	2.65

[a]Data presented as mean ± standard deviation of six replicate injections at each concentration; [b]Data obtained after standard addition method was utilized.

List of Contributors

Ahmed M. Soliman
Department of Pharmacology, Faculty of Veterinary Medicine, Cairo University, Giza, Egypt

Mohamed Aboubakr
Department of Pharmacology, Faculty of Veterinary Medicine, Benha University, Qaliobiya, Egypt

Mohamed El-Hewaity
Department of Pharmacology, Faculty of Veterinary Medicine, University of Sadat City, Minoufiya, Egypt

Yasuhiko Kawasaki, Tsugumi Fujita, Kun Yang and Eiichi Kumamoto
Department of Physiology, Saga Medical School, Saga, Japan

Leila Adibi and Maryam Khosravi
Biology Department, Faculty of Biological Sciences, Islamic Azad University North Tehran Branch, Tehran, Iran

Shahrzad Khakpour and Mahsa Hadipour Jahromy
Herbal Pharmacology Research Center, Tehran Medical Sciences Branch, Faculty of Medicine, Islamic Azad University, Tehran, Iran

Hedayat Sahraei
Neuroscience Research Center, Baghiatallah University of Medical, Tehran, Iran

Toni Homberg, Erika Vera, Oscar Pineda and Julio Ayala-Balboa
Clinical Trials Branch and Clinical Immunology Service, Unit of External Services and Clinical Research (USEIC), National School of Biological Sciences, National Polytechnic Institute, Mexico City, Mexico

Violeta Sáenz, Jorge Galicia-Carreón and Iván Lara
Unit of Pharmacovigilance, Unit of External Services and Clinical Research (USEIC), National School of Biological Sciences, National Polytechnic Institute, Mexico City, Mexico

Edgar Cervantes-Trujano and Maria C. Andaluz
Clinical Trials Branch and Clinical Immunology Service, Unit of External Services and Clinical Research (USEIC), National School of Biological Sciences, National Polytechnic Institute, Mexico City, Mexico
Unit of Pharmacovigilance, Unit of External Services and Clinical Research (USEIC), National School of Biological Sciences, National Polytechnic Institute, Mexico City, Mexico

Alejandro Estrada-García and Sergio Estrada-Parra
Department of Immunology, National School of Biological Sciences, National Polytechnic Institute, Mexico City, Mexico

Mayra Pérez-Tapia
Unit of R&D in Bioprocesses (UDIBI), National School of Biological Sciences, National Polytechnic Institute, Mexico City, Mexico

Maria C. Jiménez-Martínez
Department of Biochemistry, Faculty of Medicine, National Autonomous University of Mexico, Mexico City, Mexico

Udeme Owunari Georgewill, Iyeopu Minakiri Siminialayi and Atuboyedia Wolfe Obianime
Department of Pharmacology, Faculty of Basic Medical Sciences, College of Health Sciences, University of Port Harcourt, Port Harcourt, Nigeria

Georgewill Udeme Owunari, Siminialayi Iyeopu Minakiri and Obianime Atuboyedia Wolfe
Department of Pharmacology, Faculty of Basic Medical Sciences, College of Health Sciences, University of Port Harcourt, Port Harcourt, Nigeria

Rika Shimada
Department of Critical Care Nursing, Graduate School of Nursing, Nagoya City University, Nagoya, Japan

Yasuaki Dohi
Department of Cardio-Renal Medicine and Hypertension, Graduate School of Medicine, Nagoya City University, Nagoya, Japan

Kazunori Kimura
Pharmaceutical Department, Nagoya City University Hospital, Nagoya, Japan

Satoshi Fujii
Department of Laboratory Medicine, Asahikawa Medical University, Asahikawa, Japan

Ruth Gallily and Zhannah Yekhtin
The Lautenberg Center for General and Tumor Immunology, The Hadassah Medical School, The Hebrew University of Jerusalem, Jerusalem, Israel

Lumír Ondřej Hanuš
Department of Medicinal and Natural Products, Institute for Drug Research, The Hadassah Medical School, The Hebrew University of Jerusalem, Jerusalem, Israel

Tanbir Ahammad
Department of Pharmacy, BRAC University, Dhaka, Bangladesh

Marium Begum, Md. Iftekhar Hussain and Mohammad Mizanur Rahman
Department of Pharmacy, Primeasia University, Dhaka, Bangladesh

A. F. M. Towheedur Rahman
Department of Pharmaceutical Sciences, North South University, Dhaka, Bangladesh

Moynul Hasan
Department of Pharmacy, Dhaka International University, Dhaka, Bangladesh

Saikat Ranjan Paul
Department of Pharmacy, Southeast University, Dhaka, Bangladesh

Shaila Eamen
Department of Pharmacy, Jahangirnagar University, Dhaka, Bangladesh

Md. Hazrat Ali
Department of Pharmacy, International Islamic University of Chittagong, Chittagong, Bangladesh

Md. Ashraful Islam
Department of Biomedical Imaging, Faculty of Bioscience, Abo Akademi University, Turku, Finland

Mamunur Rashid
Department of Pharmacy, University of Rajshshi, Rajshahi, Bangladesh

Byung-Yoon Cha, Takayuki Yonezawa and Toshiaki Teruya
Research Institute for Biological Functions, Chubu University, Matsumoto, Japan

Wen Lei Shi
Department of Biological Chemistry, Chubu University, Matsumoto, Japan

Kotaro Watanabe, Kiyotake Suenaga, Yuichi Ishikawa and Shigeru Nishiyama
Department of Chemistry, Faculty of Science and Technology, Keio University, Yokohama, Japan

Kazuo Nagai and Je-Tae Woo
Research Institute for Biological Functions, Chubu University, Matsumoto, Japan
Department of Biological Chemistry, Chubu University, Matsumoto, Japan

Suleiman I. Sharif*, Aseel H. Nassar, Fatima K. Al-Hamami, Maha M. Hassanein, Ashkur H. Elmi and Rubian S. Sharif
Department of Pharmacy Practice & Pharmacotherapeutics, College of Pharmacy, University of Sharjah, Sharjah, United Arab Emirates

Andang Miatmoko, Kumi Kawano and Yoshiyuki Hattori
Department of Drug Delivery Research, Hoshi University, Shinagawa, Japan

Etsuo Yonemochi
Department of Physical Chemistry, Hoshi University, Shinagawa, Japan

Yoshinari Taguchi, Shinji Arakawa, Natsukaze Saito and Masato Tanaka
Graduate School of Science and Technology, Niigata University, Niigata, Japan

Silvia Reina and Enri Borda
Pharmacology Unit, School of Dentistry, University of Buenos Aires, Buenos Aires, Argentina
National Research Council of Argentina (CONICET), Buenos Aires, Argentina

Cecilia Pisoni, Alicia Eimon, Carolina Carrizo and Roberto Arana
Section of Rheumatology and Immunology, Department of Internal Medicine, CEMIC, Buenos Aires, Argentina

Md. Abdus Salam and Md. Rokonujjaman
Department of Chemistry, University of Dhaka, Dhaka, Bangladesh

Asma Rahman, Ummay Nasrin Sultana and Md. Zakir Sultan
Centre for Advanced Research in Sciences (CARS), University of Dhaka, Dhaka, Bangladesh

Froylán Ibarra-Velarde, Yazmin Alcala-Canto and Yolanda Vera-Montenegro
Department of Parasitology, Faculty of Veterinary Medicine and Zoothecnics, National University Autonomous of Mexico, Mexico City, Mexico

Esraa Elsayed Ashry, Rasha Bakheet Abdellatief, Abeer Elrefaiy Mohamed and Hassan Ibrahim Kotb
Faculty of Medicine, Assiut University, Assiut, Egypt

Nikoloz V. Gongadze and Makrine Mirziashvili
Department of Medical Pharmacology and Pharmacotherapy, Tbilisi State Medical University, Tbilisi, Georgia

Galina V. Sukoyan
Department of Medical Pharmacology and Pharmacotherapy, Tbilisi State Medical University, Tbilisi, Georgia
International Scientific Centre of Introduction of New Biomedical Technology, Tbilisi, Georgia

Zaza Chapichadze
Department of Pharmacology, State Regulation Agency for Medical Activities Ministry of Health and Social Affairs of Georgia, Tbilisi, Georgia

Tamara D. Kezeli, Nino M. Dolidze and Mariam ChipashviliA
Department of Pharmacology, Faculty of Medicine, I. Javakhishvili Tbilisi State University, Tbilisi, Georgia

Jeffrey H. Burton, William D. Johnson and Frank L. Greenway
Pennington Biomedical Research Center, Baton Rouge, USA

Rafeeq Alam Khan, Maryam Aslam and Shadab Ahmed
Department of Pharmacology, Faculty of Pharmacy and Pharmaceutical Sciences, University of Karachi, Karachi, Pakistan

Jane J. Xu
Alberta Health Services, Pharmacy Services, Edmonton, Canada

Ilene Burton
Alberta Health Services, Transplant Services, Edmonton, Canada

Wayne J. Tymchak and Glen J. Pearson
University of Alberta, Division of Cardiology, Edmonton, Canada
Mazankowski Alberta Heart Institute, Edmonton, Canada

Sarah Madeline Brown and Philip Jeremy Hampton
Department of Dermatology, The Newcastle upon Tyne Hospitals NHS Foundation Trust, Royal Victoria Infirmary, Newcastle, UK

N. Tanna and J. Pitkin
London North West Healthcare NHS Trust, London, UK
School of Science & Medicine, Imperial College, London, UK

T. Tatla, T. Winn, S. Chita, K. Ramdoo and C. Batten
London North West Healthcare NHS Trust, London, UK

Xiaoyan Chen, Roy A. Lysaa, Ragnhild Jaeger, Emanuel Boadu and Georg Sager
Medical Pharmacology and Toxicology, Department of Medical Biology, Faculty of Health Sciences, Arctic University of Norway, Tromso, Norway

Takahiro Mizoguchi, Mitsue Ishisaka, Masamitsu Shimazawa and Hideaki Hara
Molecular Pharmacology, Department of Biofunctional Evaluation, Gifu Pharmaceutical University, Gifu, Japan

Yui Kobatake and Hiroaki Kamishina
Department of Veterinary Medicine, Faculty of Applied Biological Sciences, Gifu University, Gifu, Japan

Yasuhiko Nishioka and Tsukasa Kirimoto
Taiho Pharmaceutical Co., Ltd., Tokushima, Japan

Ahmed M. Soliman
Department of Pharmacology, Faculty of Veterinary Medicine, Cairo University, Giza, Egypt

Mahmoud Sedek
Department of Poultry and Fish Diseases, Faculty of Veterinary Medicine, Damanhour University, Damanhour, Egypt

Nahal Beik, Katelyn Sylvester and Megan Rocchio
Department of Pharmacy, Brigham and Women's Hospital, Boston, USA

Michael B. Stone
Department of Emergency Medicine, Brigham and Women's Hospital, Boston, USA

Jacqueline Trivedi, Firuza Kharas, Sapna Parikh, Roda Dalal, Aurelio Lobo, Lyle Fonseca, Mahesh Jadhav, Shruta Dadarkar, Asha Almeida, Ankita Srivastava and Ashish Suthar
Department of Herbal Development, Piramal Life Sciences India Limited, Mumbai, India

Aruna Dontabhaktuni and David R. Taft
Long Island University, Brooklyn, USA

Mayankbhai Patel
Long Island University, Brooklyn, USA
Current Address: Takeda Pharmaceuticals International Co., Cambridge, USA

Permissions

www.ingramcontent.com/pod-product-compliance
Lightning Source LLC
Chambersburg PA
CBHW080248230326
41458CB00097B/4084